DEPRESSION – CAUSES, DIAGNOSIS AND TREATMENT

ANTIDEPRESSANTS: TYPES, EFFICIENCY AND POSSIBLE SIDE EFFECTS

DEPRESSION – CAUSES, DIAGNOSIS AND TREATMENT

Additional books in this series can be found on Nova's website at:

https://www.novapublishers.com/catalog/index.php?cPath=23_29&seriesp=Depression-+Causes,+Diagnosis+and+Treatment

Additional e-books in this series can be found on Nova's website at:

https://www.novapublishers.com/catalog/index.php?cPath=23_29&seriespe=Depression-+Causes,+Diagnosis+and+Treatment

DEPRESSION – CAUSES, DIAGNOSIS AND TREATMENT

ANTIDEPRESSANTS: TYPES, EFFICIENCY AND POSSIBLE SIDE EFFECTS

JAYDEN T. VAN LEEUWEN
EDITOR

Nova Science Publishers, Inc.
New York

For permission to use material from this book please contact us:
Telephone 631-231-7269; Fax 631-231-8175
Web Site: http://www.novapublishers.com

LIBRARY OF CONGRESS CATALOGING-IN-PUBLICATION DATA
Available upon request

ISBN: 978-1-61668-581-2

Published by Nova Science Publishers, Inc. ✦ New York

CONTENTS

PREFACE

An antidepressant is a psychiatric medication used to alleviate mood disorders, such as major depression and dysthymia. These medications are among those most commonly prescribed by psychiatrists and other physicians, and their effectiveness and adverse effects are the subject of many studies and competing claims. This new book presents topical data on antidepressants including neuroplasticity hypothesis and depression; monitoring antidepressant therapy using heart rate variability; the role of antidepressant pharmacotherapy in the prevention of suicide; a new approach to treatment strategy of depressive disorders based on modulation of PEP activity with synthetic inhibitors and understanding the pathogenesis of depression and the mechanism of action of clinically effective antidepressants.

Chapter 1 – Our knowledge about brain functions is still limited in the era of knowledge and communication. Consequently, rational drug treatment for diseases that are directly related with brain functions like Alzheimer's disease, schizophrenia, Parkinson's disease, substance dependence has not yet been possible. Recently more resources are allocated in technologically and scientifically developed countries to the treatment of brain related diseases. Many scientists also state that this period will be dominated by scientific brain research.

Depression is a mood disorder that may appear in any part of life and its prevalence is increasing. Impairment of life quality at the level that causes loss of workforce and suicidal outcome in some cases increases its importance. Monoamine hypothesis that was proposed to be related with the cause of depression is still valid today although there are problems to be solved regarding definitive diagnosis of depression and rational pharmacotherapy. This forces the scientists to form alternative and more valid hypothesis about the etiology of depression.

Neuroplasticity can be defined shortly as the adaptability of neuron to internal and external stimuli. It was believed formerly that neurons can not regenerate. Recent studies on central nervous system have clearly found that neurons have the property to regenerate and repair themselves as other cells do. This observation makes the major contribution to the emergence of neuroplasticity hypothesis as well as it is a critical point for the diagnosis and treatment of diseases related with central nervous system.

In recent years, contribution of especially stress induced neuroplastic changes in the brain to depression besides other diseases with central origin is indicated. Intensity and importance of research on this topic is increasing. Neuroplasticity hypothesis of depression has the potential to make important contributions to the diagnosis of depression as well as it may be helpful in the explanation of the drug effects can not be explained by neurochemical mechanisms. Also, it seems that it may lead to the development of new and more effective drugs for depression and entrance of this drug to treatment in a short time.

In this chapter the authors tried to acquaint readers about the neuroplasticity hypothesis especially in the context of depression. Knowledge covered in this chapter is as much as the literature reviewed about this topic. Neuroplasticity is a dynamic topic. It is possible that additional concepts emerge in parallel to new developments and this subject is reshaped.

Chapter 2 - The world-wide annual suicide rate currently averages approximately 13/100,000 (0.013%/year), with higher average rates for men than women in all but a few countries, very low rates in children, and relatively high rates in elderly men. Suicide rates vary markedly among regions of the world, countries, and locales, in part reflecting differences in case-identification and reporting procedures. Rates of attempted suicide average 20–30 times higher than rates of completed suicide in the general population, but are probably under-reported. A highly controversial question is whether antidepressant treatment modifies the risks of various aspects of "suicidality" among patients with major depressive disorders. Research on the relationship between pharmacotherapy and suicidal behavior was virtually unknown until a decade ago. A minority of ecological studies and most large clinical studies have found that decreases of suicide rates by region or time are correlated with higher rates of prescribing modern antidepressants. However, other studies and data from brief, randomized, controlled trials in patients with acute major depression have found increases for patients of some ages, particularly for the risk of suicide attempts, as well as increases in suicidal ideation in the young. Although other pharmacological treatments, such as clozapine and lithium, appear to have sound evidence for reducing the risk of attempted and completed suicide, in this paper the authors proposed to analyze the relationship between suicidality in depressed adults and only antidepressants.

Chapter 3 - The cardiac autonomic nervous system is typically impaired in patients with major depression and panic disorder. Furthermore, this unfavorable condition will be dose dependent intensified by antidepressant drugs. This increases the cardiovascular risk and can be currently and non-invasively estimated by analysis of heart rate variability (HRV). The reduction of HRV is less expressed by SSRI than by TCA. This is in accordance to better acceptance of SSRI as published in the literature. The parasympathetic determinated components of HRV are in therapeutic doses more impaired than the rather sympathetic determinated components. This reduction is dependent on plasma concentration.

Under doxepin in toxic doses, a level dependent suppression of sympathetic parts (LF power) is added overtopping the suppression of vagal parts (HF power). The minimum of HRV was at that time attained that is associated in the literature with greatest mortality. This can be exlained by cardiac depression as a result of a quinidine-like effect. But the also described supraventricular and ventricular arrhythmias occur more frequently with time delay and seem to be less associated with the absolute level of developed sympathetic predominance, but rather with the dynamic of the increasing sympathetic influence in first recovery. The authors' results show a good Spearman correlation of (1) incidence of all arrhythmias within 48 h vs. (2) LF/HF after 48h / LF/HF in HRV minimum if frequency components of spectral analysis (LF and HF Power) are transformed into logarithms before ($p<.001$).

The already published results in the literature give sufficient information that HRV influences are agent specific and this may be important for prognosis. Because also starting conditions of patients are differing from each other, (1) a determination of agent specific profile of HRV changes as well as (2) a determination of basic HRV values of treated patients are desirable. If both parameters are known, the therapy could be better monitored in the future.

Chapter 4 - Retrospective diagnosis of suicide victims has revealed that about half of them have suffered from a depressive disorder. Treatment of depression with antidepressants would therefore be expected to prevent suicide but the role of antidepressant pharmacotherapy in the prevention of suicide has been difficult to evaluate.

Randomised double-blind placebo-controlled studies could be considered the best way of evaluating the effect on suicidal behaviour, but those studies have only been performed as secondary analyses examining the effect of pharmacotherapy on depressive symptoms. They have been performed on low-risk populations, and suicidal patients have been excluded for ethical reasons. Retrospective and pseudo-prospective case-control studies inherit the risk of confounders, as treatment was not randomised. Ecological studies of trends cannot investigate other factors related to a decrease in suicide rates. Descriptive studies on treatment before suicide may show low rates of treatment, but still do not prove that treatment would have been effective if given. Furthermore, complications of the prescription of antidepressants include non-compliance and risk of overdoses in suicidal people.

Apart from evaluating the possible effect of antidepressants in the prevention of suicide, certain questions need to be answered concerning the relationship between depression and suicide. Not all depressives suffer from an uncomplicated major depressive disorder. Sometimes depression is secondary to substance abuse and sometimes depression has melancholic or psychotic features. Furthermore, some investigators have postulated existence of a suicidal syndrome independent of depression, which may have implications for the efficacy of antidepressant pharmacotherapy on suicidal behaviour. Finally, a third way to investigate possible risk or benefit of antidepressants on non-fatal and fatal suicidal behaviour may be to identify certain risk groups for suicidal behaviour despite antidepressant pharmacotherapy.

Suicide and depression only partly overlap. Knowledge about this overlap may have implications for the role of antidepressant pharmacotherapy in the prevention of suicidal behaviour.

Chapter 5 - Current theories of antidepressant action are substantially based on increasing the availability of the monoamine neurotransmitters. A new trend in antidepressant medication includes mechanisms connected with neuropeptides and peptide hormones lacking in side effects. Increasing evidence proves the involvement of neuropeptides in the development of depression and anxiety. However, there is a lack of data on the enzymes cleaving neuropeptides mediating depression and anxiety. Many neuropeptides involved in emotional responses are enriched in proline residues. The unique conformation of the prolyl bond protects peptides that contain proline residues from enzyme degradation. Thus, the enzymes cleaving prolyl bonds in neuropeptides are of particular interest.

Abnormal serum and plasma activities of the serine peptidases prolyl endopeptidase (EC 3.4.21.26) and dipeptidyl peptidase IV (EC 3.4.14.5) have been consistently observed in patients with mood disorders (Maes et al., 1994-2004). In the authors' early experiments, synthetic inhibitors of PEP have been shown to have antidepressant-like activity in mice in a forced swimming test. The authors have found that the development of experimental dopamine deficit-dependent MPTP-induced depressive syndrome in rats is accompanied by activation of PEP and DPPIV in the brain frontal cortex and in the striatum. Recently the authors have elaborated a new model of anxiety-depression state in rats exposed to irreversible synthetic inhibitor of DPPIV methionyl-2(S)-cyano-pyrrolidine in the early postnatal period. Adolescent and adult rats demonstrate increased anxiety, depression-related behavior in forced swimming test and anhedonia in sucrose preference test. Anxiety-depression state in males and females is associated with the increase of DPPIV/CD26 and PEP activity in frontal cortex, striatum, nucleus accumbens, hippocamp and hypothalamus in rat brain.

Competitive PEP inhibitor benzyloxycarbonyl-alanyl-proline promoted faster reduction of depression-like behavior in rats after MPTP withdrawal. Non-competitive PEP inhibitor benzyloxycarbonyl-methionyl-2(S)-cyano-pyrrolidine prevented the development of "behavioral despair" and disturbances in rhythmic organization of swimming behavior in forced swimming test both in rats with MPTP-induced depressive syndrome and in rats with DPPIV inhibitor-induced anxiety-depression state similar to NE/5-HT reuptake inhibitor imipramine.

The results obtained in two rat models of depression prove PEP inhibitors benzyloxycarbonyl-methionyl-2(S)-cyano-pyrrolidine and benzyloxycarbonyl-alanyl-proline to have antidepressant-like properties. Data afford grounds for a new approach to treatment strategy for depressive disorders based on modulation of PEP activity with synthetic inhibitors.

Chapter 6 - Understanding the pathogenesis of depression and the mechanism of action of clinically effective antidepressants are of considerable interest. Early clinical observations pointed to a decreased monoamine function, which has resulted in the "monoamine hypothesis" of depression. However, as helpful as this hypothesis was for the development of amine-based potent antidepressants, crucial discrepancies, e.g., delayed clinical onset of mood-enhancing effects and the lack of major mood alteration after monoamines depletion, made it rather unlikely that the cause of depression is a simple deficiency of central monoamines. Furthermore, in recent years a growing body of evidence highlighted the possibility that genome regulation, epigenetic modifications or alterations in differential neuronal cell type responsiveness could play a key role in the origin and development of mood disorders.

Therefore, providing an integrative theory of the neurobiology of depression may help to explain some of the complexities of this disorder and discover novel pharmacological targets. On the basis of current knowledge the authors want to discuss an extended "monoamine hypothesis" and propose possible new fields/ideas/concepts which need to be explored for the development of more effective antidepressant treatments.

Chapter 7 - According to the World Health Organization depression and anxiety are most frequently coexisted disturbances in the system of primary medical care (World Health Organization, 1999). These two conditions to a considerable extent overlap each other on clinical symptoms and a number of pathophysiological mechanisms (Nuller and Mikhalenko, 1988; Hamilton, 1988; Kasper, 2001). Hamilton marks that the anxiety at recurrent depression reveals in 96% of cases (1988). Clayton (1990), Cloninger (1990), Rodney et al. (1997), Tollefson et al. (1993) note that the anxiety can be found at 44-91% of patients with depression.

Depressed patients with symptoms of anxiety represent a special case of treatment with necessity of a choice of medicinal preparations that have both thymoleptic and marked anxiolytic effects (Avrutski and Neduva, 1988; Bakish, 1999). Introduction in clinical practice of antidepressants with a selective spectrum of action on serotonergic system – selective serotonin reuptake inhibitors (SSRI) or activators – can considerably increase efficiency of treatment of patients and improve the quality of life. However it requires a specification of indication to prescription of either preparation, investigation of clinical and metabolic pictures during the treatment and neurochemical mechanisms of their action. As shows the analysis of the literature the neurochemical mechanism of action of antidepressants influencing on serotonin reuptake is investigated insufficiently. For example Ansseau (1993) writes that paradoxical finding that both tianeptine and selective serotonin reuptake inhibitors exhibit antidepressant activity despite clearly antagonistic mechanisms is rather puzzling.

Thus in this study the authors want to discuss from clinical and biochemical points of view some aspects of dynamics of anxious depression under the treatment with serotonergic antidepressants with different mechanisms of action on serotonin reuptake. Besides that as a consequence of the study there will be reviewed different problems such as interactions between monoaminergic and hormonal systems, contribution of endogenous intoxication in the pathophysiology of mental disorders, in particular depression. One of the main results of this study is the development of the hypothesis of neurochemical mechanism of tianeptine action – selective serotonin reuptake enhancer.

Chapter 8 - Epidemiological studies have consistently shown that depression is approximately twice as common in females as in males. There is also some evidence that there are gender differences in the clinical manifestations. Some studies have addressed the epidemiological and pharmacological implications of gender-associated differences in the overall treatment response to antidepressants in clinical practice. Recently, several new antidepressants have become available. However, antidepressants do not have the same effect in all patients all the time. It is important to be able to predict which patients would most likely benefit from particular antidepressants. To examine gender differences in treatment remission in depressed patients treated with fluvoxamine, paroxetine, sertraline, milnacipran, or maprotiline, a retrospective cohort analysis was carried out. Three hundred and sixty-eight patients were identified who had been treated with one of fluvoxamine, paroxetine, sertraline, milnacipran, or maprotiline for depression. This study was done to explore the gender differences in the effect of these antidepressants. It was found that there was no difference in the overall treatment response among these antidepressants in male patients (x^2=7.650, df=4, P=0.1053). However, there was a significant difference in the overall treatment response among these antidepressants in female patients (x^2=17.959, df=4, P=0.0013). Among female patients with depression, the remission rate was higher with sertraline and maprotiline than with fluvoxamine, paroxetine, and milnacipran. Furthermore, there was no difference in the treatment response among these antidepressants for males with their first episode of depression (x^2=6.194, df=4, P=0.1851), males with a recurrent episode of depression (x^2=9.101, df=4, P=0.0586), and females with their first episode of depression (x^2=3.725, df=4, P=0.4446). However, there was a significant difference in the treatment response among these antidepressants in females with a recurrent episode of depression (x^2=19.528, df=4, P=0.0006). Among females with a recurrent episode of depression, the remission rate was higher with sertraline and maprotiline than with fluvoxamine, paroxetine, and milnacipran. Therefore, sertraline and maprotiline are more effective than fluvoxamine, paroxetine, and milnacipran, particularly in females with a recurrent episode of depression.

Thus, gender should be considered when selecting antidepressants. These results will be useful for helping guide clinicians treating female depression.

Expert Commentary - The neurogenic theory of depression remains the source of controversies and debates, and must be further confirmed. More data and evidence are needed to confirm the involvement of adult neurogenesis in depression. Nonetheless, the evidence that increased neurogenesis contributes to the effects of antidepressants may hold the key for the understanding of the long-term consequences of the effects of antidepressants of the physiopathology of the central nervous system. It may lead to new drug design and new strategies to treat depressive disorders. To this aim, the mechanism underlying the involvement of adult neurogenesis in the etiology of depression and the activity of antidepressants remain to be fully understood.

In: Antidepressants: Types, Efficiency …
Editor: Jayden T. Van Leeuwen, pp.1-66

ISBN 978-1-61668-581-2

Chapter 1

NEUROPLASTICITY: A NEW APPROACH TO TREATMENT OF DEPRESSION

Tayfun Uzbay
Gulhane Military Medical Academy, Department of Medical Pharmacology, Psychopharmacology Research Unit, Ankara, Turkey

ABSTRACT

Our knowledge about brain functions is still limited in the era of knowledge and communication. Consequently, rational drug treatment for diseases that are directly related with brain functions like Alzheimer's disease, schizophrenia, Parkinson's disease, substance dependence has not yet been possible. Recently more resources are allocated in technologically and scientifically developed countries to the treatment of brain related diseases. Many scientists also state that this period will be dominated by scientific brain research.

Depression is a mood disorder that may appear in any part of life and its prevalence is increasing. Impairment of life quality at the level that causes loss of workforce and suicidal outcome in some cases increases its importance. Monoamine hypothesis that was proposed to be related with the cause of depression is still valid today although there are problems to be solved regarding definitive diagnosis of depression and rational pharmacotherapy. This forces the scientists to form alternative and more valid hypothesis about the etiology of depression.

Neuroplasticity can be defined shortly as the adaptability of neuron to internal and external stimuli. It was believed formerly that neurons can not regenerate. Recent studies on central nervous system have clearly found that neurons have the property to regenerate and repair themselves as other cells do. This observation makes the major contribution to the emergence of neuroplasticity hypothesis as well as it is a critical point for the diagnosis and treatment of diseases related with central nervous system.

In recent years, contribution of especially stress induced neuroplastic changes in the brain to depression besides other diseases with central origin is indicated. Intensity and importance of research on this topic is increasing. Neuroplasticity hypothesis of depression has the potential to make important contributions to the diagnosis of depression as well as it may be helpful in the explanation of the drug effects can not be explained by neurochemical mechanisms. Also, it seems that it may lead to the development of new and more effective drugs for depression and entrance of this drug to treatment in a short time.

In this chapter we tried to acquaint readers about the neuroplasticity hypothesis especially in the context of depression. Knowledge covered in this chapter is as much as the literature reviewed about this topic. Neuroplasticity is a dynamic topic. It is possible that additional concepts emerge in parallel to new developments and this subject is reshaped.

GENERAL CONCEPTS AND INFORMATION ABOUT CENTRAL NERVOUS SYSTEM

Neuron and its Structure

Neruon is the functional and structural unit of the nervous system. It is a specialized cell that receives, transmits and emits neuronal stimuli. It has special features in regards to both structure and functions, different from other cell types. Neuron, as shown in Figure 1, is comprised of a cell body, and extensions from the cell body, the dendrites and the axon. Structures like nucleus, endoplasmic reticulum, golgi apparatus and mitochondria lie in the cell body of the neuron. Neuron is connected to other neurons via dendrites extending from the axons. The dendrite is the region involved with the reception of the information and the stimuli, and direction of those to the cell body, whereas the cell body is the site of information processing, and the axon and apical part of the axon are the regions of information transmission to other neurons. The cell body is responsible from all activities necessary for its survival (Minneman, 1991). Dendrites are also called the "afferent fibers". Axons carry the received information away from the cell body. Axons are also called the "efferent fibers". Neuron cell bodies form the gray matter in brain and medulla spinalis, and rest of the neurons form the white matter (Uzbay, 2004).

Neurons are cells, which gather internal and external stimuli, analyze those stimuli and give a response accordingly, this way neurons contribute to the adaptation of the organism to internal and external environment. Neurons also can themselves generate impulses, like myocardial cells. Until recently, neurons were believed to reach a certain amount in number following birth and decrease with age, and were also believed to be the only group of cells which doesn't have the repair capacity in case of structural damage or degeneration. Today, these beliefs have lost their scientific validity. Especially in the hippocampus of rat and human, neurons were shown to be able to regenerate, and new neuron formation was also shown (Erickson et al., 1998; McKim, 2000). Nowadays, not only degenerative diseases like Parkinson's and Alzheimer's disease, but also depression are proposed to result from degeneration of especially hippocampal neurons, and there are some evidences suggesting that antidepressants act through prevention of neuronal degeneration as well as genesis of healthy new neurons (Vogel, 2000, Czeh et al., 2001; Duman, 2002). These evidences strengthen the idea that neurons can regenerate themselves, like other cells in human body.

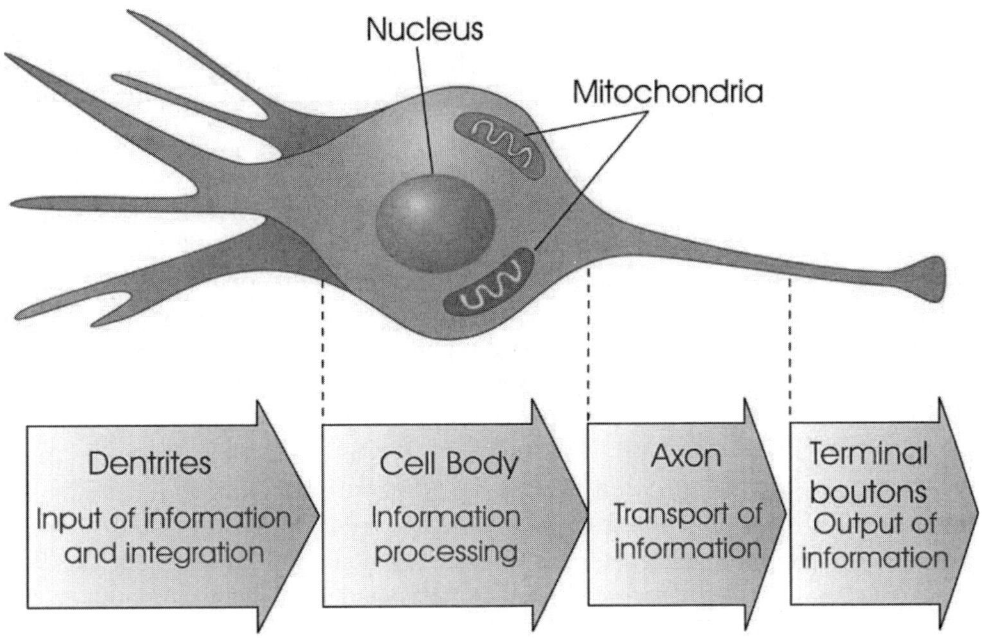

Figure 1. Structure of the neuron.

Concept of Synapse and Neurochemical Transmission

In order for the living organism to adapt the internal and external environment, signals from those sources should be received, transmitted from one neuron to another, modified, evaluated, and stored, if necessary. All these processes take place through neuronal junctions present in the nervous system. Synapse is the principal region in those junctions, where the stimulus or the information is transmitted. Synapse has three compartments morphologically: presynaptic terminal, synaptic cleft and postsynaptic area (Brown and McKim, 2000; Uzbay, 2004) (Figure 2).

Axons approaching to the cell membrane targeted for signal transmission (postsynaptic membrane), branch into less than 1 micron thick extensions. These extensions become rounded as they approach to the postsynaptic membrane and form button like expansions, which are called presynaptic terminals (Figure2). Neurotransmitters, which are chemical transmitters synthesized in the neurons, are stored in those terminals in "vesicles". During the neurotransmitter release process, these vesicles approach to the presynaptic membrane and open releasing the neurotransmitter into the synaptic cleft (Uzbay, 2004) (Figure2).

Postsynaptic area is the place where the neuronal signals are transmitted or received. In synapses between two neurons, postsynaptic area is usually on the dendrites of the receptive neuron. Any effector cell (like muscle cells or glandular cells) in contact with the neuron can also form the postsynaptic area. The dendrites receiving the stimulus or the effector cell membrane is called the postsynaptic membrane. Postsynaptic membrane is approximately 70 angstron thick and has the lipid-protein-lipid structure. On this membrane lie the receptors which are proteins binding the chemical transmitters (neurotransmitters) released from the presynaptic membrane (Uzbay, 2004) (Figure2).

Synaptic cleft is the approximately 250 angstron long gap between the presynaptic and postsynaptic membranes. Neurotransmitters released from the presynaptic terminal, cross the cleft via diffusion, and bind their specific receptors on postsynaptic membrane. Following this, neurotransmitters interact in a specific manner with the protein structures on the postsynaptic membrane, which are called the receptors; this way they transmit the stimulus or the neuronal impulse. As a result, receptive (postsynaptic) cell responds according to the quality of the impulse (Mann and Brown, 1985; Brown and McKim, 2000; Uzbay, 2004) . This sequence of events, which is called neurochemical transmission, is the basic process of central nervous system. The behavior of the species in which a nervous system is developed also depends on the neurochemical transmission. Functioning level of this transmission plays important roles in the pathophysiology and pharmacotherapy of many disorders of nervous system.

Postsynaptic receptors can be conceptualized as detectors which constantly sense the existence of chemicals specific to them, and bind when they found any. Neurotransmitter-receptor binding is formed via electrostatic bonds. The receptor is inactive in the absence of agonists (transmitters, drug molecules or other endogenous molecules which can bind the receptor). The catalytic enzymes present in the postsynaptic membranes play a role in the mediation of the effects of receptors on postsynaptic area. Best known of those catalytic enzymes are "adenylate cyclase", "guanylate cyclase", "phospholipase C" and "phospholipase A2". There are also regulatory proteins in the postsynaptic membrane which regulate the interaction between the catalytic enzymes and the receptors. These proteins are called G proteins. Postsynaptic receptors are localised on the external surface of the membrane. The catalytic enzymes and the regulatory proteins which interact with the receptors lie on the inner surface of the membrane. Initially, chemical transmitter and the receptor form the transmitter-receptor complex. As a result of this interaction, membrane fluidity increases, and the complex approaches to the regulatory proteins and the catalytic enzymes. Then, transmitter-receptor-G protein complex is formed. Depending on the quality of the G protein in the complex, this interaction results in activation or inhibition of the adenylate cyclase. This may increase or decrease intracellular synthesis of cyclic adenosine monophosphate (cAMP), respectively. If the G protein in the complex is stimulatory (Gs) synthesis increases, if it is inhibitory (Gi), synthesis decreases. There are other types of G proteins playing important roles in intracellular biological processes. The synthesis of cAMP triggers the cascade of events in the neuron which result in emergence of the biological end response (Minneman, 1991; Ozawa et al., 1998).

Transmitters, drug molecules or endogenous molecules, act as primary messengers as they convey the biological stimulus to the cytoplasm. Other mediators in the cytoplasm, act as second messengers, further carrying the signal. The cyclic nucleotides, cAMP and cyclic guanosine monophosphate (cGMP), are important elements of second messengers. Besides, Ca/calmodulin that activates protein kinases, arachidonic acid, inositol triphosphate and diacylglycerol act as second messangers in the transmission of the biological signals (Minneman, 1991; Ozawa et al., 1998).

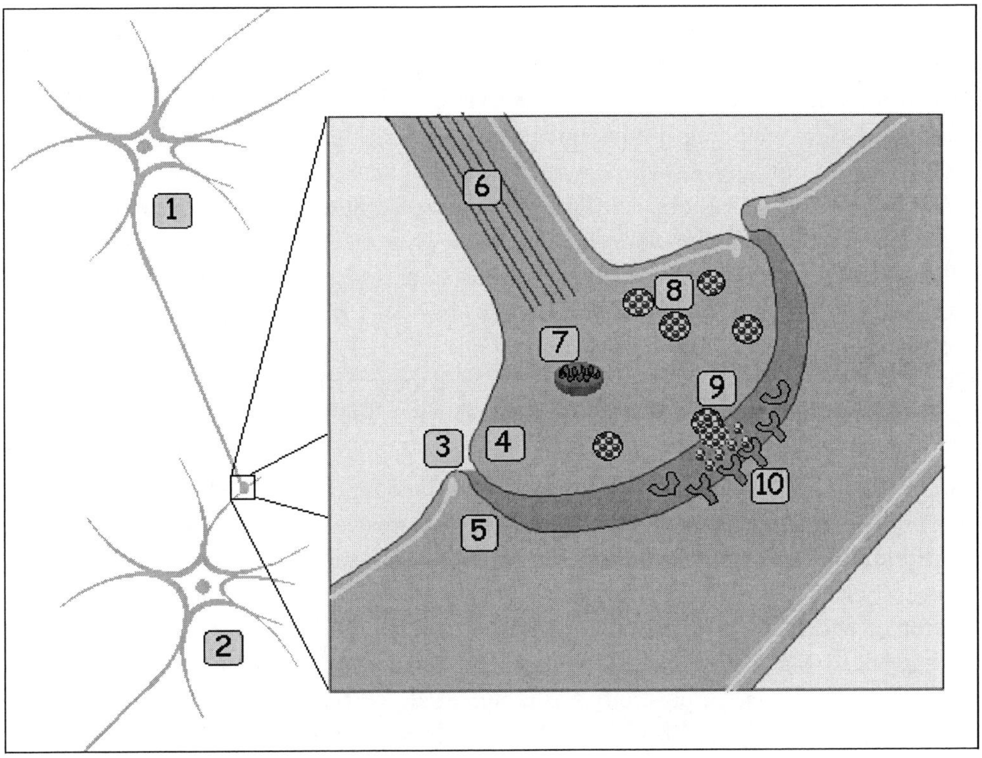

Figure 2. Morphology of synapse. 1: presynaptic neuron, 2: postsynaptic neurons, 3: synaptic cleft, 4: presynaptic terminal, 5: postsynaptic region, 6: microtubules, 7: mitochondria, 8: vesicles storing meurotransmitter, 9: neurotransmitter released from the presynaptic vesicle into the synaptic cleft, 10: receptors on postsynaptic membrane (Uzbay, 2004).

Neurotransmitters and Gene Regulation

The changes in transcription of genes may result in change in rates of synthesis of some cellular proteins, or disruption of the structure of the proteins. There is increasing evidence indicating that neurotransmitters mediating the neurochemical transmission via being released to the synaptic cleft, can regulate gene expression in the nucleus in a similar way. Gene expression has an important contribution to the adaptive responses in long term, in response to the drugs and external factors (Feldman et al., 1997; McKim, 2000).

The activation of genes occurs in two steps. Gene activation always starts with a synaptic stimulus (Armstrong and Montminy, 1993). The initiation phase, which is the first step in gene activation, occurs with the stimulation of "immediate early genes" (IEG). IEGs are in low levels when there is no cellular excitation. With the activation of synaptic input (stimulus), IEGs are induced rapidly and transiently. For example, levels of mRNA are increased significantly in 15 minutes. This increase is not permanent and persists only for 30-60 minutes. In the second step, "late initiation genes" (LIG) are activated. Since the activation of these genes depends on the activation of IEGs, their response is slower.

Substances madiating the neurochemical transmission in the synaptic cleft can regulate the gene expression, with a complex mechanism, with the contribution of "transription factors" and second messengers like cAMP, cGMP, and Ca^{2+}. Second messengers work together with some transcription factors in cases in which the neurotransmitters have a role in gene expression. For example, in the activation of the transcription via cAMP, a short segment of DNA, including 8 nucleotides, is involved, this region is called "cAMP response element" (CRE). Initially, cAMP is synthesized and activates intracellular "protein kinase A" (PKA). Following activation, catalytic subunits of PKA, are transferred into the nucleus (translocation), and here phosphorylate a nuclear protein, called CRE binding protein (CREB) (Vallejo, 1994). CREB acts as a transcription factor and mediates gene transcription. CREB can be phosphorylated with some other kinases besides PKA.

c-fos is another IEG, and is also a proto-oncogene. The transcription factor coded with c-fos is called Fos. It was shown with immunohistochemistry that Fos and c-fos mRNA are present in the brain. Like in other IEGs, levels of Fos and c-fos mRNA are low when there is no stimulation. Excitation of the neuron with the binding of a neurotransmitter to a receptor on the postsynaptic membrane increases second messengers like cAMP and Ca. The increase in the second messengers rapidly induces Fos expression, through CREB and some other transcription factors. The factor stimulating the neuron can as well be an external factor or a pharmacological factor like a drug molecule. In this case, c-fos and other IEGs serve as an indicator of neuronal activation (Morgan and Curran, 1989; Sagar and Sharp, 1993). It has been suggested that IEGs play an important role in central nervous system plasticity, and learning which is a type of plasticity (Abraham et al., 1991).

Fos expression, since it is sensitive to various drugs, is of special interest to the neuropharmacologs. There are reports of fos induction in some brain regions in response to caffein (Nakajima et al., 1989), amphetamine and cocaine (Graybiel et al., 1990), haloperidol adn some other neuroleptics (Dragunow et al., 1990), morphine (Liu et al., 1994), nicotine (Kiba and Jayaraman, 1994), and tetrahydrocannabinol -the active chemical in cannabis- (Mailleux et al., 1994). It has been proposed that, in striatum, CREB phosphorylation via dopamine D1 receptor plays an important role in Fos response to amphetamine (Konradi et al., 1994).

Fos and other IEGs are important elements which can help in exploration of the mechanisms of regulation of gene expression in the cenral nervous system through drugs and neurotransmitters. Gene expression in the central nervous system with neurotransmitters is presented in short in figure 3; and resulting plasticity is shown in Figure 4 in the example of noradrenaline and serotonine.

Principal Neuroanatomical Regions in the Central Nervous System with Functional Importance

Cerebral cortex, limbic system, diencephalon, mesencephalon, serebellum, brain stem and medulla spinalis are the principal regions in central nervous system (Figure 5). These regions and structures located within them, like medulla, reticular activating system, locus ceruleus, basal ganglia and periaquaductal grey matter reponsible from all affects and behaviors in sophisticated living things (Minneman, 1991; Brick and Erickson, 1998; McKim, 2000).

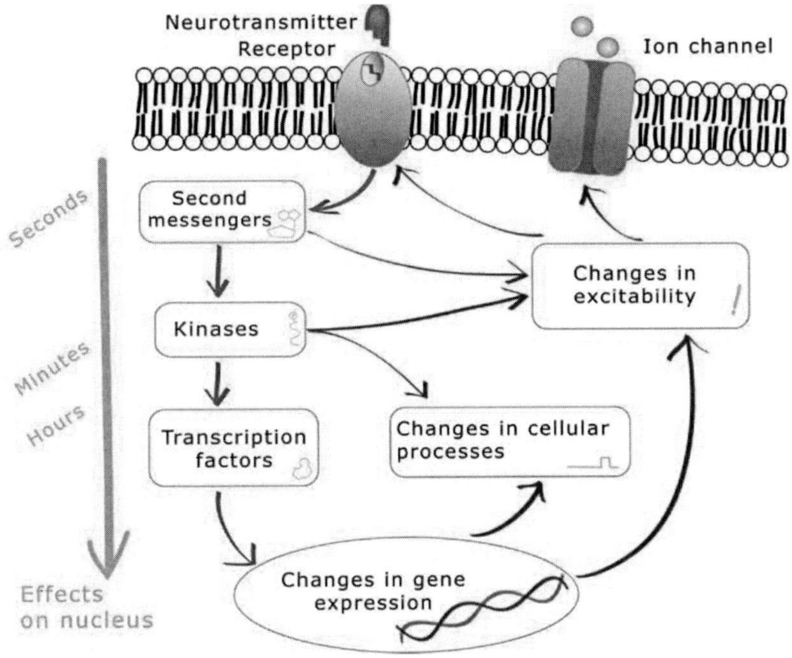

Figure 3. Gene expression through neurotransmission in the central nervous system.

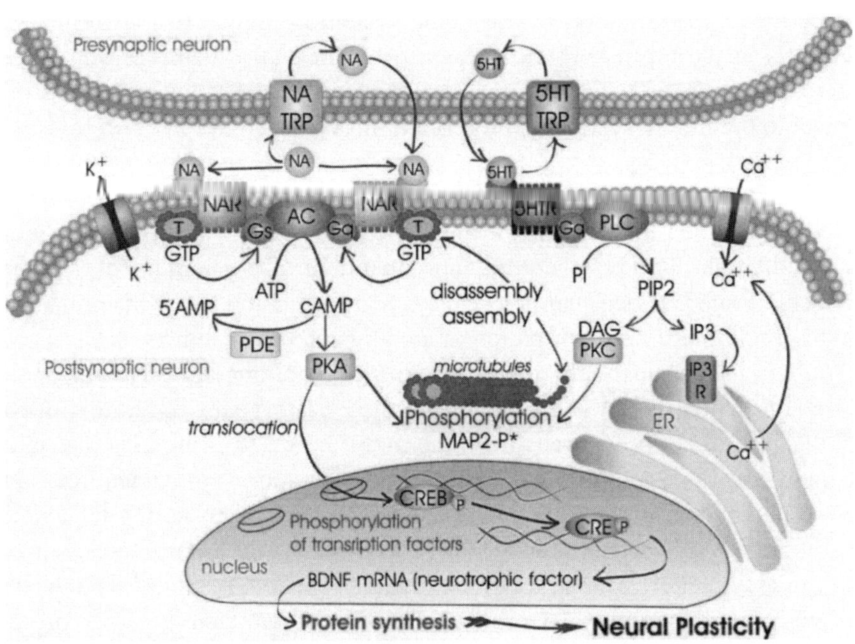

Figure 4. Gene expression through neurotransmission in the central nervous system and neuroplasticity (NA: noradrenaline, 5-HT: serotonine, AC: adenylate cyclase, PLC: phospholipase C, PKC: phosphokinase C, DAG: diacylglicerol, IP3: inositol triphosphate; Gs, Gi, and Gq: stimulator, inhibitor and q type G proteins, respectively, CREB: cAMP response element binding protein (modified from Ozawa et al., 1998).

Spinal cord serves as a relay station for the integration of the information and execution of reflex activities. It conveys information coming from sensory neurons and conveys motor commands from brain to the muscles. The central part of the spinal cord is called grey matter. The axons of the sensory neurons enter into the grey matter in spinal cord from the dorsal side, and motor fibers leave the cord from the ventral side. The ventral horn of the grey matter in spinal cord contains cell bodies of the motor neurons; these neurons are directly related to muscular activity. This region is also important in formation of many reflexes. Dorsal horn also contains neurons which transmit sensory information.

Medulla is the region lying in the base of the brain and brain stem. It begins immediately after the spinal cord. Many neurons related to autonomic nervous system enter in and exit from the brain through medulla. In medulla there are some centers related to vital functions. One of these, is the respiratory center which controls breathing. Respiratory center in the medulla is sensitive to barbiturates, opiates and alcohol which dose-dependently suppress its activity. Overdose and intoxications with those drugs, results in coma and death due to the suppression of the respiratory center. Another center in this region is the chemoreceptor trigger zone (CTZ) which is responsible from the regulation of nausea and vomitting. CTZ is sensitive to pharmacological agents like opiates and nicotine. Intaking these drugs causes nausea and vomitting via dose-dependently stimulating of CTZ.

Two dense nerve projections originating from the medulla and projecting to higher regions are "*reticular activating system*" (RAS) and "*raphe system*". One of the most important functions of the RAS is to maintain the cortical activation and control the state of arousal. Drugs which increase the activity of inhibitor neurotransmitters like GABA, depress RAS and arousal. The stimulation of the raphe system is related to the formation of sleep. Raphe nucleus is in the brainstem and serotonine is the major neurotransmitter. Drugs that modulate serotonergic activity in this region also affect sleep. Neuronal axons in the raphe nucleus project to the limbic system and forebrain through medial forebrain bundle and play a role in mood regulation.

Locus ceruleus is another nucleus located in brainstem. Projections from the neurons in locus ceruleus extend to limbic system and cortex. The major neurotransmitter in locus ceruleus is noradrenalin. It is believed that more than half of the noradrenergic neurons in the brain lie in locus ceruleus. Locus ceruleus causes fear, panic and anger in animals and human. This region has important role in formation of anxiety and panic attacks.

Cerebellum is located just above the medulla. Its functions are related to motor system. Voluntary motor action is initiated and controlled via a part of cortex, motor cortex. Serebellum receives direct projections from the motor cortex and muscles through the spinal cord. It is important in formation and regulation of voluntary motor actions. Among other functions mediated by the cerebellum are the eye movements and learning related processes.

Basal ganglia are subcortical nuclei located in the cerebral hemispheres, above the brain stem and in the grey matter. Anatomically it contains "caudate nucleus", "putamen", "globus pallidus", "amygdaloid complex". Globus pallidus and putamen together are also called "lenticular nucleus". And, lenticular nucleus and caudate nucleus are together called "corpus striatum". Putamen and caudate nucleus together are called "striatum". Striatum mainly receives projections from cerebral cortex and thalamus, and axons extend to globus pallidum. Striatum is the input area for the neuronal fibers to the basal ganglia, and globus pallidum is the output area. Basal ganglia have an essantial role in regulation of voluntary motor activity. Lesions in basal ganglia, results in diseases characterised with movement system problems, like Parkinson disease. Basal ganglia also have contribuiton to the regulation of eyemovements and spatial memory.

Periaquaductal grey matter (PGM) is a structure functioning along the cenral part of the brain. It contributes to two important functions of the central nervous system. These are the perception of pain and aversive stimuli. PGM acts as a relay station for the axons carrying noxious stimuli from the dorsal horn of the spinal cord. This region is rich in opioid receptors. Electrical stimulaiton of the PGM in animals causes the perception, differentiation and learning of the aversive stimuli.

Limbic system is mainly responsible from the regulation of mood and motivation. It contains hypothalamus, nucleus accumbens, hippocampus, amygdala, and septum. Lesions of some parts of hypothalamus may result in excessive increase or abolishing of eating and drinking behaviour in animals. Food related reinforcement in animals is believed to be mediated through hypothalamus. Mesolimbic dopaminergic system is formed by the projections from the ventral tegmental area of the midbrain to the limbic system (particularly to nucleus accumbens); and it is responsible from reward. Dysfunctions in this system may be responsible from schizophrenia.

Hippocampus is a limbic structure especially related to memory and learning. Many years before surgical removal or lesioning of hippocampus as a treatment of epilepsy, were reported to result in serious amnesia. In rats, hippocampus is closely related to spatial memory, and lesions may cause deficits in learning and memory.

Amygdala and *septum* are other two limbic structures receiving serotonergic projections from the raphe nucleus. Amygdala is especially related to formation of anxiety and aggression. Lesioning of this region abolishes aggression and anxiety, whereas electrical stimulation causes excessive increase in these behaviours in animals. Lesions of septum in laboratory animals, result in changes in affect.

Cerebral cortex is the highest and most complex part of the brain. Glutamate and GABA are the two main neurotransmitters, excitatory and inhibitory, respectively. The most important function of the cortex is the management of integration of the sensory information received from lower centers. It has important contribution to the regulation of motor activity. It has specialised parts for the recognition of spoken or written language. Besides, more importantly, it has important role in the formation of mental processes related with cognition and thoughts.

Mental Diseases, the Contribution of Stress and Hippocampal Disorders

Hippocampus: Neuroanatomy, Histology and Hippocampal Neural Pathways

Hippocampus is the most important region in the brain about neuroplasticity. There may be two reasons for this. First, it is really rich in incoming and outgoing fibers (Figure 6), and is densely connected to other parts of the limbic system, especially amygdala. Second, it is the center for basic adaptive responses: memory and learning. Thus, due to the main subject of this book, we will be reviewing neuroanatomy, neurohistology of hippocampus and stress related changes in hippocampus in more detail.

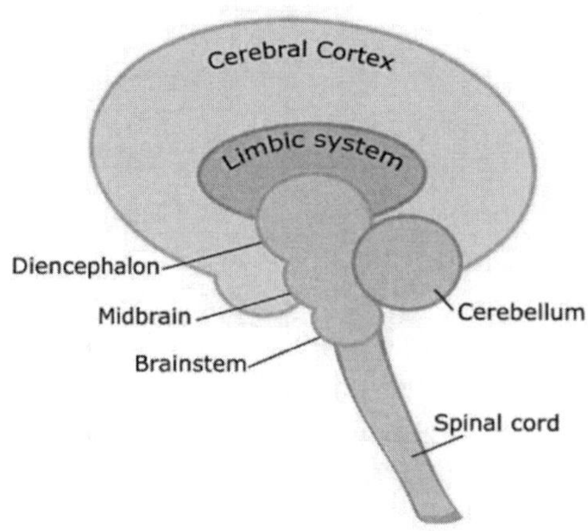

Figure 5. Principle neuroanatomic regions in central nervous system.

Hippocampus is an important neuroanatomic structure in midbrain limbic system (Figues 7).

Hippocampus is circumvented with lateral ventricule, entorhinal cortex and subiculum. Cornu ammonis and dentate gyrus are the functionally most important parts of the hippocampus (Figure 8). Cornu ammonis can be divided into 4 subregions, named CA1 to CA4. Pyramidal and granular cells that may easily be seen with microscopic examination are the most important functional elements of hippocampus. Pyramidal cells are distributed from the CA1 to CA4, wheras granular cells are localised to dentate gyrus (Figure 8, 9).

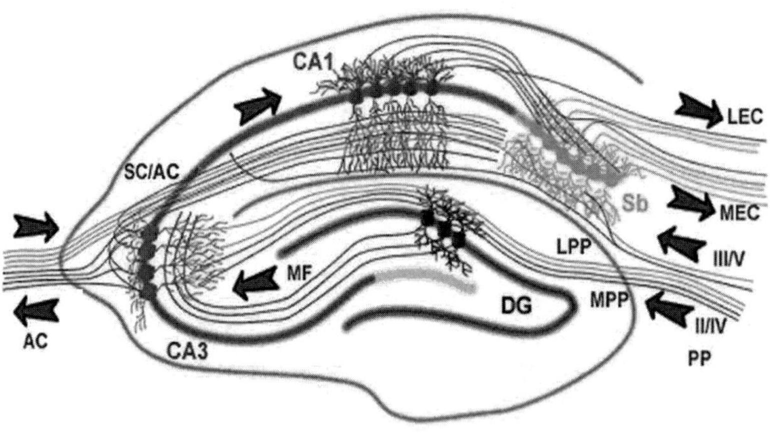

Figure 6. Hippocampal neural circuits. Nerve fibers coming to hippocampus from lateral and medial entorhinal cortex (MEC, LEC) are connected to pyramidal neurons in CA3 region of cornu ammonis (CA) and dentate gyrus (DG) through perforant pathway (PP). CA3 neurons receive neural input from DG through mossy fibers (MF), and project their axons over Schaffer collaterals (SC) and commissural pathway (CP) to CA1 regions. CA1 neurons receive direct fibers form PP and project axons to subiculum (Sb). Fibers starting from this region project back to EC forming the hippocampal output (Uzbay, 2005).

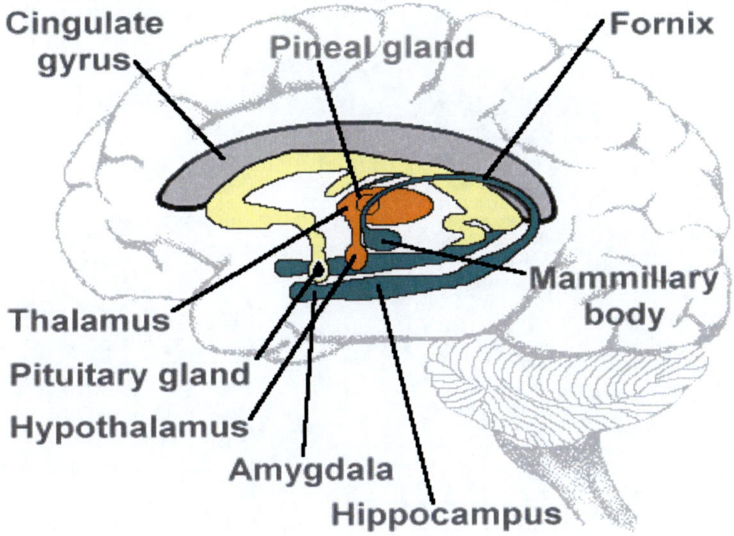

Figure 7. Hippocampus and limbic system (Uzbay, 2005).

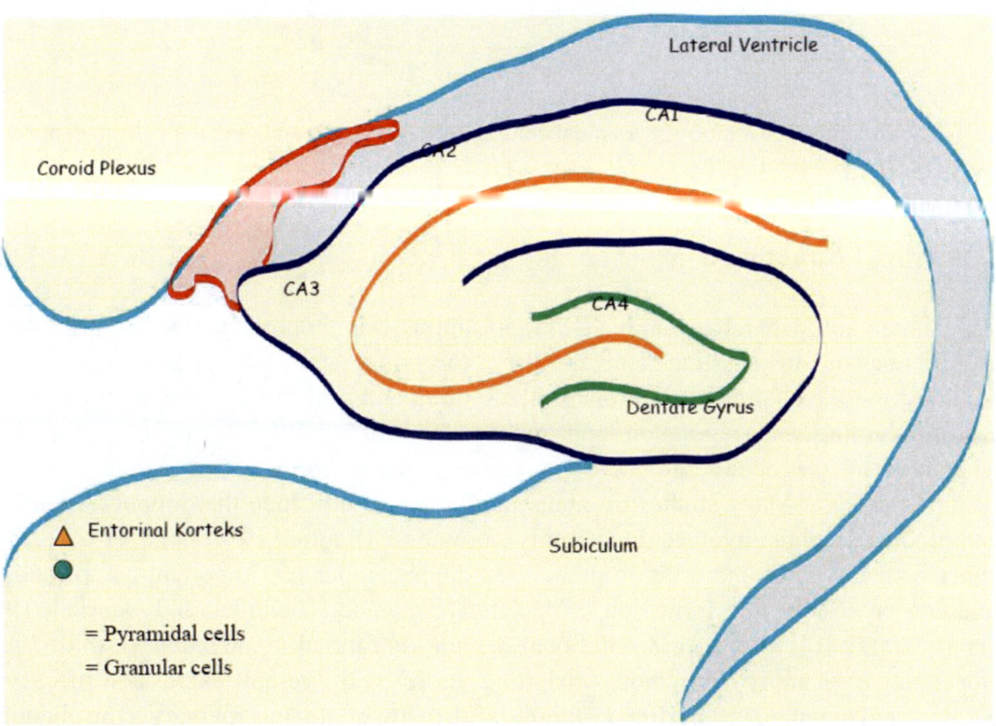

Figure 8. Neuroanatomical subregions of hippocampus in a coronal section (Uzbay, 2005).

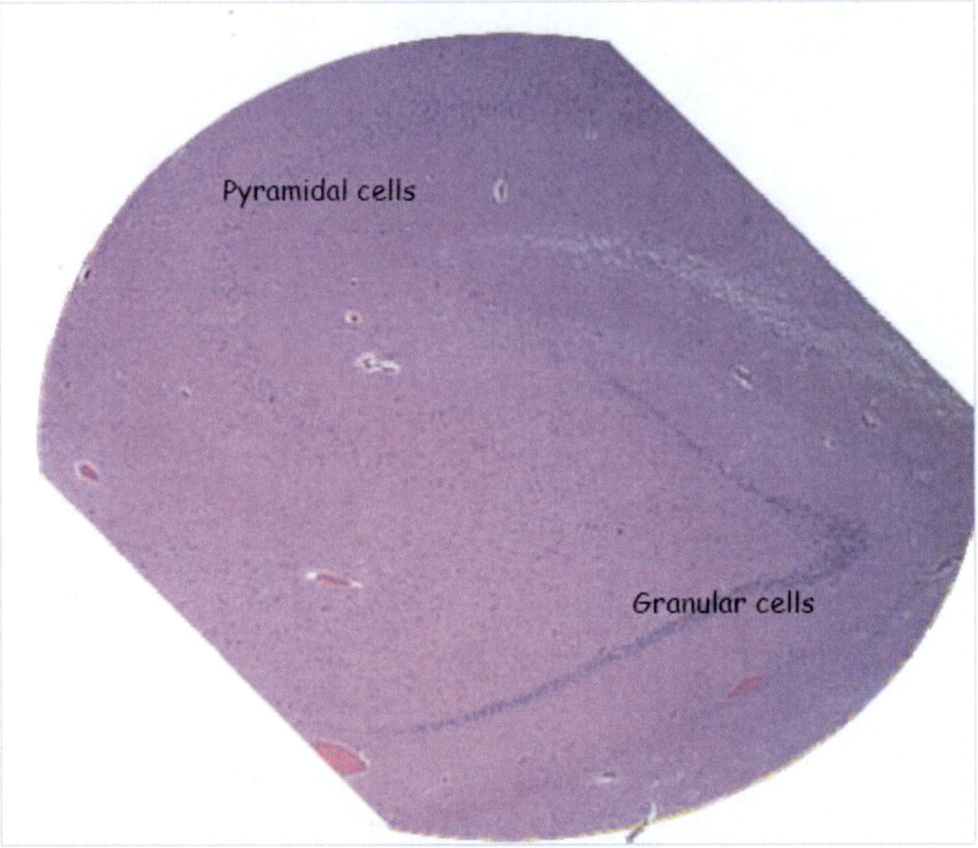

Figure 9. Microscopic appearance of pyramidal cells in cornu ammonis and granular cells in dentate gyrus, in the hippocampus (Uzbay, 2005).

Hippocampal Functions

In human and laboratory animals, hippocampus has important role in physiologic processes relevant to learning and memory formation. **"Septohippocampal pathway"**, originating from the cholinergic neurons in the septum and projecting to the hippocampus, is related to learning and regulation and management of short-term memeory functions. Degeneration of the cholinergic neurons causes various forms of demantia, including **Alzheimer's disease. Many studies on human and animals conclude that hippocampus is an** important brain region involved in memory formation (Squire, 1992; Sala et al., 2004). Together with amygdala and orbitofrontal cortex, hippocampus has important contribution in information processing and formation of declarative memory (Poldrack and Gabrieli, 1997; Shu et al., 2003). It is known that, emotional memory is formed in amygdala (Cahill, 2000), and declarative memory formation, including cases with verbal expression occurs in hippocampus (Brewin, 2001). **Hippocampus is also important in "memory consolidation"** which is the process of conversion of short-term memory to long-term memory in the neocortex. Here, hippocampus plays a critical role in supplying the first input necessary for the long-term memory, conversion of these to long-term memories, and formation and strenghtening of the synaptic connections necessary for the maintenance of long-term memory (Wittenberg and Tsien, 2002; Sala et al., 2004).

Hippocampus, working together with amygdala, is related to conditioned fear response. A stimulus that may cause fear and threat reaches to amygdala, which is the most imporant structure about these emotions; hippocampus and some other cortical structures are also stimulated independent from amygdala. Hippocampus performs the necessary function of processing and realisation of the stimulus (Sala et al., 2004). This immediately leads to better interpretation of the fearful stimulus and evaluation of the real threatening value, initiation of the memory processes necessary for taking precautions, and neglecting the stimulus if it is not a real threat. Improper functioning of the hippocampus, results in the incapability of the organism in rationally responding to the stimuli. This condition may be related to many psychiatric problems, like anxiety and suicide.

There are two stages in the process of stress related disorders. First, there is an increase in catecholaminergic activity and because of that there is an increase in amount and rate of flow of oxygen and glucose into the brain. This is a beneficial condition, in that it results in an acute increase in cognitive processes with the stimulus. This can be an example of the organism's increasing level of arousal in case of a threatening situation. Still, prolonged duration of exposure to the increased levels of catecholamines may interfere with the cognitive functions (McEwen and Sapolsky, 1995). In the second stage, HPA is stimulated in response to the stres, resulting in increased glucocorticoid release and levels. Increased levels of glucocorticoids can supress learning related neuronal processes like "long term potentiation" (LTP) in hippocampus (Sala et al., 2004). Low levels of glucocorticoids enhance neuronal processes like LTP, wheras higher levels supress. This data has been consistently proven to be true with many experiments (Diamond and Rose, 1994; McEwen and Sapolsky, 1995; Pavlides et al., 1995; Lupien and McEwen, 1997).

Another important function of hippocampus is the regulation of response to stress. It is not yet clearly known which neurotransmitter systems are involved in the regulation of responses during and after repetitive distressing stimuli in the hippocampus. Though there are clear evidences that glucocorticoids, particularly corticosterone, and excitatory aminoacids, particularly glutamate have significant contributions. Glucocorticoids are believed to act in collaboration with excitatory aminoacids, serotonine and GABA in the regulation of these responses (Sala et al., 2004).

In laboratory animals, with the first exposure to stress, there is an increase in glutamate release in prefrontal cortex and prefrontal areas; this causes increase of monoamines in brain regions like ventral striatum, amygdala and prefrontal areas (Moghaddam, 2002). Within these conditions, hippocampus regulates the activity of hypothalamohypophysealadrenal axis (HPA) through its projections to the neuroendocrine related areas of the paraventricular nuclei. In the studies of stress reactions of animals, it was suggested that increased levels of glucocorticoids decrease the capacity of hippocampus to supress HPA, and this resulted in the hypothesis of "glucocorticoid turnover". According to this hypothesis, excessive stress or glucocorticoid use damages the hippocampus and cause severe injury. This hypothesis received important support from findings of some preclinical studies (McEwen 1999a, b; Sapolsky, 2000; Sala, 2004). In several species of laboratory animals, it is shown that there may be a correlation between increased levels of glucocorticoids during distress and structural damage in the hippocampus (Uno et al., 1989; Sapolsky et al., 1990; Watanabe et al., 1992). In several studies in which high levels of glucocorticoids are applied for prolonged periods or restrain stress was applied, it has been shown that significant level of damage at cellular level occur, like increased neuronal dendritic reshaping (Woolley et al., 1990), apical atrophy in the dendrites (Magarinos et al., 1996; Watanabe et al., 1992), structural changes in synapses (Magarinos et al., 1997), suppression of neurogenesis (Gould et al., 1998; Duman et al., 2001), increase of neuronal loss (Uno et al., 1989, Mizoguchi et al., 1992), in the hippocampus.

Glucocorticoids applied exogenously, or released in increased amounts in response to the stress, increase glutamatergic activity in the hippocampus (Moghaddam et al., 1994; 2002; Stein-Behrens et al., 1994; Venero and Borrel, 1999). High levels of glutamate have disadvantageous effects on the hippocampus due to stimulation of NMDA receptors and increase in intracellular Ca (Landfield, 1994). Both inhibitors of steroid synthesis and NMDA receptor antagonists were shown to repair the dendritic atrophy caused by stress (Magarinos and McEwen, 1995a, b). These observations indicate that high levels of glucocorticoids released as a response to stress, can result in severe damage in hippocampus, through increasing inflow of Ca via stimulation of NMDA receptors.

It can be assumed that, serotonine has a role in stress-induced damage in the hippocampus due. It is reported that serotonine release is increased during stress (Chaouloff, 1993). There are studies indicating that the damage in the CA3 region of the hippocampus resulting from stress can be prevented by application of tianeptin, an antidepressant increasing serotonine reuptake (Watanabe et al., 1992; McEwen et al., 1997; Magarinos et al., 1999). Findings of these studies support that hypothesis. There is not still enough evidence to consider that serotonine or serotonergic system have as strong influence in the stress response in hippocampus as glutamate has. Yet, it is not clearly known how tianeptin affects the serotonergic system (Pineyro and blier, 1999), and there is the possibility that it may have positive effects on the hippocampal injury due to the interaction with other neurotransmitter system. Recent studies have shown that tianeptin blocks free radical nitric oxide (Wegener et al., 2003), which is known to cause neuronal injury and excitatory responses activating the glutamatergic system in the central nervous system (Garthwaite, 1991; Uzbay and Oglesby, 2001), and it directly inhibits glutamatergic activity in hippocampus (Kole et al., 2002; Reagan et al., 2004). The effects of tianeptin on the stress related damage in hippocampus and probable mechanisms of action will be explored in greater detail in later sections of this book.

There are many publications indicating that stress induced changes in hippocampus can be related to psychiatric disorders like posttraumatic stress disorder, borderline personality disorder and depression. Hippocampal changes in depression and relevance of stress induced changes in hippocampus and depression will be discussed later in this book, under the title of neuroplasticity.

Depression and Neurobiology of Depression

Depression is an important psychiatric disorder that affects individuals' quality of life and social relations directly. Depression is characterized by emotional symptoms such as hopelessness, apathy, loss of self-confidence, sense of guilt, indecisiveness, and amotivation, as well as biological symptoms like psychomotor retardation, loss of libido, sleep disturbances, and loss of appetite. When the symptoms are very severe major depression is considered. The prevalence of major depression is approximately 9% in both the United States and Europe (Fichter et al., 1996; Lepine et al., 1997).

Depression should be considered a disease to be definitely followed and treated because of its prevalence, negative effect on the workforce, and suicidal outcome. However, depression is underdiagnosed for several reasons (Richelson, 2001). One of the main reasons is the lack of objective diagnostic methods like neuroimaging techniques. Today the diagnosis of depression also depends on the information obtained from the patient and assessment of this information in the context of several scales. These assessments occasionally yield false or insufficient diagnoses due to the subjectivity of the data.

In recent years, the contribution of pharmacotherapy to depression treatment has become greater. Depression treatment mostly requires long-term, chronic antidepressant therapy, and thus the side effects and safety of available antidepressants are of great importance. A substantial proportion of the adverse effects of antidepressants are explained by their synaptic effects. Changes in the synaptic activity of many neurotransmitters, especially serotonin and noradrenalin, due to these drugs account for many of these side effects as well as their antidepressant activity (Richelson, 2001). The neurobiological mechanisms underlying depression should be clarified in order to diagnose depression more reliably and to treat it more effectively by developing more specific drugs.

Today, the most widely accepted opinion about depression concerns its direct relation with noradrenergic and serotonergic systems. The mechanism of action of available antidepressants involves one or both of these systems. Therefore, a general overview of noradrenergic and serotonergic systems will also be included in this section.

Noradrenergic System

Many of the adrenergic neuron bodies are located at a nucleus in the brainstem, namely the locus ceruleus (LC). This is a center that also executes other functions like behavior, cognition, mood, emotions, and movements. Noradrenergic fibers originating from the LC join to the medial forebrain bundle and form projections to the limbic system, hypothalamus, and cortex (Figure 10). The noradrenergic system is responsible for the modulation of arousal, modulation of mood, and central modulation of blood pressure and heart rate. Increased noradrenergic activity is associated with anxiety, mania, hypervigilance, and induction of the brain reward system. Decreased noradrenergic activity is known to be associated with depression as well as decreased attention and concentration, impairment in working memory, slowed information processing, psychomotor retardation and fatigue (Stahl, 1996).

Decreased noradrenergic transmission is proposed to contribute to some schizophrenic symptoms (Bird et al., 1979; Snyder, 1982). Noradrenalin contributes to the motor effects of dopamine. In Parkinson's disease decreased noradrenergic activity due to noradrenergic neuron damage in the brainstem also contributes to motor impairment although not as much as the dopamine system does (Marsden, 1982). Noradrenergic neuron destruction also contributes to the symptoms in Alzheimer's disease due to a cholinergic defect.

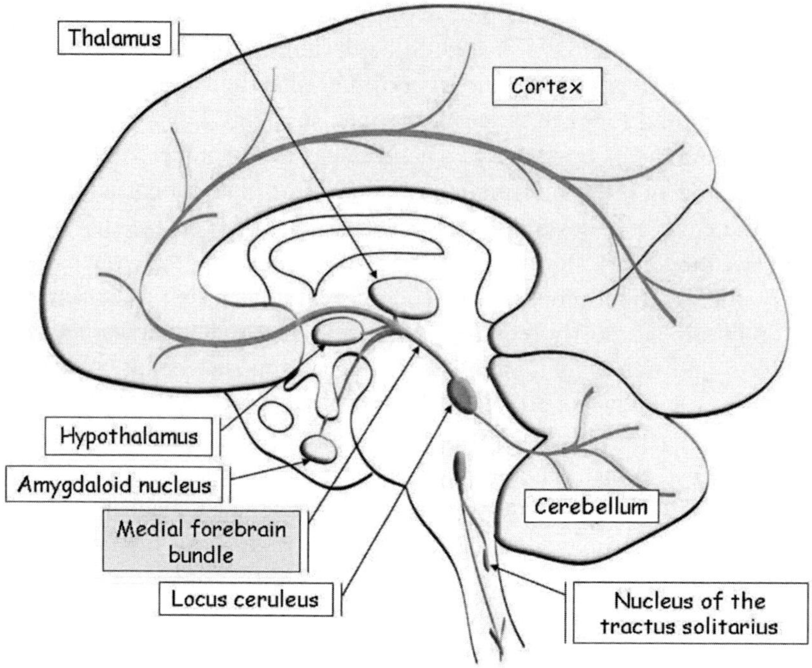

Figure 10. Brain noradrenergic system (Uzbay, 2004).

Serotonergic System

Serotonin is a neurotransmitter in the central nervous system and a transmitter that has neuromodulatory effects on different effector cells at the periphery. Neurons localized in the brainstem dorsal and median raphe nuclei are the primary sources of serotonin (Ninan, 1999). Serotonergic fibers originating from the raphe nucleus form projections to the thalamus, hypothalamus, limbic system, striatum, cerebral cortex and cerebellum (Figure 11).

The main functions of the serotonergic system in the central nervous system are listed below.

Mood

The role of serotonin in anxiety is supported by its modulatory effects over the LC and by serotonergic fibers reaching the amygdala (Dubovsky and Thomas, 1995; Ninan, 1999).

The interaction between serotonergic and noradrenergic systems may be associated with anxiety development. Research on monkey brains shows that the LC has serotonergic neurons as well as noradrenergic neurons. In addition, the brainstem raphe system, which may be regarded as the central serotonergic center, is also innervated by noradrenergic neurons and the LC receives serotonergic innervation from the brainstem raphe system (Mason and Fibiger, 1979; Hohen-Saric, 1982; Ninan, 1999).

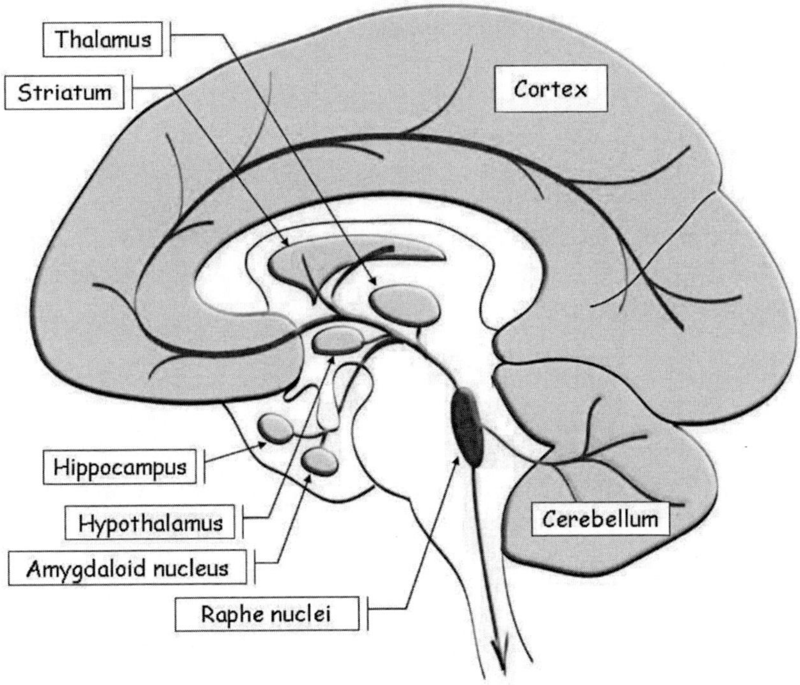

Figure 1. Brain serotonergic system (Uzbay, 2004).

It is proposed that modulation of central serotonergic activity has a role in the anxiolytic effects of benzodiazepines besides their interaction with the LC and the noradrenergic system (Stein et al., 1975; Sepinwall and Cook, 1980).

Important data indicate that among the serotonin receptors presynaptic 5-HT1A autoreceptors and postsynaptic 5-HT3 receptors are associated with anxiety. 5-HT1A receptor agonist drugs such as buspiron, ipsapiron and gepiron are used in the treatment of generalized anxiety disorder in particular (Goldberg and Finnerty, 1979; Yocca, 1990). It is also observed that serotonin 5-HT3 receptor blockage has positive effects in several experimental anxiety models. These findings suggest that 5-HT3 receptor antagonists like ondansetron may be a novel class of drugs for anxiety treatment (Rang et al., 1998; Olivier et al., 2000). Recently, selective serotonin reuptake inhibitors like fluoxetine and noradrenalin and serotonin reuptake inhibitors like venlafaxin have been observed to be effective in the treatment of different anxiety disorders (Stahl, 1996; Rang et al., 1999, Allgulander et al., 2001). However, the mechanism of action of these antidepressants on serotonin and noradrenalin in the treatment of anxiety has not been clearly identified yet.

A decrease in serotonergic activity is associated with depression. In experimental studies decreases in brain serotonergic activity due to social isolation have been known about for a long time (Garattini et al., 1967). Specifically, rodents display hyperactive and aggressive behavior during long-term social isolation that can be blocked with antidepressant treatment (Garzon and del Rio, 1981). These social isolation forms based on serotonin deficiency are used as experimental depression models in rodents (Leonard, 1998). On the other hand, selective serotonin reuptake inhibitors and some postsynaptic receptor agonists, which increase serotonergic activity in the synaptic space, are used widely and effectively for treating depression (Cowen, 1998; Vaswani et al., 2003).

Hallucinations and Behavioral Changes

Serotonin analogues like LSD depress brainstem serotonergic neurons that are responsible for inhibition in the cortical area. This loss of inhibition is thought to be responsible for hallucinogenic effects. Serotonin precursors cause 'wet dog shake' behavior in experimental animals (Rang et al., 1999).

Modulation of Sleep and Arousal

Degeneration of the raphe nucleus and serotonergic hypoactivity inhibit sleep, and serotonin microinjection to the brainstem induces sleep (Rang et al., 1999).

Nociception

Serotonin has inhibitory effects on pain conductance in the spinal channel. Depletion of serotonin via parachlorphenylalanine (pCPA) or selective lesions of serotonin containing descending neurons inhibits the analgesic effects of morphine in experimental animals (Uzbay et al., 1999).

Modulation of Eating and Drinking Behavior

Serotonergic drugs in the paraventricular nucleus of the hypothalamus contribute to the control of appetite. Anticholinergic drugs may cause weight gain by increasing appetite (Rang et al., 1999).

Other

5-HT3 receptor antagonists like ondansetron have strong antiemetic effects. They inhibit nausea and vomiting, particularly during chemotherapy. Serotonin is also associated with temperature regulation and sexual dysfunction (Rang et al., 1999).

Monoamine Hypothesis of Depression

Most information about the mechanism of depression depends on the monoamine hypothesis, which is still partially valid today. The main biochemical hypothesis proposed in depression is based on a direct relationship between the occurrence of depression and loss of monoamine neurotransmitters, especially noradrenalin and serotonin, in certain areas of the brain (Bunney and Davis, 1965; Schildkraut, 1965). In mania there is hyperfunction of these neurotransmitters in the same regions. This hypothesis is supported by the depression-treating effects of drugs like tricyclic antidepressants, monoamine oxidase inhibitors and selective serotonin reuptake inhibitors (SSRI) that increase monoaminergic transmission and effectiveness in synapses in contrast to the depression-causing effect of reserpine, a drug that has activity opposite to these drugs, in both humans and animals (Leonard, 1998; Delgado et al., 1998).

In biochemical studies of depressive patients, although not in all forms of depression, results supporting monoamine hypothesis were obtained in many patients (Bondy, 2002). The contribution of noradrenalin to depression is confirmed by the observation of significantly decreased renal excretion of its metabolite 3-methoxy-4-hydroxyphenylglycol (MHPG) in depressive patients compared with normal controls (Maas et al., 1968). Serotonin's role in depression has been subject to more detailed studies, and the view that serotonin is the major monoamine associated with the development of depression has gained importance over time. In studies, amounts of 5-hydroxyindol acetic acid (5-HIAA), the major metabolite of serotonin, in cerebrospinal fluid, and tryptophan, the free precursor of serotonin in plasma, are found to be lower in depressive patients than in controls (van Praag, 1982a). Results of postmortem examinations also show that serotonin and serotonin metabolites are significantly lower in several regions of the brain in depressive people (van Praag, 1982b). The most important data proving the importance of biogenic amines concern the antidepressant activity of drugs that increase monoamine activity in the synaptic space by inhibiting monoamine reuptake (tricyclic antidepressants) and enzymatic catabolism (MAO inhibitors).

In line with the monoamine hypothesis, predicting that drugs that increase the synaptic effectiveness of monoamines have antidepressant effects, many drug groups like tricyclic antidepressants and serotonin/noradrenalin reuptake inhibitors (SNRI) have been discovered and used for treatment. Tricyclics started to be used in the late fifties as the first antidepressants. In this period, based on the opinion that increasing monoamine levels may be successful in depression treatment, monoamine oxidase (MAO) enzyme inhibitors were started to be used along with tricyclic antidepressants. In the sixties and seventies inhibitors specific to MAO subtypes as well as inhibitors specific to noradrenalin and serotonin reuptake started to be used. The main reason for developing more specific drugs is to minimize side effects and to produce a stronger effect. In recent years drugs that are more specific to one of these monoamines like selective serotonin reuptake inhibitors such as fluoxetine and paroxetine and selective noradrenalin reuptake inhibitors such as reboxetine have become part of antidepressant treatment (Pacher et al., 2001). Studies on drugs that affect the serotonin system were not limited to serotonin reuptake inhibition in the synaptic space. Attempts were made to develop other drugs affecting serotonin receptors, especially 5-HT2 and 5-HT3, and these drugs are widely used in depression treatment (Hindmarch, 2002; Kennedy et al., 2004).

Is The Monoamine Hypothesis Alone Sufficient to Explain Depression?

Whether monoamine hypothesis can explain all parameters associated with depression has been discussed for a long time. There are two important problems regarding the monoamine hypothesis. The first is the presence of refractory depression cases that do not respond to any antidepressant. Their number is too high to be neglected. The second important and interesting problem is the antidepressant effects of some drugs that have opposite effects on monoamines and the lack of significant differences between the antidepressant effects of these drugs. The most interesting example of this is the similar antidepressant effectiveness of tianeptine, a drug defined as an atypical antidepressant by some authors, and SSRIs, which have a theoretically opposite mechanism of action. The addition of tianeptine to antidepressant treatment led to a debate on the serotonin part of the monoamine hypothesis and forced scientists to seek new insights.

The tianeptine molecule was synthesized at the Servier Institute, France, at the beginning of the eighties during research to develop new antidepressant drugs more effective and safer than tricyclics. Its molecular formulation is $C_{21}H_{24}ClN_2NaO_4S$, and its molecular structure includes a substituted dibenzotiazepine nucleus and a long aminoheptanoic acid side chain (figure 12). This 7 carbon amino acid (NH-$(CH_2)_6$-COONa) side chain distinguishes it from tricyclic antidepressants.

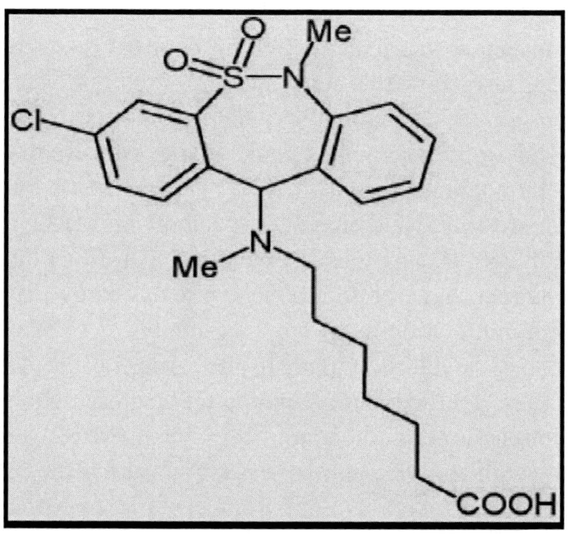

Figure 12. Chemical structure of tianeptine.

Tianeptine is an antidepressant primarily acting on the serotonergic system. It does not inhibit serotonin reuptake as many antidepressants do; instead it increases serotonin reuptake selectively in both the brain and thrombocytes. This effect occurs after both acute and chronic administration (Menini et al., 1987; Kato and Weitsch, 1988; Fattacini et al., 1990).

In contrast to tricyclic antidepressants and SSRIs, tianeptine decreases serotonin's activity and amount in serotonergic synapses of the central nervous system by increasing serotonin reuptake. The antidepressant effects and similar antidepressant effectiveness of tianeptine, and SSRIs that have opposite mechanisms of action on the serotonergic system (Loo et al., 1999; Waintraub et al., 2000) are an interesting point indicating that central mechanisms of action associated with depression should be reviewed. The following opinions attempt to explain the antidepressant effectiveness of tianeptine (Ansseau, 1993; Uzbay and Yüksel, 2002).

The first hypothesis states that diseases may be characterized more by increases in serotonergic neurotransmission than by serotonin decreases, and therefore agents decreasing serotonin levels have good antidepressant effectiveness. Indeed, it is reported that many antidepressant drugs can cause a degree of 5-HT receptor blockage, and receptor blocking effects may be dominant over serotonergic activity increasing effects. This opinion also suggests the depression hypothesis based on increased serotonergic activity due to several reasons (Aprison et al., 1982). Some antidepressants prominently block post-synaptic 5-HT2 receptors. For example, amitriptilin causes a strong blockage in 5-HT2 receptors while causing moderate inhibition of serotonin reuptake, and the net effect is a decrease in serotonergic transmission (Nagayama et al., 1980; Willner, 1985). Another finding that supports this hypothesis is the antidepressant effect of the 5-HT2 receptor blocker, ritanserin (Reyntjens et al., 1986). However, the predominant effect of 5-HT receptor blockage over serotonin reuptake inhibition is not a general property of all antidepressants (Ansseau, 1993).

The second opinion is the presence of depression subtypes characterized by an increase or decrease in serotonergic activity (Willner, 1985). Tianeptine may be effective in depressions characterized by an increase in serotonergic activity while SSRIs are effective in depressions characterized by a decrease in serotonergic activity. However, placebo-controlled double-blind studies found no difference between tianeptin and SSRIs in similar depression types and thus do not support this hypothesis.

The third opinion is that there is no relation between the clinical antidepressant effects of SSRIs and serotonin reuptake inhibition. In other words, although serotonin reuptake inhibition starts from the first day of SSRI treatment the antidepressant effects of these drugs emerge 2-3 weeks later (Quitkin et al., 1984; Kato and Weitsch, 1998). Moreover, although in vitro and acute administration of classical tricyclics like imipramin and desipramin causes serotonin reuptake inhibition, chronic administration causes serotonin reuptake to increase (Barbaccia et al., 1983). A similar effect is reported for fluvoxamine (Brunello et al., 1987). It is possible to relate these effects of antidepressants with clinical changes following antidepressant treatment. During treatment with serotonin reuptake inhibitors an increase in depression severity during the first 1-2 weeks followed by a rapid clinical improvement (Ansseau, 1998) may also confirm this opinion. This kind of biphasic clinical change is more common with SSRIs like fluvoxamine (Den Boer and Westenberg, 1998). According to this opinion, tianeptine is an antidepressant drug that produces effects from the beginning of treatment that are produced later by other drugs. No worsening of symptoms with tianeptine at the beginning of antidepressant treatment and a rapid antidepressant effect also support this opinion.

As a result, until the antidepressant effect of tianeptine was shown, it seemed more logical that decreased serotonergic neurotransmission has a role in depression, and the antidepressant effectiveness of SSRIs supported this opinion. Tianeptine, an antidepressant, that has a mechanism of action opposite to that of SSRIs, necessitated a reevaluation of the biochemical basis of depressive disorders and revealed that it cannot be explained solely by the monoamine hypothesis.

An interesting study conducted recently suggests that tianeptine has a mechanism of action similar to that of fluoxetine (Alici et al., 2006). This experimental study examined the drug preference and discrimination producing properties of fluoxetine and tianeptine in rats. The principle of the model used in this test is to overlap the discriminative effects of tianeptine and fluoxetine or the ineffectiveness of saline injections in a mechanism where test subjects may get food using a left or right pedal (Uzbay, 2004). To do this firstly the food intake of the subjects is restricted. Then they are put into cages and stay there for two days to learn to obtain food by pressing a pedal. During the first treatment session the system is adjusted so that the subject receives food when it presses either of the pedals. After the subject learns to get food by pressing a pedal the system is adjusted so that food is given after the subject presses different pedals in response to saline or tianeptine injections. For example, to get food, the subject learns to press the left pedal if saline is injected and the right pedal if tianeptine is injected. After all subjects are taught to differentiate the saline and tianeptine pedals (figure 13) they enter the principle experiment.

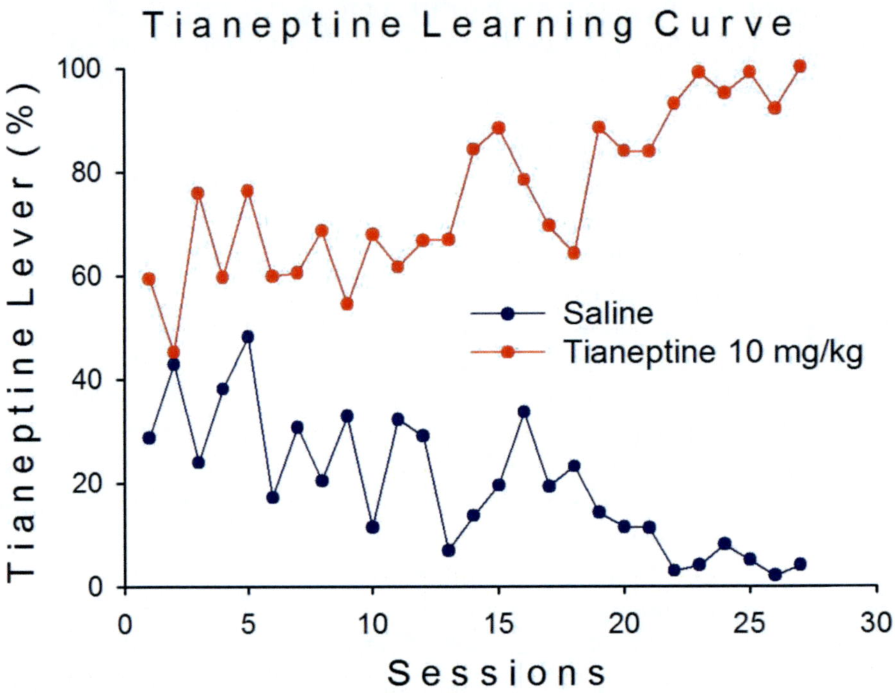

Figure 13. Discrimination of tianeptin (10 mg/kg) from saline. Although at the beginnig of the study **rats' ability to discriminate tianeptin from saline was varying between** 30-50 % at the end it reached to nearly 100%. Vertical axis of the graph shows percentage pressing of samples on tianeptin arm (n=7; TNP=Tianeptin) (Alici et al., 2006).

During the test the system is adjusted again as the beginning so that food is given if the subject presses either of the pedals. This time fluoxetine is given instead of tianeptin to the subjects that have learned to discriminate between saline and tianeptine. If the substance is tested (fluoxetine) has stimulating properties similar to those of tianeptine the subjects are expected to press the right pedal to get food. In this study the subjects experience a fluoxetine injection similar to that of tianeptine in a certain dose range. In other words, tianeptine and fluoxetine created similar discriminative properties in rats (figure 14). These results also indicate that tianeptine and fluoxetine may have important similarities in terms of their behavioral mechanisms of action.

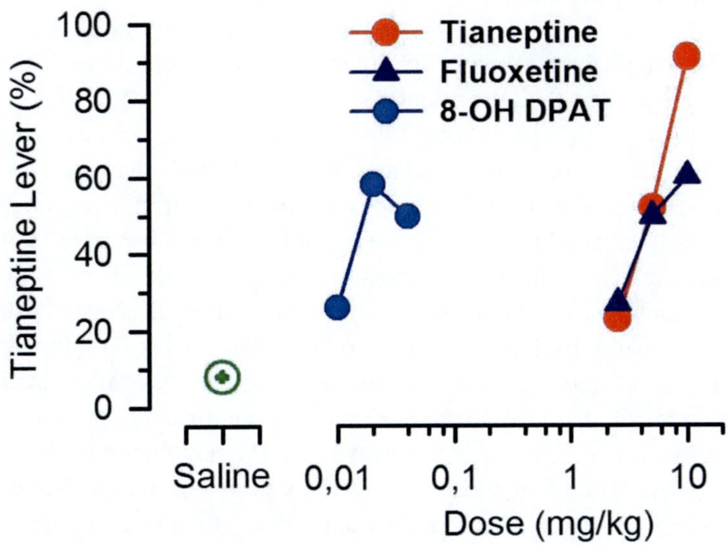

Figure 14. Figure 14: Fluoxetine shows tianeptin like effects on rats trained for tianeptin at a certain dose (n=7-9; TNP=Tianeptin) (Alici et al.., 2006).

Another interesting finding of this study is the lack of similar discriminative stimulating properties between tianeptin and venlafaxine, a serotonin and noradrenalin reuptake inhibitor, and caffeine, another stimulating substance that antagonizes adenosine (figure 15). These findings show that tianeptine's discriminative properties are not associated with caffeine-like psychostimulation. In addition, there are expected to be differences between the mechanisms of action of tianeptin and another antidepressant, venlafaxine.

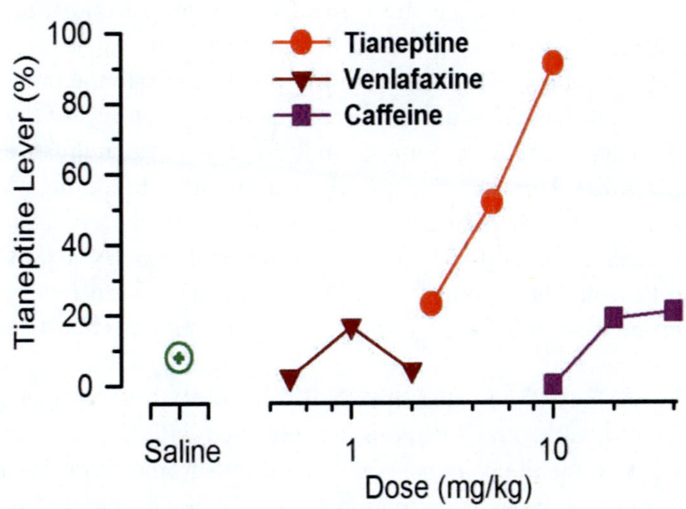

Figure 15. Venlafaxine and caffeine administration to rats trained for tianeptinedoes not show tianeptine like effect (n=7-9; TNP: Tianeptine) (Alici et al.., 2006).

Neuroplasticity Hypothesis

A decrease in hippocampal volume in patients with recurrent, refractory depressions or in those having unipolar depression or long-lasting depression, while there is no change in hippocampal volume in young patients with less depressive episodes (Sala et al., 2004), indicates that depression may be associated with structural changes and degeneration in important central regions like the hippocampus as much as with direct changes in the synaptic activities of neurochemicals like monoamines. Starting from these observations, attempts are made to explain the mechanism of depression using changes in neuroplasticity, and the neuroplasticity hypothesis of depression is proposed (Fuchs et al., 2004; Castren, 2005).

This hypothesis explains depression via structural changes in the brain and remodeling in some critical areas like the hippocampus due to these changes rather than the amounts of neurotransmitters released into the synaptic space, their metabolism and their effect on the postsynaptic region via receptors or other ways. This remodeling occurs due to a change in brain neuroplasticity. Besides monoamines like noradrenalin and serotonin, changes in the amounts of several excitatory neurotransmitters like glutamate are also associated with remodeling related functional impairment. Antidepressant treatment primarily reverses this remodeling in addition to stabilizing the impaired monoaminergic balance. During chronic antidepressant treatment a normalized state of neuron structure and synapses is maintained due to the neuroprotective effect (Fuchs et al., 2004). In the following sections of this book the development of depression and the mechanisms of action of antidepressants will be discussed in detail in the context of neuroplasticity.

NEUROPLASTICITY

What is Neuroplasticity?

Most of the neurons in humans are formed in the late second trimester in prenatal life. Neuronal migration begins in the first weeks of gestation and is nearly finished at term. Indeed, the development of the human brain is more dynamic in the prenatal period and in the early postnatal period than in adult periods. Synapse formation is very rapid from birth to approximately 6 years of age. Beginning from the age of 14 the number of synapses gradually decreases (Stahl, 2000). This decrease continues throughout life although it slows to a certain level. As the number of synapses decreases the ability of neurons to regenerate and repair themselves continues along with new neuron formation. Formerly, it was thought that besides the decrease in the number of synapses the ability of neurons to regenerate themselves was also lost and no new neurons were formed. Today the opposite has been proved to be the case.

The central nervous system has the ability to adapt both exogenous and endogenous stimuli. Many important central functions are executed with this adaptation, and insufficient adaptation causes the emergence of several diseases. Neuroplasticity can be defined shortly as changes in the brain's **neurons** and structural and functional changes in synapses formed by these neurons. If the changes are not confined to a single neuron but reach the level of a synapse **the adaptive response formed may also be called 'synaptic plasticity'. Variability** of synaptic activity plays a role in the adaptation of the nervous system. The behavioral effects of hormones may be examples of endogenous variations. It has long been known that animal sexual behavior is associated with periodically released hormones and that these hormones exert their effects by changing synaptic activity (Cotman and Nieto-Sampedro, 1984). Adaptation to environmental changes may only be accomplished by learning, and learning requires synaptic plasticity. Learning is the strongest and most important adaptive response of the central nervous system to endogenous and exogenous stimuli. LTP formation in neurons is necessary for learning. LTP formation is an adaptive response associated with neuroplasticity and synaptic plasticity. Although chronic and severe stress causes negative neuroadaptive changes like depression, short term and limited stress is necessary for LTP, which forms the basis for learning. As shown in this discussion, neuroplasticity can cause positive as well as negative changes.

The aplysia is one of the animals most commonly used to examine synaptic mechanisms of learning. This snail rapidly withdraws its gills when a tactile stimulus is applied to its tail or siphon. A decrease in response is observed if the stimulus is repeated. This habituation is explained by a decrease in the efficiency of synapses between sensory and motor neurons. If an electric shock is applied to the tail of the aplysia simultaneously with a tactile stimulus to its siphon a stronger and longer gill withdrawal response is observed with subsequent tactile stimuli. This phenomenon, namely sensitization, is explained by an increase in the efficiency of synapses between sensory and motor neurons (Feldman, 1997).

Table 1. Neuroplasticity-induced changes in the brain

Increase or decrease in dendritic branching
Breakage of dendrites
Increase in dendritic length
New synapse formation or disappearance of present synapses
Change in synaptic efficiency of present synapses (Increase or decrease)
Neurogenesis
Apoptosis
Changes in main brain metabolites
Changes in survival of present neurons (increase or decrease)
Increased resistance of neurons to breakage under stress
Changes in stimulus-induced postsynaptic potentials of present neurons
Changes in activities of neurotrophic factors (increase or decrease)

Some physical changes may appear in the whole neuron or in a part like the dendrite due to neuroplasticity. In addition, new neuron formation, changes in neurons' resistance to negative factors like chronic severe stress and an increase or decrease in synaptic activity may appear. Changes in the central nervous system associated with neuroplastic responses are seen in Table 1.

Depending on the strength and length of the stimulus and the properties of primary responding region, one, several or all of these changes may appear. The quality of the resulting neuroplasticity and remodeling due to it also depend on these factors. New neuron formation is called neurogenesis. Neurogenesis is observed most often in the hippocampus and olfactory region. Increases in hippocampal volume and neurogenesis are seen with every mental exercise and chronic stress causes decreases in hippocampal volumes and neurogenesis of hippocampal neurons (Stahl, 2000; Czeh et al., 2001).

Neurotrophic factors are always released in very low concentrations and sometimes they change neurotransmitter-mediated central neurochemical transmission. Some psychotropic drugs may act on central neurotrophic factors besides neurochemical transmission (Carvey, 1998). Some of the important neurotrophic factors known to be present in the central nervous system are seen in Table 2. Neurotrophic factors do not function as neurotransmitters in the central nervous system; primarily they help the development and regeneration of neurons and they contribute to important neuron pathways for structural health and maintaining function. Neurotrophic factors have important roles in the central nervous system for programming and execution of apoptosis. Deficiency of certain neurotrophic factors specific to certain neurons due to endogenous or exogenous reasons triggers a biological cascade resulting in the death of that neuron or group of neurons (Carvey, 1998; Stahl, 2000).

Table 2. Some of the important neurotrophic factors present in the central nervous system

Nerve growth factor (NGF)
Brain-derived neurotrophic factor (BDNF)
Neurotrophin 3 (NT-3)
Neurotrophin 4/5 (NT-4/5)
Neurotrophin-6 (NT-6)
Neurotrophin-7 (NT-7)
Transforming growth factor b3 (TGF-b3)
Basic fibroblast growth factor (bFGF)
Acidic fibroblast growth factor (aFGF)
Glia-derived neurotrophic factor (GDNF)
Ciliary neurotrophic factor (CNTF)
Cholinergic development factor (CDF)
Platelet-derived neurotrophic factor (PDNF)
Insulin-dependent growth factor (IDGF)
Epidermal growth factor (EGF)
Proapoptotic receptors (P75)
Antiapoptotic receptors (TrkA)

Adopted from Carvey, 1998; Stahl, 2000; Sah et al., 2003; Shoval and Weizman, 2005.

The oldest and most widely known neurotrophic factor is nerve growth factor (NGF), isolated in the fifties by Rita Levi Montalcini. It is the best characterized member of the neurotrophins. NGF gene is located on Chromosome 1 (p21-p22.1 region). NGF has been found in the cortex, the hippocampus, the pituitary gland and the spinal cord. It was shown to promote the survival of primary sensory neurons, and of sympathetic and cholinergic neurons of the basal forebrain (Shoval and Weizman, 2005). It has been suggested that NGF has a prominent role in the pathophysiology and pharmacotherapy of some neurodegenerative disordes such as Alzheimer type senil dementia (Allen et al., 1991; Backman et al., 1997).

Brain-derived neurotrophic factor (BDNF) is a basic dimeric protein. BDNF's gene is located on Chromosome 11, bad p13 (Maisonpierre et al., 1991). This gene has been proposed as a possible source of malfunction in signal transduction from monoamine receptors (Kuipers et al., 2005). BDNF is structurally related to NGF, but it is more widespread in the central nervous system than NGF. Like NGF, BDNF is widespread in the hippocampus (Shoval and Weizman, 2005). Hippocampal damage has been shown to upregulate BDNF level in that region (Ballarin et al., 1991). BDNF has important roles in neurons' survival, maintaining their viability and executing their functions. Normally, BDNF sustains the viability of brain neurons, but the expression of this gene is inhibited under stress. The possibility that BDNF contributes to the action of antidepressant treatment has been supported by behavioral studies of recombinant BDNF and transgenic mouse models. Microinfusion of BDNF into hippocampus produces an antidepressant response in the learned helpness and forced swimming test model of depression (Shirayama et al., 2002; Duman, 2004). The antidepressant effect of BDNF is observed after a single infusion, and is relativelylong-lasting. Transgenicoverexpression of a dominant negative mutant of the BDNF receptor, trkB, in the hippocampus and other forebrain structures is also reported to block the effect of antidepressant treatment, demonstrating that BDNF signalling is necessary for an antidepressant response (Saarelainen et al., 2003). As more importantly, decreased plasma BDNF levels have been found in depressive patients in recent clinical studies (Aydemir et al., 2006, Kim et al., 2007). Furthermore, decreased levels of BDNF were reversed after antidepressant escitalopram therapy (Aydemir et al., 2006). Increasing BDNF expression-induced glutamate receptor activation may also be a new target for the treatment of depression. Memantine that modulates glutamate transmission increases BDNF expression. Riluzole, a sodium channel blocker, also increases BDNF expression and neurogenezis in rat hippocampus Marvanova et al., 2001; Katoh-Semba et al., 2002).

Neurotrophin-3 (NT-3)'s gene, located on Chromosome 12 band p13 (Maisone et al., 1991). NT-3 has a role in early neuronal development and that it would be a putative candidate for taking part in the pathophisiology of neurodevelopmental disorders such as schizophrenia (Shoval and Veizman, 2005). It also enhances dopaminergic neuron survival (Gall et al., 1992), indicating a possible role in the pathophysiology of other dopaminergic-related neuropsychiatric disorders such as Parkinson's disease and Tourette's syndrome.

Neurotrophin-4/5 (NT-4/5)'s gene is localized in human chromosome 19 band q 13.3 (Ip et al., 1992). It consists of two identical 130 amino acid subunits sharing 48% sequence identity to NGF and also related to BDNF. It is involved in the promotion of nerve growth and hippocampal cultures synaptic activity (Yin et al., 2001a,b; Schwyzer et al., 2002; Shoval and Weizman, 2005).

Neurotrophin-6 (NT-6) and neurotrophin-7 (NT-7) have been identified only in lower vertebrates. Any relevance of NT-6 and NT-7 to human neurophysiology, neuropathology or possible role in treatment is yet to be elucidated (Shoval and Weizman, 2005).

Neurotrophin receptors are widely expressed in the central nervous system and in the peripheral nervous system, both during brain development in adults. There are two known classes of neurotrophin receptors: The neurotrophin tyrosine kinase receptors (Trk) (high affinity) and the neurotrophin receptor $p75^{NTR}$ (low affinity) (Levin and Barde, 1996; Shoval and Weizman, 2005).

Trks are transmembranal proteins, prosesing and intirinsic tropomyosin related kinase activity. Three different Trks have been found. They are TrkA, TrkB and TrkC. TrkA has the highest affinity for NGF, TrkB has the highest affinity for BDNF and NT-4/5, while TrkC has the highest affinity for NT-3 (Chao et al., 1998; Shoval and Weizman, 2005).

Neurotrophins also bind, with lower affinity, to the $p75^{NTR}$ receptor. Its exact role is not clear, but it has been found to mediate the migration of Schwan cells explants. Interestingly TrkA and $p75^{NTR}$ were shown to collaborate to generate high affinity binding sites for NGF (Chao and Hempstead, 1995). $p75^{NTR}$ seems to act as a co-receptor modulating Trk signalling. Ths functional croostalk between Trk and $p75^{NTR}$ appears to be a key prosesses in the role of neurotropins in the nervous system (Kaplan and Miller, 2000).

Various psychotrop drugs have neuroprotective effects via affecting some neurotrophic factors and elements involved in signal transduction in neuronal membranes. Some of them are listed in Table 3.

Table 3. Neuroprotective effects of drugs

Drugs	Neuroprotection from	Neuropotection suggested to involve
Lithium	Glutamate toxicity β-Amyloid toxicity Oxidative stress MPP^+	Bcl2, GSK-3, CREB, BDNF
Valproate	MPP^+	Bcl2, GSK-3, BDNF, MAPK
Atypical Neuroleptics	Stress Oxidative stress	BDNF, FGF-2, SOD-1
Dopamine Receptor Agonists	Oxidative stress L-DOPA-induced apopitosis	Bcl2, SOD, gluthatione, caspase3
Antidepressants	Stress Glutamate toxicity	cAMP, CREB, BDNF, GDNF
Antibiotics	Stroke Glutamate toxicity	Caspase1, nitric oxide synthase

Adopted from Shamir et al., 2005; Bcl2: B-cell lymphoma, BDNF: Brain-derived neurotrophic factor; cAMP: Adenosine 3', 5'-cyclic monophosphate; CREB: cAMP response element binding protein; FGF-2: Fibroblast growth factor 2; GDNF: Glia-derived neurotrophic factor; GSK-3: Glycogen synthase kinase-3; MAPK: Mitogen-activated protein kinase; SOD: Superoxide dismutase.

Association between Stress and Depression

Publication of the first report and the beginning of the discussion of the detrimental effects of stress took place in the first quarter of the last century. Firstly, it was shown that chronic and heavy stress causes gastric ulceration and hypertrophy of the adrenal gland (Selye, 1976). The detrimental effects of stress on the brain and behavior started to be discussed in the sixties. In the late sixties the suggestion that the hippocampus, a medial temporal structure, is the most sensitive region in the brain regarding binding of glucorticoids to receptors specific for them both in humans and rats formed the basis for the association between stress and psychiatric disorders (McEwen, 1968; McEwen and Weiss, 1970). Glucocorticoids are released in response to stress. Glucocorticoid release is also elevated in major depression and in Cushing's disease (Brown et al, 1999; Starkman et al, 2003). These findings indicate that conditions that cause stress to living organisms may be associated with depression. Recent studies clearly showed that hippocampal functions are modulated by hormones and neurotransmitters like glutamate, and both glucocorticoid and glutamate levels are increased during conditions that cause stress (McEwen et al, 2002; Moghaddam, 2002; Popoli et al, 2002). Recent studies also suggested that increased glucocorticoid levels and stressful living trigger depressive symptoms (Bayer, 2000; Moghaddam, 2002; Parker et al, 2003).

Depression affects many brain structures. Brain changes with major depression have been reported for the hippocampus amygdale, caudate nucles putamen and frontal cortex, structures that are all extensively interconnected. They comprise a neuroanatomical circuid called the limbic-cortical-striatal-pallidal-thalamic tract. In view of this, the hippocampal changes have to be seen in a broader context, since it is unlikely that disturbed neurogenezis and structural changes in the hippocampus under the stress will fully explain a disorder as complex as major depression (Fuchs, 2009). It has been suggested that the pathogenesis of depression involves injured hippocampal neurogenezis. In animal models, chronic stress dramatically reduces hippocampal neurogenezis and increases apoptosis in the hippocampal and cortical neurons. It has also been shown that some antidepressants prevented these effects of chronic stress in animals (Czeh et al., 2001; Schmidt and Duman, 2007; Zoladz et al., 2008). On the other hand, stress is known to significantly affect learning and memory processes. These effects are dependent on the type, duration and intensity of the stressor. Emotional arousal may enhance learning and memory through synaptic activity of amygdale-related pathways and this is thougt to be the basis of intense, long term memories of traumatic events and posttraumatic stress disorder (Duman, 2004).

Given that the hippocampus is sensitive to stress and glucocorticoids are released during stress, stress-induced hippocampal changes are very important in depression development and as a target of antidepressant drugs. Using these findings as a basis, experimental models based on stress have been formed and both stress-induced changes in elements of neuroplasticity and the effects of antidepressant treatment on these changes have been rigorously examined. Research on this topic is increasing day by day and is growing in importance.

Synaptic Plasticity, Stress and the Effects of Antidepressant

Stress is one of the most important stimuli affecting the central nervous system. The brain has the capacity to adapt to stress-induced changes. Only under chronic stress is the brain's capacity to adapt insufficient at several levels. This insufficiency may cause diseases that originate from the central nervous system (e.g., depression) due to negative remodeling of neuronal quality and neuronal organization. However, the development of important central functions like learning and recovery from diseases (by reversion of remodeling) also requires neuroplasticity. Three weeks of chronic restrain stress may cause breakage of the dendritic structures in the rat hippocampus (figure 16). In parallel with this, impaired neurogenesis characterized by decreases in hippocampal volume and neurotrophic factors (like BDNF), neuronal atrophy and death may be observed. This may also be interpreted as negative neuroplasticity.

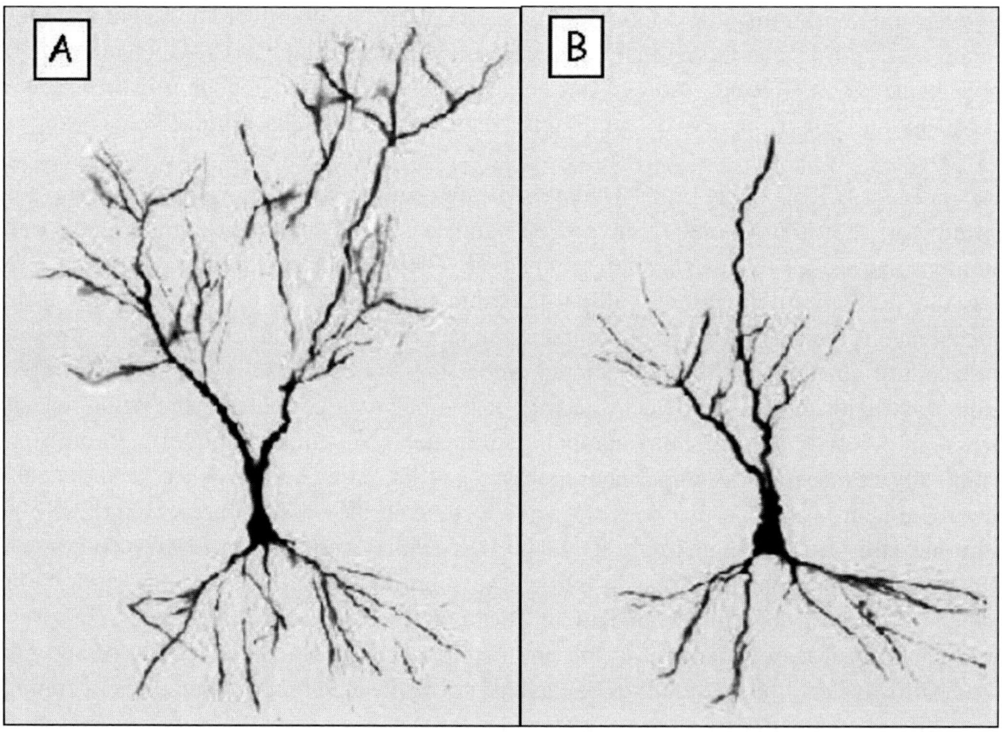

Figure 16. Dendritic changes in rat hippocampal neurons before (A) and after (B) exposure to stress for three weeks (McEwen, 2004).

This negative neuroplasticity in the brain may be reversed by chronic antidepressant treatment. According to this view, under chronic stress structural defects in the hippocampal CA3 region (neuronal atrophy) and dentate gyrus and a decrease in neurogenesis also occur besides an increase in glucocorticoid levels. This negative neuroplasticity causes depression, and antidepressant treatment ameliorates depression by decreasing neuronal atrophy and increasing neurogenesis (figure 17).

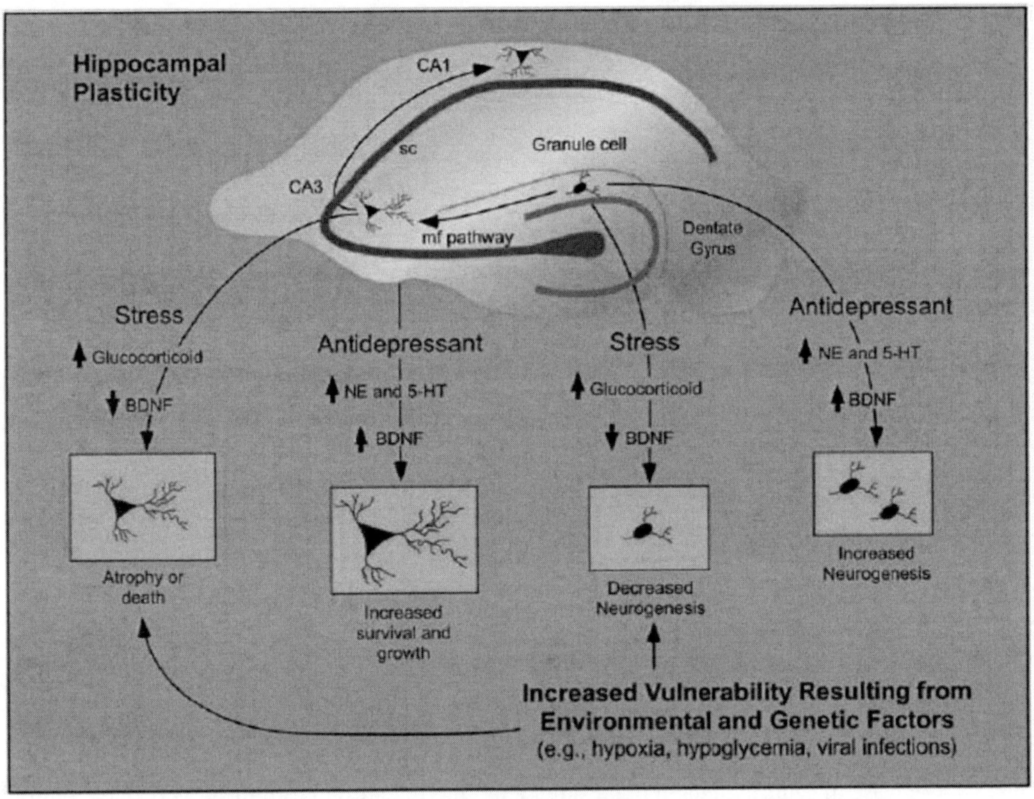

Figure 17. Hippocampal neuroplasticity in depression and effects of the antidepressants (Duman, 2004).

Significant increases occur in dendritic lengths, hippocampal volume, BDNF amount and neurogenesis with antidepressant treatment (Magarinos et al., 1999; Czeh et al., 2001; Duman, 2002; Fuchs et al., 2002; McEwen et al., 2002). Positive effects of antidepressants on neuroplasticity in the rat hippocampus, especially CA3 neurons, after chronic stress are shown in figure 15, 16 and 17.

Breakage of Dendrites Due to Stress and the Effects of Antidepressants

Magarinos et al. (1999) observed shortening of dendritic length in pyramidal neurons of the CA3 region of rats exposed to stress caused by restrain stress for three days. Then fluoxetine and tianeptin was applied to rats exposed to similar stress of the same severity and duration. In contrast to the observation that dendritic lengths return to normal in tianeptine administered rats, fluoxetine was not found to be effective. The results of this study indicate that stress-induced remodeling of dendrites may be reversed by an antidepressant, tianeptine. The lack of effect with another depressant, fluoxetine, in this study suggests that the two antidepressants differ with regard to the mechanisms of action of their effects on stress-induced remodeling of dendrites (Figure 18).

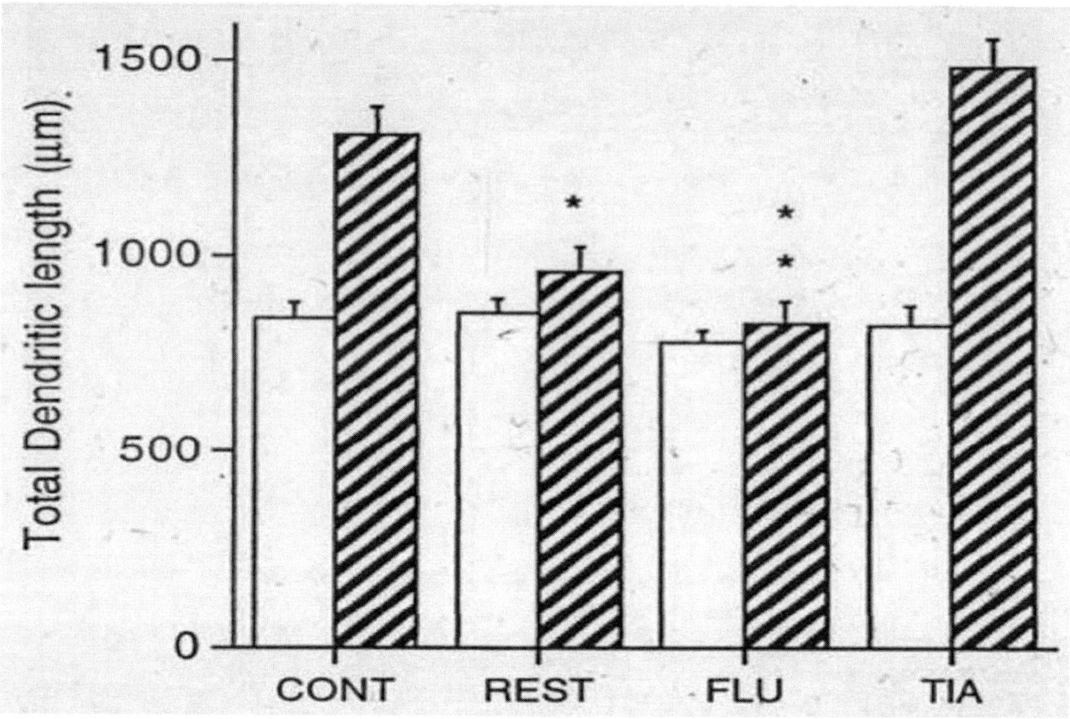

Figure 18. Decrease in dendritic length in rats after exposure to chronic restrain stress (Cont=Control; Rest=Restrain stress; Flu=Fluoxetine; Tia=Tianeptin; *$p<0.05$ (statistically significant) (Magarinos et al., 1989).

Stress, Hippocampal Volume and the Effects of Antidepressants

Another form of stress-induced neuroplastic remodeling in the central nervous system is volume changes. In studies using magnetic resonance imaging, selective volume decreases were detected in the hippocampus (Sheline, 2000; Sheline et al., 2003; Manji et al., 2003). Ohl et al. (2000) showed in a study on three shrews that chronic psychosocial stress and long-term cortisol administration cause important changes in hippocampal volume. Several subsequent experimental studies also supported the view that chronic exposure to stress causes decreases in hippocampal volume in experimental animals. A more important and interesting result is the reversion to normal of the changes in hippocampal volume due to stress with antidepressant drugs (Figure 19) (Czeh et al., 2001; van der Hart et al., 2002).

These findings are also consistent with studies on other species that found no association between hypercortisolemia and hippocampal neurotoxic effects (Vollman-Hansdorf et al., 1997; Levrenz et al., 1999; Sousa et al., 2000). When we take all these findings into account we conclude that hippocampal volume changes observed in depression cannot be associated with increased corticosteroid release.

Another possible explanation for hippocampal volume changes involves the impairment of neurogenesis under stress. However, hippocampal neurogenesis occurs in a relatively small number of neurons and only at a level that compensates for the neurons that died in the granular layer (Fuchs et al., 2004).

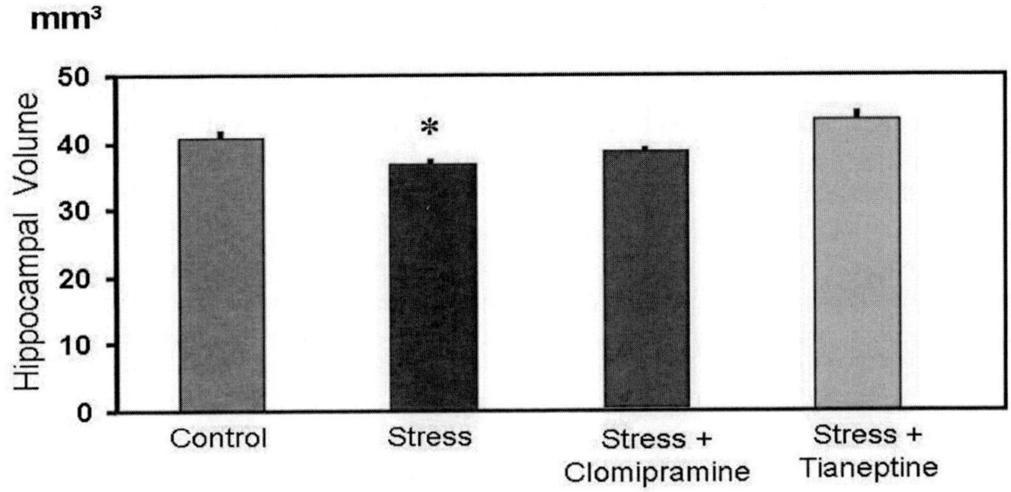

Figure 19- Decrease in rat hippocampal volume due to chronic stress and effect of clomipramine and tianeptin treatment on this (Czeh et al., 2001; van der Hart et al., 2002).

If amount and location are taken into account, stress-induced impairment of hippocampal volume will not be expected to occur at a level large enough to be detected by the available methods. However, it is possible that long exposure to stress or impairment in neurogenesis accompanying severe and long-lasting depression may cause this kind of change over time. This hypothesis needs to be supported by thorough experimental and clinical studies. Stress-induced changes in the glial cells of the hippocampal neuron network or dendritic, axonal and synaptic components may also contribute to hippocampal volume loss. In addition, a more mechanistic approach may show that stress-induced changes in the fluid balance between ventricles and brain tissue also cause volume loss. Although studies that suggest ventricular enlargement and loss in several brain tissues in patients with different psychiatric disorders partially support this hypothesis, it would be very speculative to try to explain hippocampal volume loss solely with changes in the fluid balance between the ventricles and brain tissue. As a result, time and further studies are required to explain the causes of hippocampal volume loss in depression or due to stress more clearly.

Stress, Brain Metabolites and the Effects of Antidepressants

Locally applied proton magnetic resonance spectroscopy (MRS) can be used in the research and evaluation of neuropsychiatric disorders. A major advantage of this method is its noninvasiveness (Kato et al., 1998). Proton MRS permits the in vivo measurement of brain metabolites. With this method concentrations of N-acetyl-aspartate (NAA), a neuroaxonal marker of viable and functional capacity of neurons; creatine and phosphocreatine (Cr), an important energy substrate for all cells; compounds including choline (Cho) such as phosphocholine, an important element of cell membrane; and cerebral metabolites such as myo-inositol (ins), an important marker of astrocytes, can also be measured (Birken and Oldendorf, 1989; Urenjak et al., 1993; Brand et al., 1993).

Czeh et al. (2001) examined the effects of one week of chronic psychosocial stress on cerebral metabolites such as NAA, Cr, Cho and Ins in tree shrews using proton MRS. They found significant decreases in NAA, Cr and Cho concentrations due to chronic stress. These decreases suggest mainly a decrease and/or functional impairment in neuroaxonal cell density accompanied by a significant impairment in synaptic plasticity. Applying antidepressants together with stress is shown to normalize decreases in NAA, Cr and Cho levels (fig 20). These observations suggest that cerebral metabolites such as NAA, Cr and Cho may be used for the assessment of stress-induced synaptic plasticity impairment. In addition, these findings support the neuroplasticity hypothesis of depression. Moreover, monitorization of NAA, Cr and Cho levels via MRS appears to indicate the effectiveness of antidepressant therapy.

Czeh et al. (2001) observed no significant changes in Ins level either with stress or during antidepressant therapy. Given that Ins is an important marker for astrocytes chronic stress,and depression may be thought to have no significant effect on astrocytes.

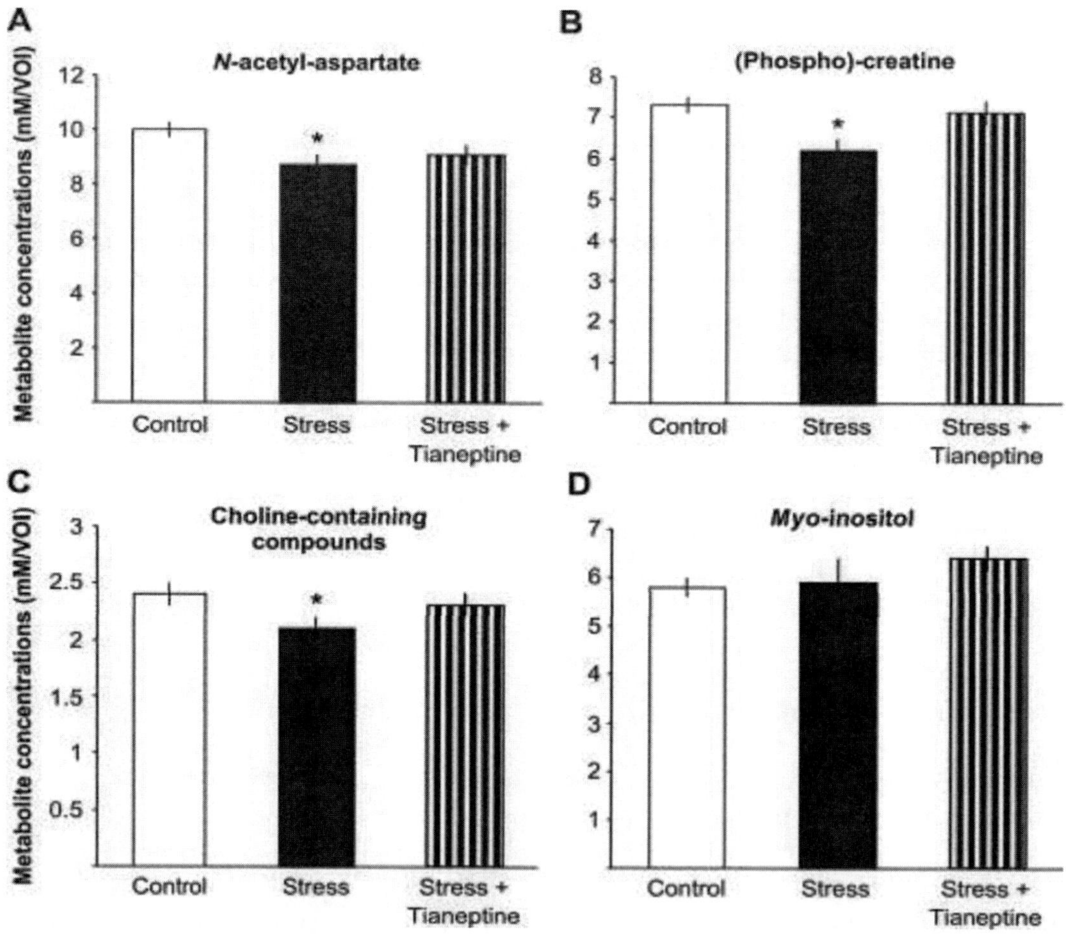

Figure 20. Cerebral metabolite concentrations in three shrews; (A) N-acetyl aspartate; (B) phospho creatine; (C) choline containing compounds and (D) myo-inositol. Control (n=6), stress (n=6) and stress+tianeptin (n=6). Metabolite concentration şs **given as mean ±standard deviation** (mM/VOI). *p<0.05 differecnce from he control is statistically significant (Czeh et al., 2001).

Astrocytes, together with oligodendrocytes and microglia, are important elements of the brain's glia. Their proportion in the glia is higher than that of oligodendrocytes and microglia. They form about one third of brain tissue. Astrocytes play roles in the regulation and execution of many functions very important for synaptic plasticity such as establishing ionic homeostasis in extracellular space, neurotransmitter metabolism, neuronal feeding, providing energy to neurons, regulation of neuronal migration, and secretion of neurotrophic factors. Astrocytes also have an important role in blood brain barrier formation. A new and exciting discovery about astrocytes is their possession of receptors for neurotransmitters and steroid hormones. These receptors do not have many features different from receptors located in neuron membranes, and if they are stimulated with appropriate steroids or neurotransmitters postreceptor biological and electrical events are triggered inside astrocytes. Astrocytes may also coordinate Ca mediated signal transduction (Fuchs et al., 2004).

As Czeh et al. (2001) found no significant changes in Ins due to chronic stress it is not possible to determine whether antidepressant treatment is effective at the astrocyte level or not. The resistance of the glia and especially astrocytes to chronic stress should also be kept in mind. Assessment of cerebral Ins levels with more severe stress models other than psychosocial stress or more prolonged psychosocial stress may bring more clarity to this subject.

Stress, Hippocampal Neurogenesis and the Effects of Antidepressants

The dentate gyrus region of the hippocampus displays an adult neurogenesis characterized by cell death and neogenesis replacing death cells. In this region there is a continuous turnover due to death and regeneration of cells (Biebl et al., 2000; Kuhn et al., 2001). Premature cells produced in the subgranular layer of the hippocampus migrate to the granular layer, where they transform into mature cells. These neurons newly generated in the granular layer have morphologic and physiologic features similar to those of mature neurons previously found in the granular layer (van Praag et al., 2002). Adult hippocampal neurogenesis is shown in many warm-blooded animals and mammals, including humans (Groos, 2000). Interestingly, hippocampal neurogenesis is affected by pharmacological stimulants as well as stimulants from inside and outside (peripheral) the organism (Fuchs and Gould, 2000; Eisch, 2002). For example, stress, as a stimulant both inner and outer or peripheral, may suppress the viability and reproduction of hippocampal granular neurons (Gould et al., 1997; Czeh et al., 2002; Pham et al., 2003; Heine et al., 2004).

Marking with 5-bromo-2'deoxyuridine (BrdU) is used to assess hippocampal neurogenesis. Twenty-four hours after the intraperitoneal application of 100 mg/kg BrdU to rats, staining of healthy dendrites in hippocampal slices with BrdU may easily be seen (fig 21). Decreases in neurotrophic factors and dendritic extensions of neurons or atrophies characterized by dendritic breakage result in decreases in neuron numbers that may be marked by BrdU. This method can be used to show increases or decreases in neurogenesis (Gould et al., 1997; Gould, 1999; Czeh et al., 2001).

In rats chronic stress causes prominent decreases in the number of BrdU stained cells, especially in the hippocampal CA3 region, suggesting a significant decrease in neurogenesis in this region.

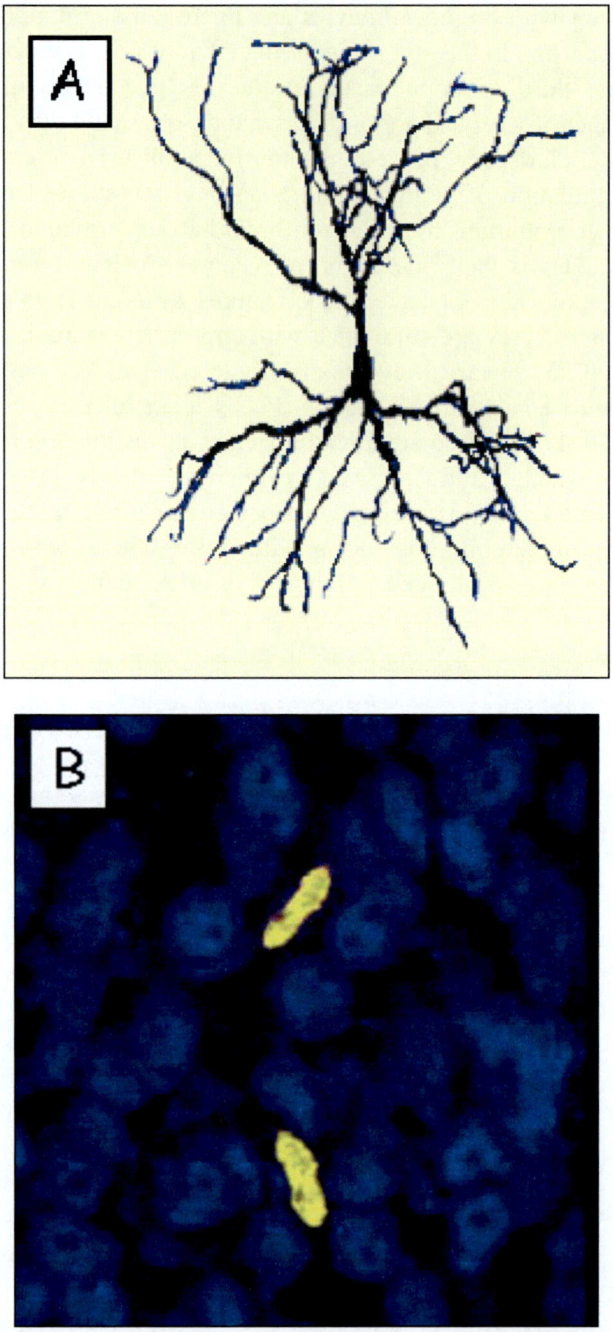

Figure 21. Image of healthy dendrites (A) and a healthy neuron stained with bromodeoxyuridine (B) (Czeh et al., 2001).

In 2001 Czeh showed that in rats decreased neurogenesis in the hippocampal region due to stress caused by chronic movement restriction can be normalized by an antidepressant, tianeptine (Czeh et al., 2001).

In a subsequent study using the same design, van der Hart tested the effects of another antidepressant, clomipramine, and obtained the same results (van der Hart, 2002) (Fig 22).

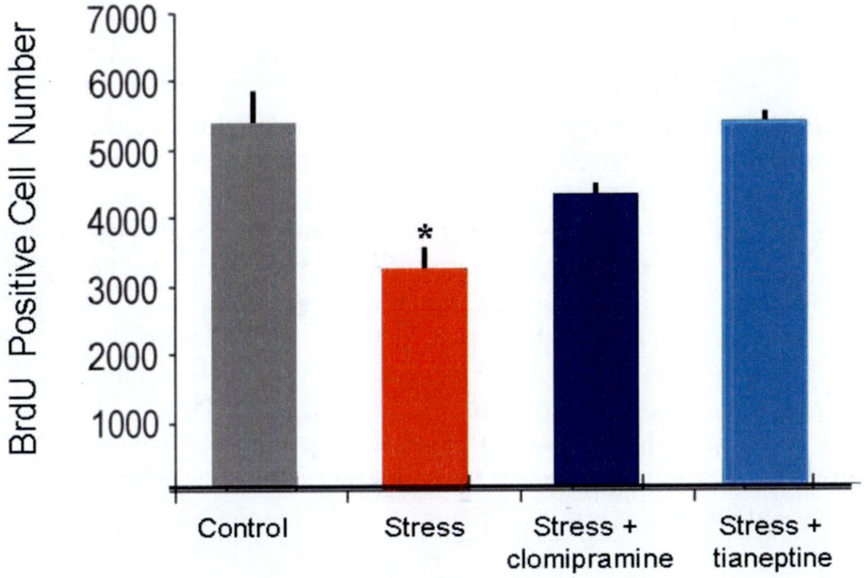

Figure 22. Antidepressant drugs prevent stress induced decrease in neurogenesis in hippocampal CA3 region (BrdU= Bromodeoxyuridine; Czeh et al., 2001; van der Hart et al., 2002).

The results of both studies suggest impairment of the healthy dendrite structure in hippocampal formation due to stress and its amelioration with antidepressant therapy. They also prove that antidepressants can be used effectively to treat stress-induced impairment of neurogenesis. Other authors also suggest that stress-induced impairment plays an important role in the etiology of depression (Jacobs et al., 2000; Eisch, 2002; Kronenberg, 2003). Many classic treatments of depression, like lithium and electroconvulsive therapy, and many new generation antidepressant drugs have been shown to induce cytogenesis and neurogenesis in the dentate gyrus. It should be noted that improvements in neurogenesis are achieved not with acute but with chronic treatment (Chen et al., 2000; Madsen et al., 2000; Malberg et al., 2000; Scott et al., 2000). Although these studies strongly suggest an important role of hippocampal neurogenesis in depression and antidepressant treatment, we should keep in mind that for now the evidence is restricted to animal studies. The clinical value of this subject will be better understood with large-scale clinical studies.

Stress, Hippocampal Apoptosis and the Effects of Antidepressant

Apoptosis can be defined briefly as cell death. In brain tissue apoptosis is physiologically the reverse of neurogenesis. Normally, apoptosis and neurogenesis work in concert to enable stability. An increase in one may trigger the other and vice versa. Environmental factors such as stress and endogen factors such as increases in free radicals and glucocorticoids not only decrease neurogenesis but also induce apoptosis. At any site in the brain an increase in apoptosis without accompanying neurogenesis or regression of neurogenesis with ongoing apoptosis results in degeneration and functional losses.

Apoptotic cells may be defined and evaluated using immunohistochemical methods. Taking into account that in major depression an increase in apoptosis may also occur along with neurogenesis, whether neuronal apoptosis occurred and whether this apoptosis responded to antidepressant therapy are also examined in animal models. The most important and comprehensive study on this subject was performed recently by Lucassen and study group, who applied chronic psychosocial stress to tree shrews (Lucassen et al., 2004). The tree shrews were put in cages in pairs, one of which was aggressive and dominant and the other passive and recessive. Thus passive and recessive animals were exposed to psychosocial stress in the form of dominant and aggressive ones for seven days. At the end of the study samples exposed to and not exposed to (controls) stress were sacrificed under ethical conditions and apoptotic cell numbers were detected in the temporal cortex and cornu ammonis and dentate gyrus regions of the hippocampus using in situ end labelization (ISEL) under a microscope after staining with diaminobenzidine (Figure 23). The effect of antidepressant treatment on the observed increase in apoptotic cells induced by stress was also examined. Tianeptine was chosen as the antidepressant and the effects of 28-day chronic treatment were evaluated.

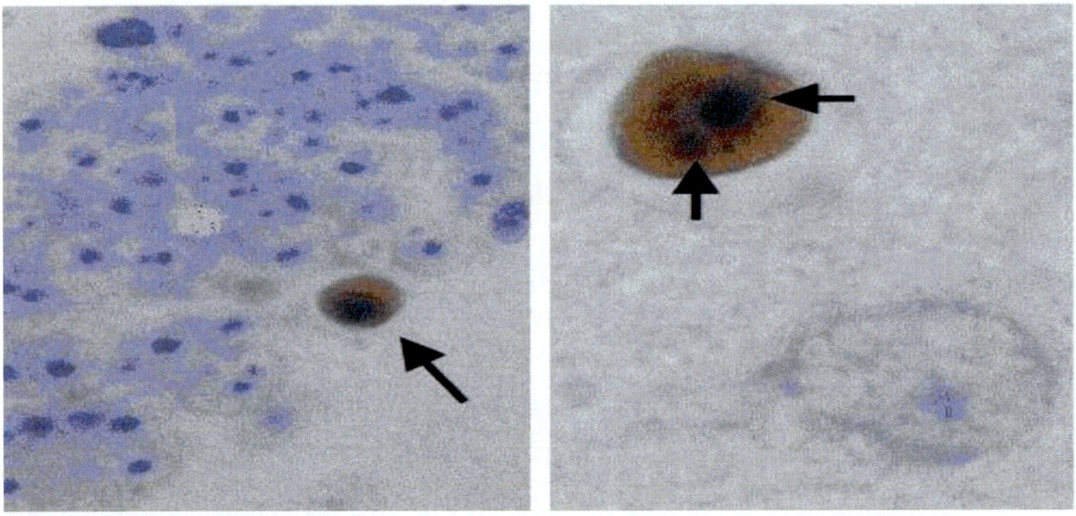

Figure 23. TUNEL-positive apopitotic cells painted with diaminobenzydine in the tree shrew hippocampus (arrows) (adopted from Fuchs et al., 2004).

The results suggest that 7 days of psychosocial stress caused increased apoptosis in the hippocampal formation of tree shrews. Chronic antidepressant therapy significantly decreased both apoptosis aggravated by stress and apoptosis in normal samples in the temporal cortex and hippocampus. However, tianeptine did not affect apoptosis increasing with stress in normal samples in the cornu ammonis of the hippocampus or the granular layer of the dentate gyrus (fig 24).

These results indicate that apoptosis of neurons in the temporal cortex and subgranular region is more sensitive to chronic tianeptine treatment. On the other hand, antidepressant treatment had positive effects on apoptosis in addition to increasing neurogenesis and correcting dendritic structural defects.

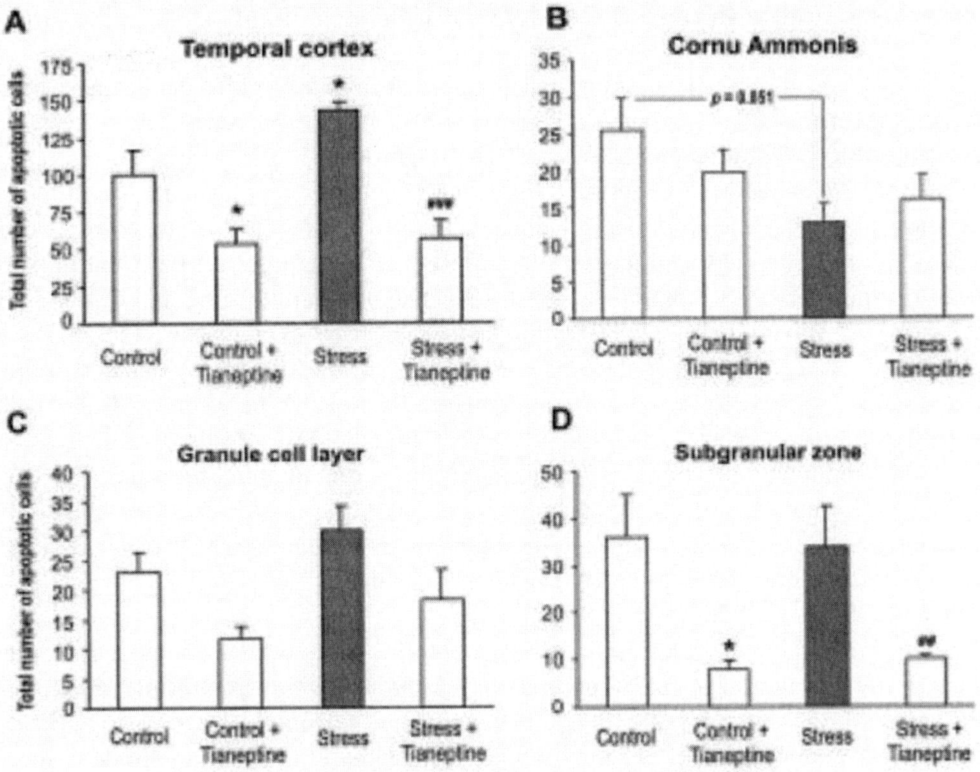

Figure 24. Effects of seven days psychosocial stress on total apoptotic cell numbers in the temporal cortex (A), the cornu ammonis (B), granular layer (C) and subgranular layer (D) of the dentate gyrus. Stress increases apoptosis in the temporal cortex and the dentate gyrus. Chronic tianeptin administration inhibits apoptosis both stress induced and seen in normal controls in the temporal cortex and subgranular dentate gyrus although it is ineffective in other areas (* p<0.05 statistically significant difference from control) (Lucassen et al., 2004)

Chronic tianeptine therapy also inhibited apoptosis in the cornu ammonis of normal samples but this effect did not reach statistical significance. The insufficient sample size may have had an effect on this. However, one of the most interesting findings of this study was the significant decrease in the total number of marked apoptotic cells in the cornu ammonis compared with controls in contrast to the expected decrease (figure 24). This decrease may also be the cause of tianeptine's ineffectiveness in the cornu ammonis. The available data did not make it possible for a reasonable explanation to be made for the decrease in apoptosis in the cornu ammonis with stress while it is increasing in other areas. Stress-induced apoptosis may be said to display regional differences. It is clear that more studies are needed for a better understanding of this subject. However, the results of this study definitely show that chronic antidepressant therapy inhibits regionally specific increases in apoptosis.

Another important point that emerged from Lucassen's study is that chronic tianeptine treatment not only inhibited apoptosis induced by stress but also apoptosis in normal samples. This suggests a potential negative effect on organisms' normal apoptosis functions. Inhibition of normal apoptosis may also be associated with increases in certain cells and a carcinogenic effect. Although this approach is highly speculative, antiapoptotic effects should also be considered from this perspective.

Stress, Postsynaptic Potential Changes and the Effects of Antidepressant

As previously discussed, learning and memory formation is one of the most effective adaptation mechanisms of organisms against inner and outer stimuli and it is closely associated with long-term potentiation (LTP) emergence, particularly in hippocampal formation. LTP is induction of excitatory postsynaptic plasticity produced by high frequency stimulation of afferent nerve fibers (Diamond et al., 2004). One of the most important observations about the LTP and learning relationship is suppression of LTP and impairment of learning and memory formation by stress longer than a certain time and above a certain severity (Foy et al., 2004). This observation is confirmed by many subsequent studies (Kim and Diamond, 2002; Diamond et al., 2004). When we consider the importance of learning and memory as a neuroplasticity response, examining the relationship between stress and LTP and the effects of antidepressants on this is a must, regarding the neuroplasticity of depression and the contribution of neuroplasticity to the mechanism of action of antidepressants.

The most comprehensive study examining the effect of stress on LTP and the efficiency of antidepressants on this was conducted by Rocher and his study group (Rocher et al., 2004). In this study rats were kept waiting on a platform elevated 1 meter to induce height anxiety-related acute stress (Fig 25).

In rats waiting on an elevated, narrow platform there was an acute stress reaction characterized by a significant rise in plasma corticosterone levels. As a result, an inhibition in LTP in fibers projecting from the hippocampus to the prefrontal cortex characterized by a decrease in the amplitude of EPSPs was observed. A decrease in EPSP amplitude despite high frequency electrical stimulation indicates disturbance of synaptic plasticity. However, in samples given tianeptine EPSP amplitudes recovered in relation with dose (fig 26).

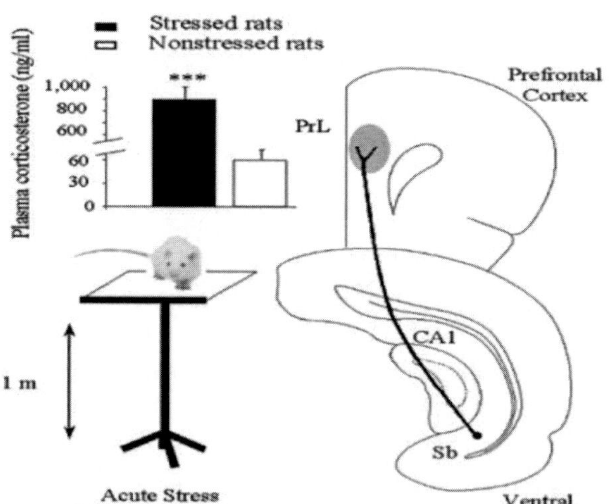

Figure 25. Induction of acute stress reaction in rats in elevated and narrow platforms. Changes in plasma corticosterone levels in rats exposed to stress. The pathway at which excitatory postsynaptic potentials (EPSP) are measured by excitation with high frequency stimulus are seen in the section on right side of the figure. Assessments are made on glutamatergic fibers that projects directly prelimbic region of prefrontal cortex from CA1 (Sb=Subiculum; PrL= Prelimbic area; CA1 = CA1 region of cornu ammonis) (Lucassen et al., 2004).

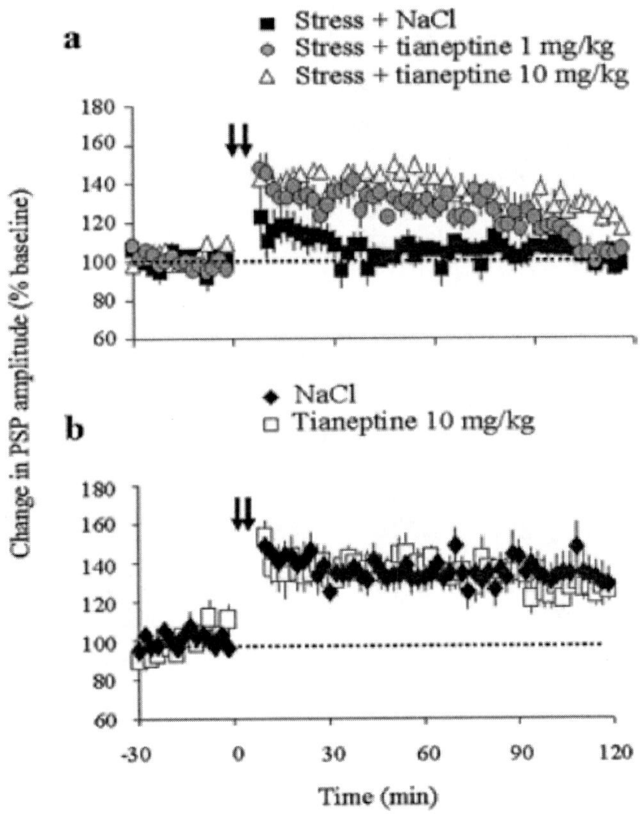

Figure 26. Effects of the antidepressants over stress induced impairment of EPSP amplitudes in fibers that Project from hippocampus to prefrontal cortex. (a) = rats exposed to stress (b) rats not exposed to stress (Rocher et al., 2004).

In this study the maximum tianeptine dose applied did not cause a significant change in high frequency-induced EPSPs in controls not exposed to stress (Fig 27). This suggests that tianeptine's effect is specific to stress-induced changes in neuroplasticity.

Rocher et al. (2004) evaluated the effects of not only tianeptine but also of fluoxetine. In this part of the study a 10-mg acute dose of either tianeptine or fluoxetine was injected into the nerve pathway between the hippocampus and prefrontal cortex 40 minutes before high frequency electrical stimulation. Changes in EPSPs were evaluated at 30-minute intervals for 2 hours after high frequency stimulation (Fig 27).

As seen in the figure, both fluoxetine and tianeptine before LTP induction with a high frequency electrical stimulus corrected stress-induced EPSP decreases without causing a change in EPSPs in the examined pathway between the hippocampus and prefrontal cortex. Since neither drug caused a significant change in postsynaptic potentials (PSP) before electrical stimulation their effect is specific to stress-impaired LTP and thus to synaptic plasticity. One of the interesting observations of this study is the longer duration of action of tianeptine on stress-impaired LTP compared with fluoxetin (fig 26). This suggests that there may be therapeutic differences between antidepressants regarding their effects on LTP. Another most important inference from this study is that it forms a basis for explaining stress-induced cognitive impairments with LTP disturbances in neuron networks between the hippocampus and prefrontal cortex.

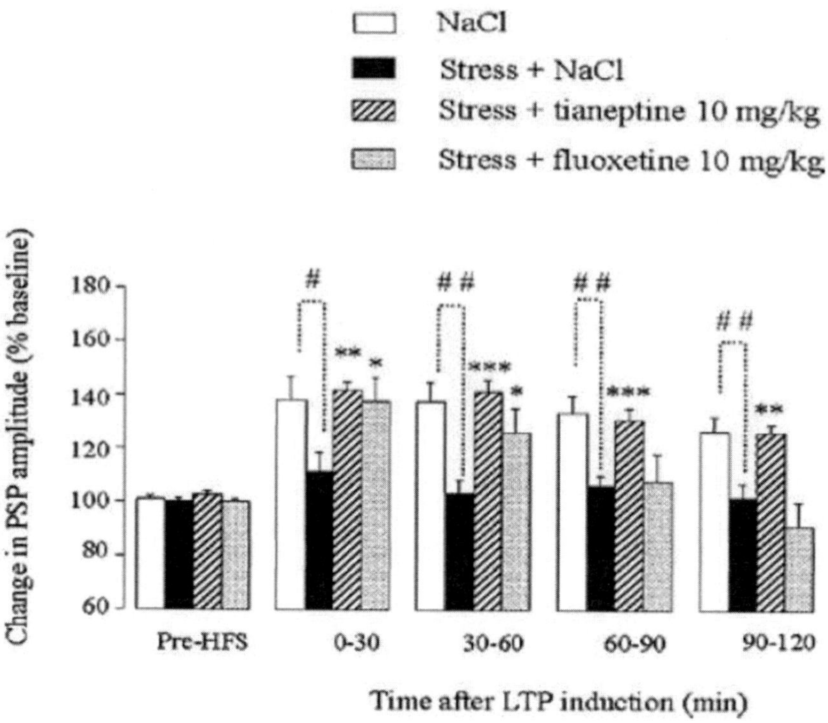

Figure 27. Stress induced changes in EPSP amplitudes due to high frequency electrical stimulus and effects of the antidepressants (Rocher et al., 2004).

Although hippocampal LTP formation is very important for learning and memory, LTP formation is not restricted to the hippocampal formation. Many studies have clearly shown that LTP is formed in many nuclei of the hippocampus (Maren and Fanselow, 1995; Chapman et al., 2003; Yaniv et al., 2003a). Nevertheless, in the amygdala, in contrast to the hippocampus and prefrontal cortex, there is an increase in synaptic transmission and PSP amplitudes of formed EPSPs related to emotional stimuli (Rogan et al., 1997; Blair et al., 2001). A recent experimental study also found that in rats exposed to stress due to staying in an unfamiliar environment despite the decrease in LTP magnitudes in the amygdala low threshold LTP formation was blocked in the hippocampus (Yaniv et al., 2003b). Given that anxiety and fear emerge in conditions at which the amygdala is stimulated, an increase in LTPs in the amygdala with inhibition in the hippocampus and prefrontal cortex may be explained as necessary for survival under stress.

Some preliminary behavioral and electrophysiological studies interestingly indicate that treatment with antidepressants like tianeptine is ineffective on stress-induced LTP changes in amygdala. For example, Burghardt et al. (2004) has shown that fear conditioning, a strong form of emotional learning, is not affected by acute tianeptine administration. Vouimba et al. (2003) also showed that a stress-related amygdaloid LTP increase that may be regarded as a reflection of fear conditioning is not changed by tianeptine treatment. According to these data the effects of tianeptine on stress-related LTP change may be thought to be restricted to the hippocampus and prefrontal cortex without affecting the amygdaloid complex. Nevertheless, the effects of other antidepressants on the LTP increases observed under stress should also be examined and taken into account during evaluation.

Some clinical studies indicate that tianeptine effectively treats somatic anxiety symptoms accompanying depression and may have anxiolytic effects (Defrance et al., 1988; Guelfi et al., 1989; Wilde and Benfield, 1995). In this case, the ineffectiveness of tianeptine on increases in LTP induced due to fear and stress may seem controversial. However, measured PSP increases in the amygdala due to fear and stress may be associated with normal anxiety rather than being pathologic. Examining LTP changes in the amygdala and the effects of tianeptine on this in models measuring pathologic anxiety will help us to understand this subject better. However, although some studies indicate that tianeptine has an anxiolytic effect, this study assessed tianeptine's effects on somatic anxiety accompanying major depression rather than its effects solely on anxiety. Controversial results were also obtained in studies conducted on experimental animals with models of solely different types of anxiety (Zethof et al., 1995; Cutler et al., 1997). Effects of tianeptin and other antidepressants on amygdala neuroplasticity should be assessed with further and more detailed studies.

Contribution of Glutamate in Stress Induced Neuroplasticity and the Effects of Antidepressants on Glutamatergic System

Chronic stress not only triggers glucocorticoid release. Recent studies have clearly shown that excitatory amino acidergic system is also stimulated under stress and increases in glucocorticoid release occur in many brain regions especially in hippocampus (Lowy et al., 1993; 1995; Maghaddam et al., 1994). N-methyl-D-aspartate receptors are abundant in the central nervous system and they are among the most important receptors mediating the excitatory effects of glutamate. NMDA receptor antagonists have been shown to increase neurogenesis in dentate gyrus of hippocampus (Cameron et al., 1995) and prevent dendritic remodelling assumed to appear due to stress induced increase in glucocorticoid release (Magarinos et al., 1999; McEwen 1999b). These observations indicate that glutamatergic system may have a key role in the regulation of synaptic plasticity and antidepressants may affect not only monoamines but also other neurotransmitters like glutamate.

Excitatory neuotransmitters like glutamate suppress neurogenesis in dentate gyrus of hippocampus and have a key role breakage of stress induced breakage in hippocampal dendrites. Regulation of the extracellular glutamate levels may be a potential cause of remodelling because of the dendritic disruption and breakage of CA3 region hippocampal neurons induced by chronic stress. Regulation and distribution of glia glutamate transporter (GLT-1) and its isoforms may give an idea about glutamate activity as well as structural disruptions of dendrite and suppression of neurogenesis. A detailed study testing this hypothesis was conducted recently by Reagan and his study group (Reagan et al., 2004). In this study regulation and distribution of glia GLT-1 and one of its isoforms GLT-1b in rat hippocampus that are exposed to chronic restrain stress for 21 days through the restriction of their movements 6 hours a day. In this study, effects of an antidepressant, tianeptin, over chronic stress induced changes in the expression of GLT-1 and GLT-1b is also examined to answer the question whether antidepressants affect the glutamate mediated changes in synaptic plasticity after stress.

Tianeptine was given to the treatment groups (together with stress) by intraperitoneal route at a dosage of 10 mg/kg chronically for 21 days.

Stress application based on chronic movement restriction (restrain stress) results in a significant increase in GLT-1 mRNA levels and protein expression in the hippocampal CA3 region and dentate gyrus of the rat. An important aspect of this study is the assessment of stress-induced changes at different sites and in some detail in the cornu ammonis and dentate gyrus. Indeed, significant increases in GLT-1 mRNA levels and protein expression appeared only in the CA3 region of the cornu ammonis and molecular layer of the dentate gyrus. When the effects of stress in the CA3 region are evaluated in detail, stress-induced increases are seen to be limited to the stratum oriens and stratum radium. No stress-induced change occurred for GLT-1 in the CA3 region of the stratum pyramidalis. Likewise, no stress-induced change was detected in the granular layer of the dentate gyrus or hilus (Figure 28 A and B). These observations suggest that several regions such as CA3 of the hippocampal formation and the molecular layer of the dentate gyrus are more sensitive to chronic stress induced by movement restriction and to changes in glutamate activity due to this. Whether any change in unaffected regions may be seen by using other stress models or by using the same model for longer may only be clear after further studies.

The most important finding of this study is that stress-induced glutamate activity increases can be suppressed by antidepressant treatment (Figure 28 A and B). Tianeptine treatment did not change the GLT-1 mRNA levels or protein expression in hippocampal layers not affected by stress. This finding is important because it shows that antidepressant drugs ameliorate the neuroplastic changes induced by glutamate. It follows from this that antidepressants can affect not only monoamines like noradrenalin and serotonin but also excitatory neurotransmitters like glutamate.

In this study, stress induced by chronic movement restriction did not cause any significant change in GLT-1b (an isoform of GLT-1) mRNA levels in any region of the hippocampus. Moreover, no significant effect of chronic tianeptine (10 mg/kg, ip) treatment was observed (Figure 29). These findings indicate that changes induced by glutamate transporters in the hippocampal formation and tianeptine effects are only limited to GLT-1, and isoforms like GLT-1b are not affected by stress or tianeptine.

Thus, stress causes glutamatergic activity to increase, particularly with GLT-1 increases. This can be prevented by tianeptine and this effect occurs in the hippocampal formation, especially in the CA3 region and dentate gyrus. In addition, it is seen that GLT-1 plays an important role in the effect of tianeptine on glutamatergic regulation.

Modulation of glutamatergic transmission by tianeptine is confirmed by the results of electrophysiological studies that investigated the effects of stress-induced changes in the glutamatergic synapses. For example, Kole et al. (2002) showed that tianeptine normalizes NMDA currents augmented by stress in the CA3 region of the hippocampal formation in rats subjected to chronic stress.

Nitric oxide (NO) may also make a modulatory contribution to the effects of antidepressants through glutamate. NO is a labile, free radical gas with a very short half-life (6-10 sec) that has important biological activity both in the periphery and in the central nervous system. It is synthesized by a reaction that uses L-arginine as a precursor and is catalyzed by NO synthase (Snyder and Bredt, 1992). There are three different isoforms of NOS: endothelial (eNOS), inducible (iNOS) and neuronal (nNOS) (Moncada et al., 1997).

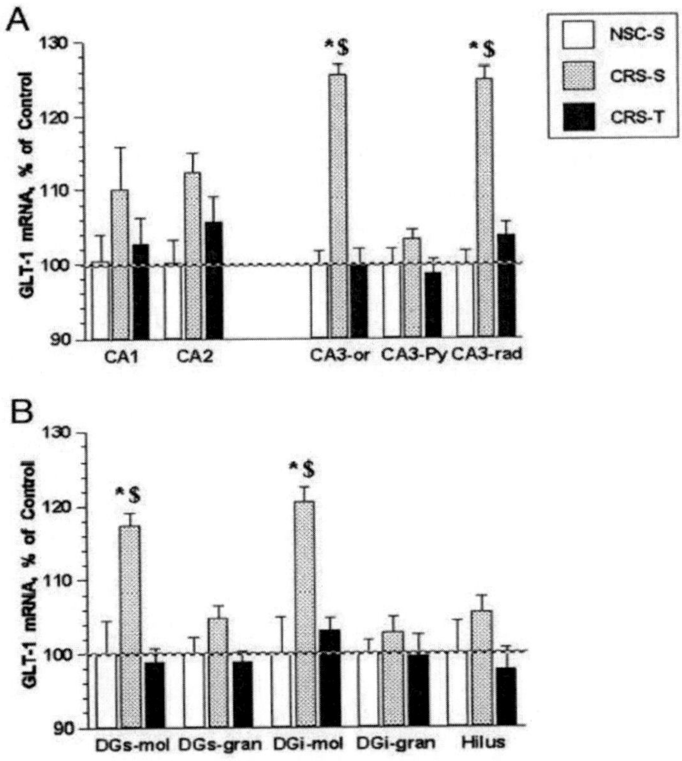

Figure 28. Changes in GLT-1 mRNA expression in rats exposed to restrain stress and effect of tianeptin tretment. (A) Cornu ammonis region; or = stratum oriens, py = stratum pyramidale, rad = stratum radiatum. (B) Dentate gyrus, mol= molecular layer, gran= granular layer, s= superior, i= inferior. NSC-S= non-stress + saline control; CRS-S= chronic stress + tianeotin. * p<0.05 statistically significant from chronic stress + tianeptin (Reagan et al., 2004).

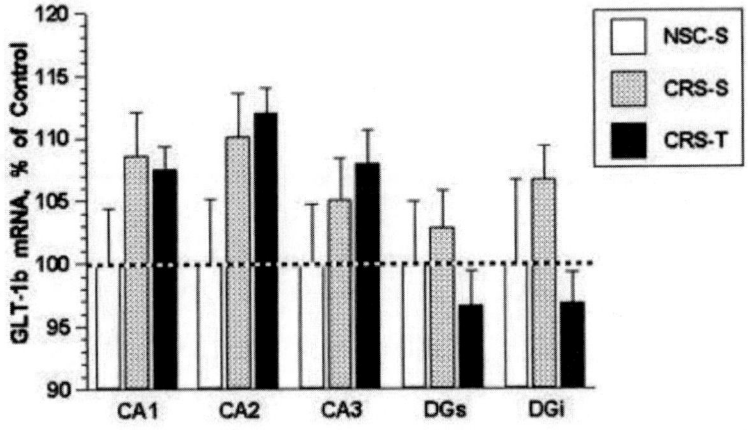

Figure 29. GLT-1b mRNA expression changes in rats exposed to restrain stress and effects of the antidepressants. No significant change is observed in he levels of hippocampal GLT1-b mRNA levels of rats exposed to stress. (CRS-S = Chronic stress + saline; CRS-T = Chronic stress + tianeptin; NSC-S = non stress + saline) (Reagan et al., 2004).

It is shown that NOS activity is found in many brain regions, including the hippocampus (Forsterman et al., 1990). In addition, based on data showing that NO can be a new and unusual neurotransmitter, the existence of a central L-arginine-NO pathway is suggested (Moncada and Higgs, 1993).

Results of several clinical and experimental studies indicate that NO may play a role in other neuropsychiatric diseases like the physical component of alcohol and substance addiction (Uzbay and Oglesby, 2001), schizophrenia (Zoroglu et al., 2002; Yanik et al., 2003), bipolar affective disorders (Savas et al., 2002) and obsessive compulsive disorder (Zoroglu et al., 2003).

It is proposed that in the central nervous system NO interacts with the glutamatergic system and second messenger cGMP contributing to the emergence of excitatory responses like alcohol deprivation syndrome (Uzbay and Oglesby, 2001). According to this view, stimulation of excitatory amino acid receptors, especially NMDA receptors with glutamate, causes Ca^{2+} /calmoduline mediated activation of NOS by increasing the entrance of Ca^{2+} into the cell at the postsynaptic neuronal membrane. Activation of NOS also causes NO synthesis and increases NO production. NO synthesized and released at the postsynaptic neuron diffuses to the presynaptic neuron retrogradely and provokes the glutamate release at the presynaptic terminal by stimulating guanilate cyclase (GC) (Garthwaite et al., 1989; Garthwaite, 1991; Uzbay and Oglesby, 2001) (Figure 30).

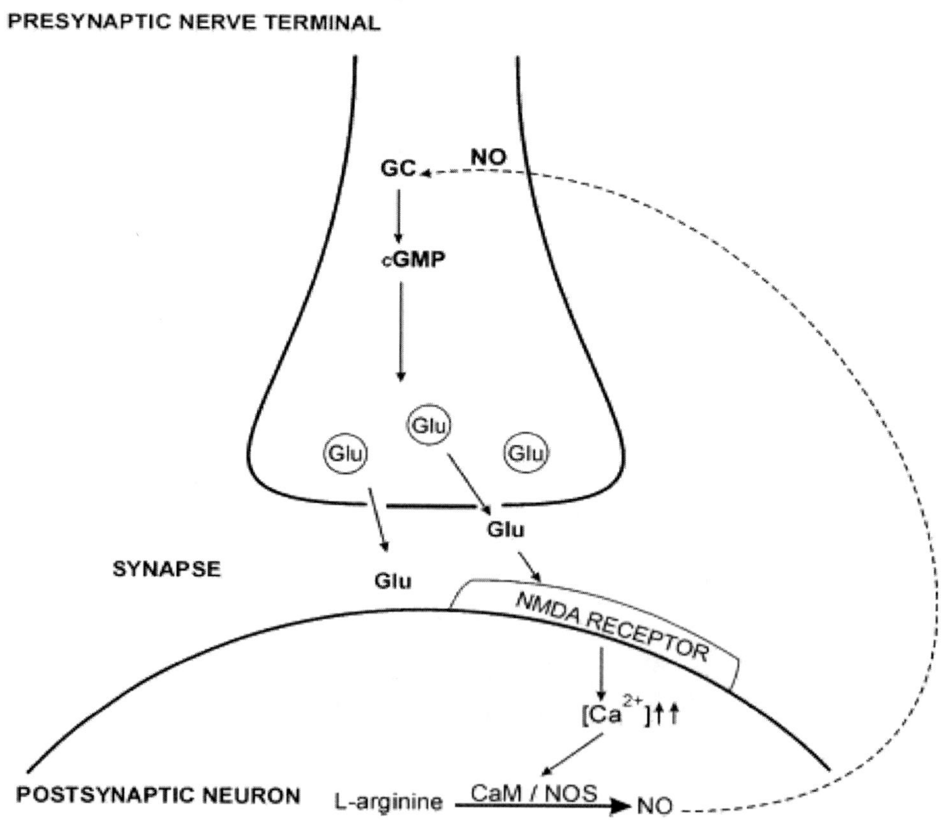

Figure 30. NO- Glutamate-NMDA relation in the central nervous system (Uzbay and Oglesby, 2001).

Increases in striatal L-sitrulline levels in the rat brain (Gören et al., 2001) during alcohol deprivation and significant increases in cGMP levels especially in the hippocampus and striatum during both chronic alcohol intake and alcohol deprivation (Uzbay et al., 2004) are findings that support the contribution of NO to the excitatory symptoms during alcohol deprivation syndrome. Wegener et al. (2003) showed that antidepressants like fluoxetine and tianeptine inhibit NOS, a NO synthesizing enzyme in the central nervous system, and NO activity, especially in the hippocampus. NOS-inhibiting effects of antidepressants in the hippocampus may indirectly augment their inhibitory effect on glutamate activity. Given that NO is a free radical and that excessive NO facilitates cell degeneration, it is expected that the NO-activity-decreasing effects of antidepressants may help to protect neurons. It is known that antidepressants like tianeptine exert their neuroprotective effects by also blocking the increase in lactate dehydrogenase activity induced by hypoxia (Plaisant et al., 2003).

All these observations indicate that antidepressant drugs have some beneficial effects on disorders associated with depression and/or neuronal disorders that cause depression inhibition of the glutamatergic system directly or indirectly. Positive effects on free radicals can also contribute to the neuroprotective effects. Examining the interaction of antidepressants with glutamate and NO will also be of great assistance in the development of more effective psychotropic drugs.

Stress, Neurotrophic Factors and the Effects of Antidepressants

During chronic stress formation and corticosterone administration, an increase in glucocorticoid release is observed, especially in the CA1 and CA3 regions of the hippocampal formation of the brain, while concentrations of important neurotrophic factors like BDNF decrease. These decreases are characterized by a decrease in BDNF mRNA expression (Scaccionoce et al., 2003). A decrease in neurotrophic factor release reduces the resistance of neurons to stress. Besides neuronal atrophies due to breakage of dendrites, the balance between neurogenesis and apoptosis is also impaired. As a result, impairment of synaptic plasticity and synaptic transmission is seen (Fossati et al., 2004) (Figure 17). The cause of the BDNF level decrease under stress is suppression of BDNF gene promoter transcription through corticosteroid receptor stimulation (Schaaf et. al., 2000). Dysfunction of cAMP response element (CRE) binding protein (CREB) may also contribute to BDNF deficiency (Dowlatshahi et al., 1998). Goggi et al. (2002) showed that BDNF acutely affects both the electrophysiological aspect of LTP-induced synaptic plasticity and neurochemical aspects through release of neurotransmitters like serotonin and glutamate. Deficiency of BDNF has an important role in the pathology of many affective disorders including depression and schizophrenia (Angellucci et al., 2004). These findings indicate that BDNF is a very important neurotrophic factor both in the development of depression and in antidepressant treatment.

Treatment with antidepressant drugs increases the levels of monoaminergic neurotransmitters like serotonin and noradrenaline at synapses. The neurotransmitters released into the synaptic space activate the signal transduction system between cells by binding to specific receptors. BDNF and CREB are essential elements of this signal transduction system. However, Thome et al. (2000) performed an experimental study with mice and showed that CRE mediated gene expression (Figure 31) and CREB phosphorylation

(Figure 32) increased in various regions of the brain when desypramine (a selective noradrenaline reuptake inhibitor), fluoxetine (a selective serotonin reuptake inhibitor), and tranylcypromin, a monoamine oxidase enzyme inhibitor, were given chronically.

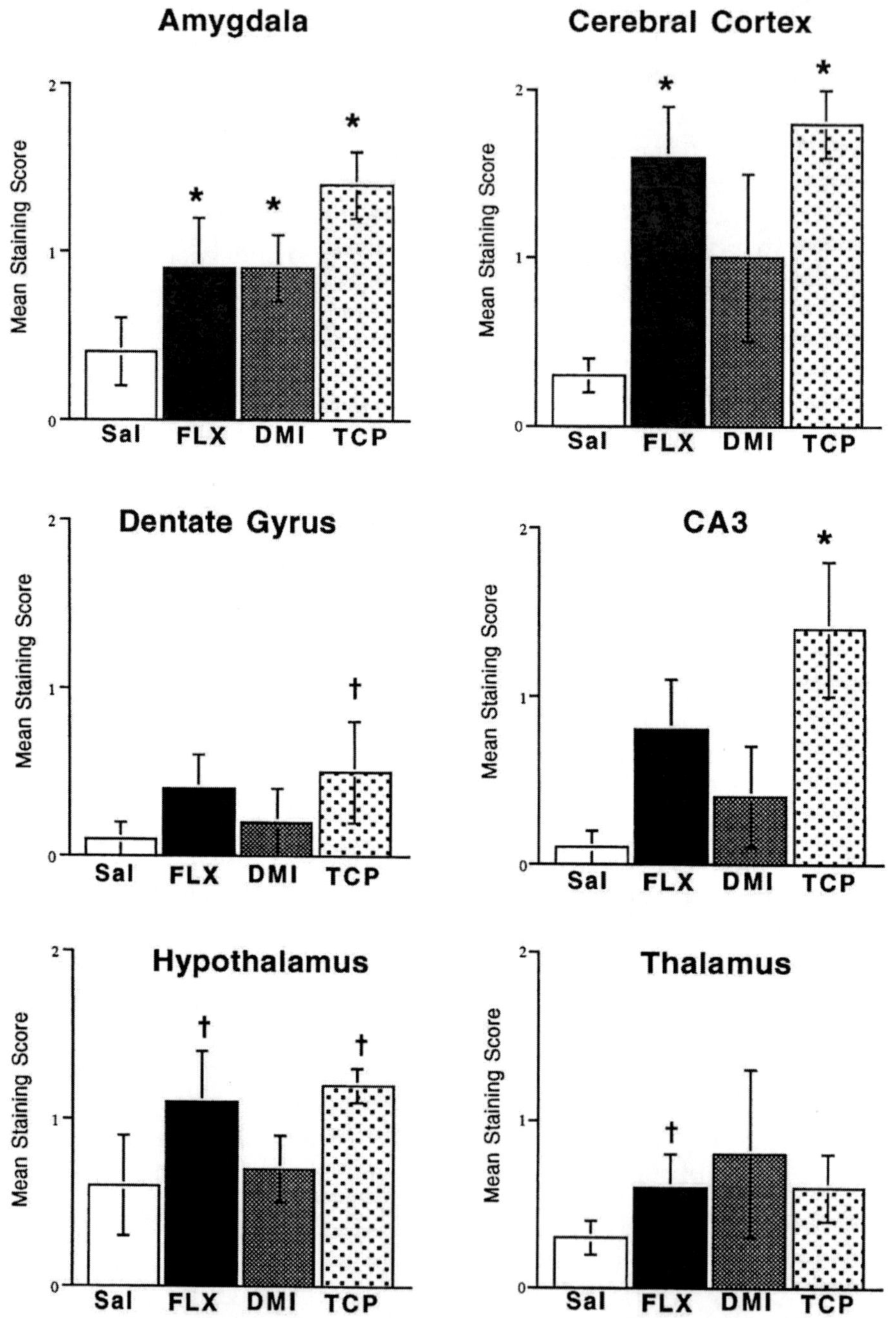

Figure 31. Chronic antidepressant treatment increases CYE-mediated gene expression in rat brain (Flx = fluoxetine; DMI= desipramine; TCP= tranylcypromin is administered once a day for 14 days and staining score is detected immunohistochemically by β galactosidase 6 hours after the last injections. * $p<0.05$; t$p<0.10$; different from saline; Kruskal-Wallis) (Thome et al., 2000).

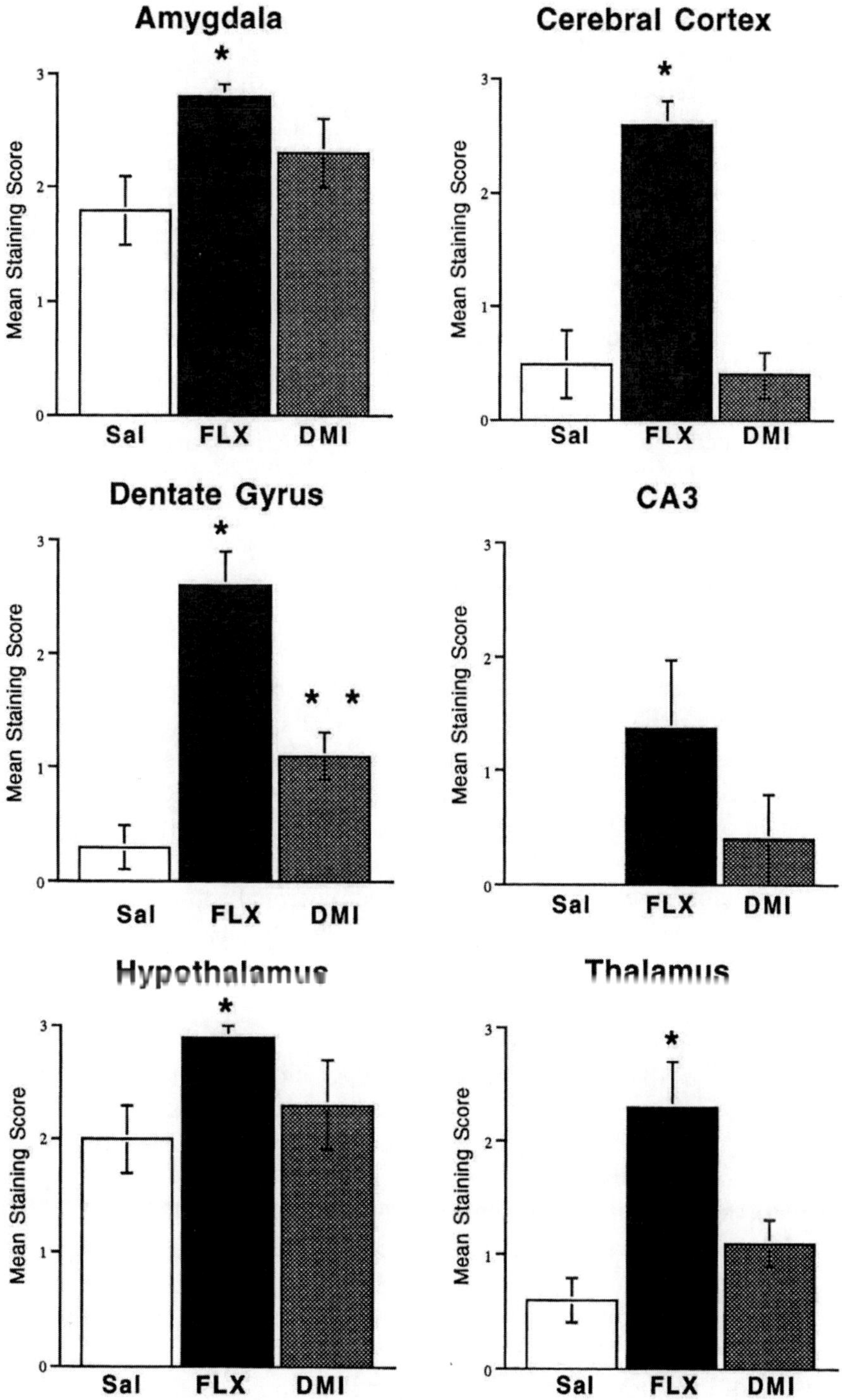

Figure 32. Chronic antidepressant treatment increases CREB phosforylation in rat brain (Flx= fluoxetine; DMI= desipramine; TCP= tranylcypromin is administered once a day for 14 days and staining score is detected immunohistochemically 6 hours after the last injections. * $p<0.05$; significantly different from saline; Kruskal-Wallis) (Thome et al., 2000).

Among the three different antidepressants used in this study, fluoxetine is found to be most effective in terms of its influence on CREB phosphorylation. Nevertheless, it is interesting that fluoxetine is ineffective on both CRE-mediated gene expression and CREB phosphorylation in the CA3 region of the hippocampal formation. This may be because this layer of hippocampus does not contribute to the effects of fluoxetine emerging through CRE.

CREB can be activated in vitro by cAMP-protein kinase A (PKA) pathway through the stimulation of 5-HT receptors (Duman et al., 1998) and noradrenergic receptors (Roseboom and Klein, 1995).

CREB activity can also be directly induced by Ca^{2+} dependent protein kinases stimulated by adrenergic receptors and serotonergic 5-HT_2 receptors (Duman, 1998). CREB activation and subsequent increases in BDNF gene expression have an important role in the antidepressant mechanism of action. Other studies also show that the cAMP/CREB/BDNF system is stimulated and activated by several antidepressants and during electroconvulsive therapy (Nibuya et al., 1995, 1996).

Stress, Hippocampal Gene Expression and the Effects of Antidepressants

Using complementary DNA (cDNA) subtractive libraries from cortisol-treated tree shrews, it has been recently identified four genes differentially expressed in the hippocampus of male tree shrews subjected to chronic psychosocial stress. These genes encode the nerve growth factor (NGF), the membrane glycoprotein 6a (M6a), the guanine nucleotide binding protein (G protein) alpha q polypeptide (GNAQ), and a CDC-like kinase 1 (CLK-1). Downregulation of M6a, GNAQ, and CLK-1 messenger RNA (mRNA) expression could be reversed by clomipramine treatment (Alfonso et al. 2004). Interestingly, these four genes have been previously related to neurogenesis, neuronal differentiation, and/or neurite outgrowth (Heasley et al. 1996, McAllister et al. 1999, Mukobata et al. 2002 and Myers et al. 1994).

In a recent study, Alfonso et al. (2006) evaluated whether these alterations in gene expression are conserved in a different stress animal model. They measured NGF, M6a, GNAQ, and CLK-1 expression levels in the hippocampus of male and female mice from BALB/c and C56BL/6 strains subjected to repeated restraint stress for 3 weeks. In this study, the authors also determined expression levels for other neuronal and synaptic plasticity-related genes such as BDNF, CREB, synaptic associated protein synapsin I, protein kinase C alpha (PKC-α), neural cell adhesion molecule 140 (NCAM-140), and growth associated protein 43 (GAP-43). Finally, to study whether antidepressant treatment can reverse the changes in gene expression observed after exposure to repeated stress, they also subjected animals to chronic restraint stress and daily tianeptine administration, an atypical antidepressant.

The results of the study indicated that Chronically stressed mice displayed a reduction in transcript levels for NGF, M6a, GNAQ, and CLK-1. In addition, other genes implicated in neuronal plasticity, such as BDNF, CREB, PKC, NCAM, and synapsin I were downregulated in stressed mice. Tianeptine treatment reversed the stress effects for the genes analyzed. Alterations in gene expression were dependent on the duration of the stress treatment and, in some cases, were only observed in male mice (Figure 33, 34 and 35).

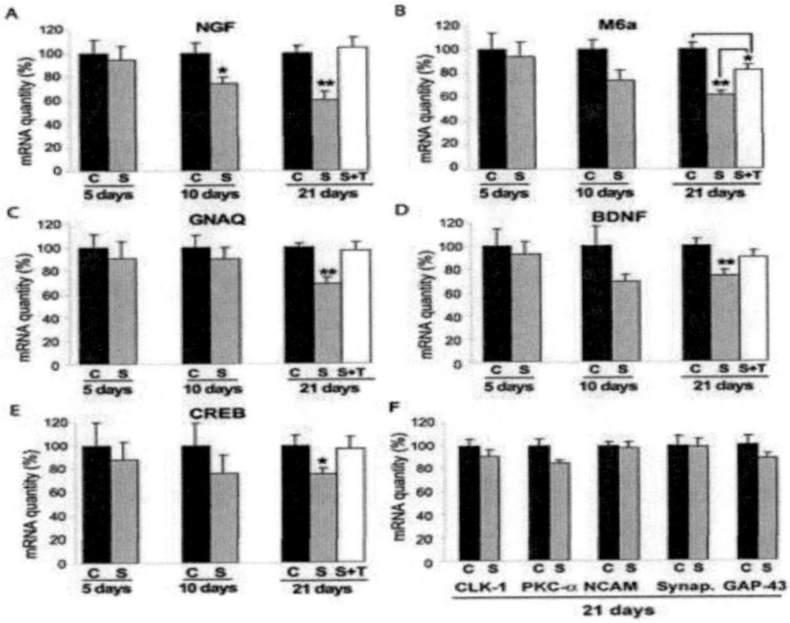

Figure 33. Differential gene expression in the hippocampus is induced only by chronic stress and is reversed by tianeptine treatment. Female BALB/c mice were either untreated control subjects ("C," black bars), subjected to 5, 10, or 21 days of restraint stress ("S," gray bars), or treated with tianeptine concomitantly to the stress procedure ("S+T," white bars). Messenger RNA samples from the hippocampal formation were used for quantification of NGF (A), M6a (B), GNAQ (C), BDNF (D), CREB (E), CLK-1, PKC-α, NCAM-140, synapsin I, and GAP-43 (F) expression levels using real time RT-PCR. Values for each individual were normalized with the reference gene cyclophilin. *p < .05, **p < .01. S+T group value for M6a expression levels is statistically different to both C and S group values. NGF, nerve growth factor; M6a, membrane glycoprotein 6a; GNAQ, guanine nucleotide binding protein (G protein) alpha q polypeptide (Alfonso et al., 2006).

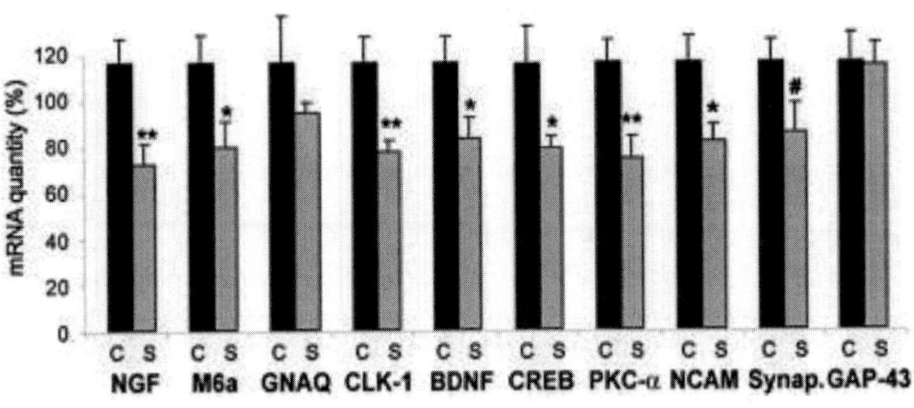

Figure 34. Regulation of gene expression in the hippocampus of chronically stressed male BALB/c mice. Male BALB/c mice were subjected to 21 days of restraint stress ("S," gray bars) or left undisturbed (control subjects: "C," black bars). Messenger RNA samples from the hippocampal formation were used for quantification of NGF, M6a, GNAQ, BDNF, CREB, CLK-1, PKC-α, NCAM-140, synapsin I, and GAP-43 cDNA amounts using real time RT-PCR. Values for each individual were normalized with the reference gene cyclophilin. Plotted data shows mean group values +SEM expressed as a percentage of the respective control group (Alfonso et al., 2006).

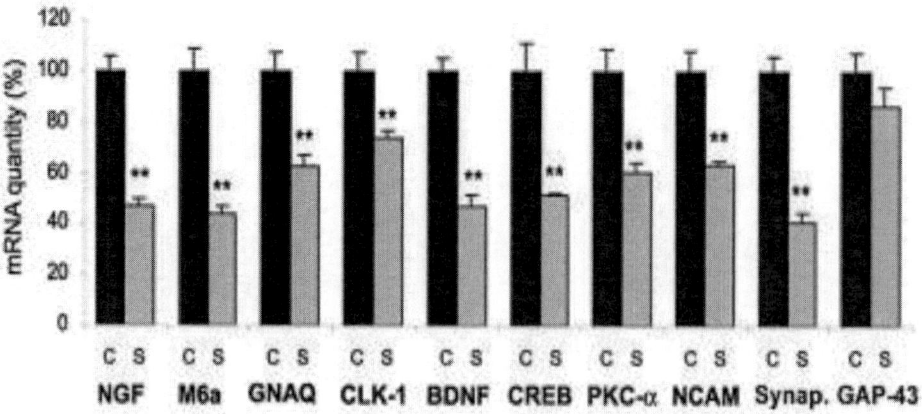

Figure 35- Neuronal remodeling-related genes are downregulated in the hippocampus of chronically stressed mice. Male C57BL/6 mice were subjected to restraint stress during 21 days ("S," gray bars) or left undisturbed (control subjects: "C," black bars). Messenger RNA samples from the hippocampal formation were used for cDNA quantification of NGF, M6a, GNAQ, BDNF, CREB, CLK-1, PKC-α, NCAM-140, synapsin I, and GAP-43 using real time RT-PCR. Values for each individual were normalized with the reference gene cyclophilin and mean group values + SEM expressed as a percentage of the respective control group are shown (Alfonso et al., 2006).

Conclusion

Despite acute regulation of monoaminergic neurotransmission, resulting in a significant increase of synaptic monoamine concentrations, most antidepressants still require several weeks before clinical effects occur. This delayed therapeutic action may results from either the indirect regulation of other neuronal signal transduction systems or the regulation of gene transcription. An "initial and adaptation" model has recently been proposed to describe the drug-induced changes of neuronal plasticity associated with the long-term actions of antidepressants in the brain (Hyman and Nestler, 1996; Kuipers et al., 2005).

In the light of the data discussed so far, it is seen that changes in synaptic plasticity that occur in the brain under stress play an important role in the development of neuropsychiatric disorders like depression. The neuroplasticity hypothesis of depression appears to explain depression more accurately than does the monoamine hypothesis. Recently, it was shown that antidepressants like tianeptine that have significant effects on neuroplasticity also have other useful effects such as being anticonvulsants associated with the excitatory amino acidergic system in experimental animals (Ceyhan et al., 2005). This observation highlights the reality that the field of neuroplasticity is widening to include other psychiatric and neurological disorders. It may be expected that drugs that have an effect on neuroplasticity treat not only depression but also other diseases related to the central nervous system and having a neurodegenerative course. This can provide a more effective treatment with fewer drugs for patients who have depression and other diseases with a central origin. Therefore, it will be inevitable to reshape the strategies of psychotropic drug development to concentrate on the development of molecules that affect neuroplasticity to include these mechanisms rather than drugs that modulate the interaction between neurotransmitter release, reuptake and receptor systems (Uzbay, 2008).

An important point concerning neuroplasticity and the effects of psychotropic drugs that should not be neglected is that available studies were conducted on experimental animals and are limited in number. Moreover, most of the studies evaluate the effects of tianeptine only. Although there are some data about fluoxetine and tricyclics, they are not sufficient for an accurate interpretation. It is necessary to test the reproducibility of data from tianeptine studies with other antidepressant drugs. In addition, it is necessary to support the experimental animal data with clinical trials. Neuroplasticity studies in humans were unable to go beyond morphological studies examining hippocampal formation and other important brain structures using magnetic resonance imaging techniques. It is certain that the development of non-invasive techniques that permit efficient assessment of central elements related to neuroplasticity in humans and comparison of these studies with clinical ones will herald a new era in the diagnosis and treatment of brain diseases.

ACKNOWLEDGMENT

Dr. Hakan Kayir has made valuable contributions during the writing process of this chapter. I thank Dr. Kayir for his eager efforts during its composition and publication.

REFERENCES

Abraham, W.C., Dragunow, M., Tate W.P. (1991). The role of immediate early genes in the stabilization of long-term potentiation. *Mol. Neurobiol.* 5: 297-314.

Alfonso, J., Pollevick, G.D., Van Der Hart, M.G., Flugge, G., Fuchs, E., Frasch, A.C. (2004). Identification of genes regulated by chronic psychosocial stress and antidepressant treatment in the hippocampus. *Eur. J. Neurosci.* 19: 659-666.

Alfonso, J., Frick, L.R., Silberman, D.M., Palumbo, M.L., Genaro, A.M., Frasch, A.C. (2006). Regulation of hippocampal gene expression is conserved in two species subjected to different stressors and antidepressant treatments. *Biol. Psychiatry* 59: 244-251.

Alici, T., Kayir, H., Aygoren, M.O., Saglam, E., Uzbay, IT. (2006). Discriminative stimulus properties of tianeptine: partial substitution by fluoxetine and 8-OH-DPAT. *Psychopharmacology*183: 446-451.

Allen, S.J., MacGowan, S.H., Treanor, J.J., Feeney, R., Wicock, G.K., Dawbarn, D. (1991). Normal beta-NGF content in Alzheimer's disease cerebral cortex and hippocampus. *Neurosci. Lett.* 131: 135-139.

Allgulander, C., Hackett, D., Salinas, E. (2001). Venlafaxine extended release (ER) in the treatment of generalised anxiety disorder. Twenty-four-week placebo-controlled dose-ranging study. *Br. J. Psychi*atry 179:15-22.

Angelucci, F., Mathe, A.A., Aloe, L. (2004). Neurotrophic factors and CNS disorders: finding in rodent models of depression and schizophrenia. *Prog. Brain Res.* 46: 151-165.

Ansseau, M. (1988). Les antidépresseurs. *Méd. et Hyg.* 46: 2314-2321.

Ansseau, M. (1993). The paradox of tianeptine. Eur Psychiat 8 (Suppl. 2): 89S-93S.

Aprison, M.H., Hintgen, J.N., Nagayama, H. (1982). Testing a new theory of depression with an animal model; neurochemical-behavioral evidence for postsynaptic serotonergic receptor involvement. In: Langer, S.Z., Takahashi, R., Segawa, T., Briley, M. (Eds.), New Vistas in Depression, New york, Pergamon Press, pp.171-178.

Armstrong, R.C., Montminy, M.R. (1993). Transsynaptic control of gene expression. *Annu. Rev. Neurosci.* 16: 17-29.

Aydemir, C., Yalcin, E.S., Aksaray, S., Kisa, C., Yildirim, S.G., Uzbay, T., Goka, E. (2006). Brain-derived neurotrophic factor (BDNF) changes in the serum of depressed women. *Prog. Neuropsychopharmacol. Biol. Psychiatry*, 30: 1256-1260.

Backman, C., Rose, G.M., Bartus, R.T., Hoffer, B.J., Mufson, E.J., Granholm, A.C. (1997). Carrier mediated delivery of NGF: Alterations in basal forebrain neurons in aged rats revealed using antibodies against low and high affinity NGF receptors. *J. Comp. Neurol.* 387: 1-11.

Ballarin, M., Emfors, P., Lindefors, N., Persson, H. (1991). Hippocampal damage and kainic acid injection induce a rapid increase in mRNA in the rat brain. *Exp. Neurol.* 114: 35-43.

Barbaccia, M.L., Gandolfi, O., Chuang, D.M., Costa, E. (1983). Modulation of neuronal serotonin uptake by a putative endogenous ligand of imipramine recognition sites. *Proc. Natl. Acad. Sci. USA* 80:5134-5138.

Biebl, M., Cooper, C.M., Winkler, J., Kuhn, H.G. (2000). Analysis of neurogenesis and programmed cell death reveals a self-renewing capacity in the adult rat brain. *Neurosci. Lett.* 291: 17-20.

Bird, E.D., Spokes, E.G., Iversen, L.L. (1979). Brain norepinephrine and dopamine in schizophrenia. *Science* 204: 93-94.

Birken, D.L., Oldendorf, W.H. (1989). N-acetyl-L-aspartic acid: a literature review of a compound prominent in ^{1}H-NMR spectroscopy studies of the brain. *Neurosci. Biobehav. Rev.* 13: 23-31.

Blair, H.T., Schafe, G.E., Bauer, E.P., Rodrigues, S.M., LeDoux, J.E. (2001). Synaptic plasticity in the lateral amygdala: a cllular hypothesis of fear conditioning. Learn Mem 8: 229-242.

Bondy, B. (2002). Pathophysiology of depression and mechanisms of treatment. Dialogues in Clinical Neuroscience. 4: 7-20.

Boyer, P. (2000). Do anxiety and depression have a common pathophysiological mechanism? *Acta Psychiatr. Scand.* (Suppl. 406): 24-29.

Brand, A., Richter-Landsberg, C., Leibfritz, D. (1993). Multinuclear NMR studies on the energy metabolism of glial and neuronal cells. *Dev. Neurosci.* 15: 289-298.

Brewin, C.R. (2001). A cognitive neuroscience account of posttraumatic stress disorder and its treatment. *Behav. Res. Ther.* 39: 373-393.

Brown, E.S., Rush, A.J., McEwen, B.S. (1999). Hippocampal remodelling and damage by corticosteroids: implications for mood disorders. *Neuropharmacology* 21: 474-484.

Brown, R.A.M., McKim, W.A. (2000). Neurophysiology, neurotransmitters, and the nervous system. In: McKim WA (Ed.), Drugs and Behavior, An Introduction to Behavioral Pharmacology. Printice Hall, New Jersey, pp. 56-81.

Brunello, N., Riva, M., Volterra, A., Racagni, G. (1987) Effect of some tricyclic and non tricyclic antidepressants on [3H] imipramine binding and serotonin uptake in rat cerebral cortex after prolonged treatment. *Fundam. Clin. Pharmacol.* 1: 327-333.

Bunney, W.E., Davis, J.M. (1965). Norepinephrine in depressive reactions. *Arch. Gen. Psychiatry* 13: 483-494.

Burghardt, N.S., Sullivan, G.M., McEwen, B.S., Gorman, J.M., LeDoux, J.E. (2004). The selective serotonin reuptake inhibitor citalopram increases fear after acute treatment but reduces fear with chronic treatment: a comparison with tinaeptine. *Biol. Psychiatry* 55: 1171-1178.

Cahill, L. (2000). Neurobiological mechanisms of emotionally influenced long-term memory. *Prog. Brain Res.* 126: 29-37.

Cameron, H.A., McEwen, B.S., Gould, E. (1995). Regulation of adult neurogenesis by excitatory input and NMDA receptor activation in the dentate gyrus. *J. Neurosci.* 15: 4687-4692.

Carvey, P.M. (1998). Drug Action in the Central Nervous System. Oxford University Press, New York.

Castrén, E. (2005). Is mood chemistry? *Nature Rev.* 6: 241-246.

Ceyhan, M., Kayir, M., Uzbay, I.T. (2005). Investigation of the effects of tianeptine and fluoxetine on pentylenetetrazole-induced seizures in rats. *J. Psychiatric. Res.* 39: 191-196.

Chao, M., Casaccia-Bonnefil, P., Carter, B., Chittka, A., Kong, H., Yoon, S.O. (1998). Neurotrophin receptors: mediators of life and death Brain res Brain res Rev 26: 295-301.

Chao, M.V., Hempstead, B.L. (1995). P75 and Trk: a two-receptor system. *Trends Neurosci.* 18: 321-326.

Chaouloff, F. (1993). Psychopharmacological interactions between stress hormones and central serotonergic systems. *Brain Res. Rev.* 18: 1-32.

Chapman, P.F., Ramsay, M.F., Krezel, W., Knevett, S.G. (2003). Synaptic plasticity in the amygdala: comparisons with hippocampus. *Ann. NY Acad. Sci.* 985: 114-124.

Chen, G., Rajkowska, G., Du, F., Seraji-Bozorgzad, N., Manji, H.K. (2000). Enhancement of hippocampal neurogenezis by lithium. *J. Neurochem.* 75: 1729-1734.

Cotman,. CW., Nieto-Sampedro, M. (1984). Cell biology of synaptic plasticity. *Science* 225: 1287-1294.

Cowen, P.J. (1998). Pharmacological challenge tests and brain serotonergic function in depression during SSRI treatment. In: Briley, M., Montgomery, S. (Eds.), Antidepressant Therapy, Martin Dunitz Ltd, London, pp. 175-189.

Cutler, M.G., Rodgers, R.J., Jackson, J.E. (1997). Behavioural effects in mice of subchronic buspirone, ondansetron and tianeptine. I. Social interactions. *Pharmacol. Biochem. Behav.* 56: 287-293.

Czéh, B., Michaelis, T., Watanabe, T., Frahm, J., de Biurrun, G., van Kampen, M., Bartolomucci, A., Fuchs, E. (2001) Stress-induced changes in cerebral metabolites, hippocampal volume, and cell proliferation are prevented by antidepressant treatment with tianeptine. *Proc. Natl. Acad. Sci. USA* 98: 12796-12801.

Czéh, B., Welt, T., Fischer A.K., Erhardt, A., Schmitt W., Muller, M. (2002). Chronic psychosocial stress and concomitant repetitive transcranial magnetic stimulation: effects on stress hormone levels and adult hippocampal neurogenesis. *Biol. Psychiatry* 52: 1057-1065.

Defrance, R., Marey, C., Kamoun, A. (1988). Antidepressant and anxiolytic activities of tianeptine: an overview of clinical trials. *Clin. Neuropharmacol.* 11 (Suppl. 2): 74-82.

Delgado, P.L., Moreno, F.A., Potter, R., Gelenberg, A.J. (1998). Norepinephrine and serotonin in antidepressant action: evidence from neurotransmitter depletion studies. In:

Briley, M., Montgomery, S. (Eds.), Antidepressant Therapy, Martin Dunitz Ltd, London, pp. 141-161.

Den Boer, J.A., Westenberg, H.G.M. (1988). Effect of a serotonin and noradrenaline uptake inhibitor in panic disorder; a double-blind comparative study with fluvoxamine and maprotiline. *Int. Clin. Psychopharmacol.* 3: 59-74.

Diamond, D.M., Rose, G.M. (1994). Stress impairs. LTP and hippocampal-dependent memory. Ann NY Acad Sci 746: 411-414.

Diamond, D.M., Campbell, A., Park, C.R., Vouimba, R-M. (2004). Preclinical research on stress, memory, and the brain in the development of pharmacotherapy for depression. *Eur. Neuropsychopharmacol.* 14 (Suppl. 5) : S491-S495.

Dowlatshahi, D., MacQuenn, G.M., Wang, J.F., Young, LT. (1998). Increased temporal cortex CREB concentrations and antidepressant treatment in major depression. *Lancet* 352: 1754-1755.

Dragunow, M., Robertson, G.S., Faull, R.L.M., Robertson, H.A., Jansen, K. (1990). D_2 dopamine receptor antagonists induce Fos and related proteins in rat striatal neurons. *Neuroscience* 37: 287-294.

Dubovsky, S.L., Thomas, M. (1995). Beyond specifity: effects of serotonin and serotonergic treatments on psychobiological dysfunction. *J. Psychosom. Res.* 39: 429-444.

Duman, R.S. (1998). Novel therapeutic approaches beyond the 5-HT receptor. *Biol. Psychiatry* 44: 324-335.

Duman, R.S., Nakagawa, S., Malberg, J. (2001). Regulation of adult neurogenezis by antidepressant treatment. *Neuropsychopharmacology* 25: 836-844.

Duman, R.S. (2002). Pathophysiology of depression: the concept of synaptic plasticity. *Eur. Psychiatry* 17 (Suppl. 3): 306-310.

Duman, R.S. (2004). Neural plasticity: consequences of stress and actions of antidepressant treatment. *Dialogues in Clinical Neuroscienve – Neuroplasticity*. 6: 157-169.

Eisch, A.J. (2002). Adult neurogenesis: implications for psychiatry. *Prog. Brain Res.* 138: 315-342.

Ericksson, P.S., Perfilieva, E., Björk-Eriksson, T., Alborn, A., Nordberg, C., Peterson, D.A., Gage, F.H. (1998). Neurogenezis in the adult human hippocampus. *Nature Medicine* 4: 1313-1317.

Fattaccini, C.M., Bolanos-Jimenez, F., Gozlan, H., Hamon, M. (1990). Tianeptine stimulates uptake of 5-hydroxytryptamine in vivo in the rat brain. *Neuropharmacology* 29: 1-8.

Feldman, R.S., Meyer, J.S., Qenzer, L.F. (1997). Principles of Neuropsychopharmacology. Sinauer Associates Inc., Sunderland, Massachusetts, pp. 58-491.

Fichter, M.M., Narrow, W.E., Roper, M.T., Rehm, J., Elton, M., Rae, D.S., Locke, B.Z., Regier, D.A. (1996). Prevalance of mental illness in Germany and the United States: comparison of the Upper Bavarian Study and the Epidemiologic Catchment Area Program. *J. Nerv. Ment. Dis.,* 184: 598-606.

Forstermann, U., Gorsky, L.D., Pollock, J.S., Schmidt, H.H., Heler, M., Murad, F. (1990). Regional distribution of EDRF/NO-synthesizing enzyme(s) in rat brain. *Biochem. Biophys. Res. Commun.* 168: 727-732.

Fossati, P., Harvey, P.O., Le Bastard, G., Ergis, A.M., Jouvent, R., Allilaire, J.F. (2004). Verbal memory performance of patients with a first depressive episode and patients with unipolar and bipolar recurrent depression. *J. Psychiatr. Res.* 38: 137-144.

Foy, M.R., Stanton, M.E., Levine, S., Thompson, R.F. (1987). Behavioral stress impairs long-term potentiation in rodent hippocampus. *Behav. Neural. Biol.* 48: 138-149.

Fuchs, E., Gould, E. (2000). Mini-review: in vivo neurogenesis in the adult brain: regulation and functional implications. *Eur. J. Neurosci.* 12: 2211-2214.

Fuchs, E., Czéh, B., Michaelis, T., de Biurrun, G., Watanabe, T., Frahm, J. (2002). Synaptic plasticity and tianeptine: structural regulation. *Eur. Psychiatry* 17 (Suppl. 3): 311-317.

Fuchs, E., Czéh, B., Kole, M.H.P., Michaelis, T., Lucassen, P.L. (2004). Alterations of neuroplasticity in depression: the hippocampus and beyond. *Eur. Neuropsychopharmacol.* 14: S481-S490.

Fuchs, E. (2009). Neuroplasticity – A new approach to the pathophysiology of depression. In: Costa e Silva JA, Macher JP, Olié JP (Eds.), Neuroplasticity. New Biochemicakl Mechanism. *Current Medicine Group*, London, pp. 1-12.

Gall, C.M., Gold, S.J., Isackson, P.J., Seroogy, K.B. (1992). Brain derived neurotrophic factor and neurotrophin -3 mRNAs are expressed in ventral midbrain regions containing dopaminergic neurons. *Mol. Cell Neurosci.* 3: 56-63.

Garattini, S., Giacolone, E., Valzelli, L. (1967). Isolation, agressiveness and brain 5-hydroxytriptamine turnover. *J. Pharm. Pharmacol.* 19: 338-339.

Garthwaite, J., Garthwaite, G., Palmer, R.M., Moncada, S. (1989). NMDA receptor activation induces nitric oxide synthesis from arginine in rat brain slices. *Eur. J. Pharmacol.* 172: 413-416.

Garthwaite, J. (1991). Glutamate, nitric oxide and cell-cell signalling in the nervous system. *Trends Neurosci.* 14: 60-67.

Garzon, J., del Rio, J. (1981). Hypersensitivity induced in rats by long tern isolation: Further studies on a new animal model for the detection of antidepressants. *Eur. J. Pharmacol.* 74: 287-294.

Goggi, J., Pullar, I.A., Carney, S.L., Bradford, H.F. (2002). Modulation of neurotransmitter release induced by brain-derived neurotrophic factor in rat brain striatal slices in vitro. *Brain Res.* 941: 34-42.

Goldberg, H.L., Finnerty, R.J. (1979). The comparative efficacy of buspirone and diazepam in the treatment of anxiety. *Am. J. Psychiatry* 136: 1184-1187.

Gould, E., McEwen, B.S., Tanapat, P., Galea, L.A., Fuchs, E. (1997). Neurogenezis in the dentate gyrus of the adult tree shrew is regulated by psychosocial stress and NMDA receptor activation. *J. Neurosci.* 17: 2492-2498.

Gould, E., Tanapat, P., McEwen, B.S., Flugge, G., Fuchs, E. (1998). Proliferation of granule cell precursors in the dentate gyrus of adult monkeys is diminished by stress. *Proc. Natl. Acad. Sci. USA* 95: 3168-3171.

Gould, E. (1999). Serotonin and hippocampal neurogenesis. *Neuropsychopharmacology* 21: 46S-51S.

Gross, C.G. (2000). Neurogenesis in the adult brain: death of a dogma. *Nat. Rev. Neurosci.* 1: 67-73.

Gören, M.Z., Arıcıoğlu-Kartal, F., Yurdun, T., Uzbay, I.T. (2001). Investigation of extracellular L-citrulline concentration in the striatum during alcohol withdrawal in rats. *Neurochem. Res.,* 26: 1327-1333.

Graybiel, A.M., Moratalla, R., Robertson, H.A. (1990). Amphetamine and cocaine induce drug-specific activation of the *c-fos* gene in striosome-matrix compartments and limbic subdivisions of the striatum. *Proc. Natl. Acad. Sci. USA* 87: 6912-6916.

Guelfi, J.D., Pichot, P., Dreyfus, J.F. (1989). Efficacy of tianeptine in anxious-depressed patients. Results of a controlled multicentre trial versus amitriptyline, *Neuropsychobiology* 1: 41-48.

Heasley, L.E., Storey, B., Fanger, G.R., Butterfield, L., Zamarripa, J., Blumberg, D., Maue, R.A. (1996). GTPase-deficient G alpha 16 and G alpha q induce PC12 cell differentiation and persistent activation of cJun NH2-terminal kinases. *Mol. Cell Biol.* 16: 648-656.

Heine, V.M., Malsam, S., Zareno, J., Joëls, M., Lucassen, P.J. (2004). Supressed proliferation and apoptotic changes in the rat dentate gyrus after acute and chronic stress are reversible. *Eur. J. Neurosci.* 19: 131-144.

Hindmarch, I. (2002). Beyond the monoamine hypothesis: mechanisms, molecules and methods. *Eur. Psychiatry* 17 (Suppl. 3): 294-299.

Hoehn-Saric, R. (1982). Neurotransmitters in anxiety. Arch Gen Psychiatry 39:735-742.

Hyman, S.E., Nestler, E.J. (1996). Initiation and adaptation: A paradigm for understanding psychotrophic drug action. *Am. J. Psychiatry* 153: 151-162.

Ip, N.Y., Ibanez, C.F., Nye, S.H., McClain, J., Jones, P.F., Gies, D.R., Belluscio, L., Le Beau, M.M., Espinoza III, R., Squinto, S.P. (1992). Mammalian neurotrophin-4: structure, chromosomal localization, tissue distribution, and receptor specificity. *Proc. Natl. Acad. Sci. USA* 89: 3060-3064.

Jacobs, B.L., Praag, H., Gage, F.H. (2000). Adult brain neurogenesis and psychiatry: a novel theory of depression. *Mol. Psychiatry* 5: 262-269.

Kaplan, D.R., Miller, F.D. (2000). Neurotrophin signal transduction in the nervous system. *Curr. Opin. Neurobiol.* 10: 381-391.

Kato, G., Weitsch, A.F. (1988). Neurochemical profile of tianeptine, a new antidepressant drug. *Clin. Neuropharmacol.* 11 (Suppl. 2): S43-S50.

Kato, T., Inubushi, T., Kato, N. (1998). Magnetic resonance spectroscopy in affective disorders. *J. Neuropsychiatry Clin. Neurosci.* 10: 133-147.

Katoh-Semba, R., Asano, T., Ueda, H., Morishita, R., Takeuchi, I.K., Inaguma, Y., Kato, K. (2002). *Faseb. J.* 16: 1328-1330.

Kempermann, G., Kronenberg, G. (2003). Depressed new neurons?- Adult hippocampal neurogenezis and a cellular plasticity hypothesis of major depression. *Biol. Psychiat.* 54: 499-503.

Kennedy, S.H., Lam, R.W., Nutt, D.J., Thase, M.E. (2004). Treating Depression Effectively. Applying Clinical Guidelines. Martin Dunitz Ltd, London, pp. 47-55.

Kiba, H., Jayaraman, A. (1994). Nicotine-induced *c-fos* expression in the striatum is mediated mostly by dopamine D_1 receptor and is dependent on NMDA stimulation. *Mol. Brain Res.* 23: 1-13.

Kim, J.J., Diamond, D.M. (2002). The stressed hippocampus, synaptic plasticity and lost memories. *Nat. Rev. Neurosci.* 3: 453-462.

Kim, Y.K., Lee, H.P., Won, S.D., Park, E.Y., Lee, H.Y., Lee, B.H., Lee, S.W., Yoon, D., Han, C., Kim, D.J., Choi, S.H. (2007). Low plasma BDNF is associated with suicidal behavior in major depression. *Prog Neuropsychopharmacol Biol Psychiatry* 31: 78-85.

Kole, M.H.P., Swan, L., Fuchs, E. (2002). The antidepressant tianeptine persistently modulates glutamate receptor currents of the hippocampal CA3 commissural associational synapse in chronically stressed rats. *Eur. J. Neurosci.* 16: 807-816.

Konradi, C., Cole, R.L., Heckers, S., Hyman, S.E. (1994). Amphetamine regulates gene expression in rat striatum via transcription factor CREB. *J. Neurosci.* 14: 5623-5634.

Kuhn, H.G., Palmer, T.D., Fuchs, E. (2001). Adult neurogenesis: a compensatory mechanism for neuronal damage. Eur Arch Psychiatry *Clin. Neurosci.* 251: 152-158.

Kuipers, S.D., Trentani, A., ter Horst, G.J., den Boer, JA. (2005). Looking beyond the receptor: Molecular biological approaches to antidepressant therapy. In: Den Boer, J.A., George, M.S., ter Horst, G.J. (Eds.), Current and Future Developments in Psychopharmacology. Benecke NI, Amsterdam, pp. 83-102.

Landfield, P.W. (1994). Increased hippocampal Ca^{2+} channel activity in brain aging and dementia. Hormonal and pharmacological modulation. Ann NY Acad Sci 747: 351-364.

Leonard, B.E. (1998). Animal models of depression. In: Briley, M., Montgomery, S. (Eds.), Antidepressant Therapy, Martin Dunitz Ltd, London, pp. 87-109.

Lepine, J.P., Gastpar, M., Mendelwicz, J., Tylee, A. (1997). The prevalence of depression in the community; the first pan-European study DEPRES (Depression Research in European Society). *Int. Clin. Psychopharmacol.,* 12: 19-29.

Leverenz, J.B., Wilkinson, C.W., Wamble, M., Corbin, S., Grabber, J.E., Raskind, M.A. (1999). Effect of chronic high-dose exogenous cortisol on hippocampal neuronal number in aged nonhuman primates. *J. Neurosci.* 19: 2356-2361.

Levin, G.R., Barde, Y.A. (1996). Physiology of the neurotrophins. *Annu. Rev. Neurosci.* 19: 289-317.

Liu, J., Nickolenko, J., Sharp, F.R. (1994). Morphine induces *c-fos* and *junB* in striatum and nucleus accumbens via D_1 and N-methyl-D-aspartate receptors. *Proc. Natl. Acad. Sci. USA* 91: 8537-8541.

Lŏo, H., Saiz-Ruiz, J., Costa e Silva, J.A., Ansseau, M., Herrington, R., Vaz-Serra, A., Dilling, H., De Risio, S. (2001). Efficacy and safety of tianeptine in the treatment of depressive disorders in comparison with fluoxetine. *Hum. Psychopharmacol.* 16 (Suppl. 1): S31-S38.

Lowy, M.T., Gault, L., Yamamato, B.K. (1993). Adrenalectomy attenuates stress-induced elevations in extracellular glutamate concentrations in the hippocampus. *J. Neurochem.* 61: 1957-1960.

Lowy, M.T., Wittenberg, L., Yamamto, B.K. (1995). Effects of acute stress in hippocampal glutamate levels and spectrin preteolysis in young and aged rats. *J. Neurochem.* 65: 268-274.

Lucassen, P.J., Muller, M.B., Holsboer, F., Bauer, J., Holtrop, A., Wouda, J., Hoogendijk, W.J., De Kloet, E.R., Swaab, D.F. (2001). Hippocampal apoptosis in major depression is a minor event and absent from subareas at risk for glucocorticoid overexposure. *Am. J. Pathol.* 158: 453-68.

Lucassen, P.J., Fuchs, E., Czéh, B. (2004). Antidepressant treatment with tianeptine reduces apopitosis in hippocampal dentate gyrus and temporal cortex. *Biol. Psychiatry* 55: 789-796.

Lupien, S.J., McEwen, B.S. (1997). The acute effects of corticosteroids on cognition: integration of animal and human model studies. *Brain Res.* Rev 24: 1-27.

Maas, J.W., Fawcett, J., Dekimejian, H. (1968). 3-methoxy-4-hydoxy-phenylglycol (MHPG) excretion in depressive patients. *Arch. Gen. Psychiatry* 19: 129-134.

Madsen, T.M., Trechow, A., Bengzon, J., Bolwig, T.G., Lindvall, O., Tingstrom, A. (2000). Increased neurogenezis in a model of electroconvulsive therapy. *Biol. Psychiatry* 47: 1043-1049.

Magarinos, A.M., McEwen, B.C. (1995a). Stress-induced athrophy of apical dendrites of hippocampal CA3c neurons: comparison of stressors. *Neuroscience* 69: 83-88.

Magarinos, A.M., McEwen, B.C. (1995b). Stress-induced athrophy of apical dendrites of hippocampal CA3c neurons: involvement of glucocorticoid secretion and excitatory amino acid receptors. *Neuroscience* 69: 89-98.

Magarinos, A.M., McEwen, B.S., Flugge, G., Fuchs, E. (1996). Chronic psychosocial stress causes apical dentritic athrophy of hippocampal CA3 pyramidal neurons in subordinate tree shrews. *J. Neurosci.* 16: 3534-3540.

Magarinos, A.M., Verdugo, J.M., McEwen, B.S. (1997). Chronic stress alters synaptic terminal structure in hippocampus. *Proc. Natl. Acad. Sci. USA* 94: 14002-14008.

Magarinos, A.M., Deslandes, A., McEwen, B.S. (1999). Effects of antidepressants and benzodiazepine treatments on the dendritic structure of CA3 pyramidal neurons after chronic stress. *Eur. J. Pharmacol.* 371: 113-122.

Maghaddam, B., Boliano, M.L., Stein-Behrens, B., Sapolsky, R. (1994). Glucocorticoids mediate the stress-induced extracellular accumulation of glutamate. *Brain Res.* 655: 251-254.

Maisonpierre, P.C., Le Beau, M.M., Espinosa III, R., Ip, N.Y., Belluscio, L., de la Monte, S.M., Squinto, S., Furth, M.E., Yancopoulos, G.D. (1991). Human and rat brain-derived neurotrophic factor and neurotrophin-3 : gene structures, distributions, and chromosomal localizations. *Genomics* 10: 558-568.

Malberg, J.E., Eisch, A.J., Nestler, E.J., Duman, R.S. (2000). Chronic antidepressant treatment increases neurogenezis in adult rat hippocampus. *J. Neurosci.* 20: 9104-9110.

Mailleux, P., Verslype, M., Preud'homme, X., Vanderhaeghen, J-J. (1994). Activation of multiple transcription factor genes by tetrahidrocannabinol in rat forebrain. *Neuroreport* 5: 1265-1268.

Manji, H.K., Duöam, R.S. (2001). Impairments of neuroplasticity and cellular resilience in severe modd disorders: implications for the development of novel therapeutics. *Psychopharmacol. Bull.* 35: 5-49.

Manji, H.K., Quiroz, J.A., Sporn, J., Payne, J.L., Denicoff, K.A., Gray, N., Zarate, Jr., C.A, Charney, D.S. (2003). Enhancing neuronal plasticity and cellular resilience to develop novel improved therapeutics for difficult-to-treat depression. *Biol. Psychiatry* 53: 707-742.

Mann, J.J., Brown, R.P. (1985). A clinical perspective on the role of neurotransmitters in mental disorders. *Hospital and Community Psychiatry* 36: 141-150.

Maren, S., Fanselow, M.S. (1995). Synaptic plasticity in the basolateral amygdala induced by hippocampal formation stimulation in vivo. *J. Neurosci.* 15: 7548-7564.

Marsden, C.D. (1982). Neurotransmitters and CNS disease-Basal ganglia disease. Lancet ii: 1141-1146.

Marvanová, M., Lakso, M., Pirhonen, J., Nawa, H., Wong, G., Castrén, E. (2001). The neuroprotective agent memantine induces brain-derived neurotrophic factor and trkB receptor expression in rat brain. *Mol. Cell Neurosci.* 18: 247-258.

Mason, S.T., Fibiger, H.C. (1979). Anxiety: The locus coeruleus disconnection. *Life Sci.* 25: 2141-2147.

McAllister, A.K., Katz, L.C., Lo, D.C. (1999). Neurotrophins and synaptic plasticity. *Annu. Rev. Neurosci.* 22: 295-318.

McEwen, B.S., Weiss, J.M., Schwartz, L.S. (1968). Selective retention of corticosterone by limbic structures in rat brain. *Nature* 220: 911-912.

McEwen, B.S., Weiss, J.M. (1970). The uptake and action of corticosterone: regional and subcellular studies on rat brain. *Prog. Brain Res.* 32: 200-212.

McEwen, B.S., Sapolsky, R.M. (1995). Stress and cognitive function. *Curr. Opin. Neurobiol.* 5: 205-216.

McEwen, B.S., Conrad, C.D., Kuroda, Y., Frankfurt, M., Magarinos, A.M., McKittrick, C. (1997). Prevention of stress-induced morphological and cognitive consequences. *Eur. Neuropsychopharmacol.* 7 (Suppl. 3) : S323-S328.

McEwen, B.S. (1999a). Stress and the aging hippocampus. *Front Endocrinol.* 20: 49-70.

McEwen, B.S. (1999b). Stress and hippocampal plasticity. Annu Rev Neurosci 22: 105-122.

McEwen, B.S., Magarinos, A.M., Reagan, L.P. (2002). Structural plasticity and tianeptine: cellular and molecular targets. *Eur. Psychiatry* 17 (Suppl. 3): 318-330.

McEwen, B.S. (2004). Structural plasticity of the adult brain: how animal models help us understand brain changes in depression andd systemic disorders related to depression. Dialogues in Clinical Science – *Neuroplasticity* 6: 119-133.

McKim, W.A. (2000). Drugs and Behavior: An Introduction to Behavioral Pharmacology, Fourth Edition, Prentice-Hall Inc., New Jersey, pp. 26-347.

Menini, T., Mocaer, E., Garattini, S. (1987). Tianeptine, a selective enhancer of serotonin uptake in rat brain. Naunyn-**Schmiedeberg's** *Arch. Pharmacol.* 336: 478-482.

Minneman, K.P. (1991). Pharmacological organization of the CNS. In: Wingard LB, Brody TM, Larner J, Schwartz A (Eds.), Human Pharmacology, Molecular to Clinical. Wolfe Publishing Limited, London, pp. 299-341.

Mizoguchi, K., Kunishita, T., Chui, D.H., Tabira, T. (1992). Stress induces neuronal death in the hippocampus of castrated rats. *Neurosci. Lett.* 138: 157-160.

Moghaddam, B., Bolinao, M.L., Stein-Behrens, B., Sapolsky, R. (1994). Glucocorticoids mediate the stress-induced extracellular accumulation of glutamate. *Brain Res.* 655: 251-254

Moghaddam, B. (2002). Stress activation of glutamate neurotransmission in the prefrontal cortex: implications for dopamine-associated psychiatric disorders. *Biol. Psychiatry* 51: 775-787.

Moncada, S., Higgs, A. (1993). The L-arginine-nitric oxide pathway. *N. Engl. J. Med.* 329: 2002-2012.

Moncada, S., Higgs, A., Furchgott, R. (1997). XIV. International union of pharmacology nomenclature in nitric oxide research. *Pharmacol. Rev.* 49: 137-142.

Morgan, J.I., Curran, T. (1989). Stimulus-transcription coupling in neurons: Role of cellular immediate-early genes. *Trends Neurosci.* 12: 459-462.

Mukobata, S., Hibino, T., Sugiyama, A., Urano, Y., Inatomi, A., Kanai, Y., Endo, H., Tashiro, F. (2002). M6a acts as a nerve growth factor-gated Ca(2+) channel in neuronal differentiation. *Biochem. Biophys. Res. Commun.* 297: 722-728.

Myers, M.P., Murphy, M.B., Landreth, G. (1994). The dual-specificity CLK kinase induces neuronal differentiation of PC12 cells. *Mol. Cell Biol.* 14: 6954-6961.

Nagayama, H., Hinntgen, J.N., Aprison, M.H. (1980). Pre- and post-synaptic serotonergic manipulations in an animal model of depression. *Pharmacol. Biochem. Behav.* 13: 575-579.

Nakajima, S., Daval, J-C., Morgan, P.F., Post, R.M., Marangos, P.J. (1989). Adenosinergic modulation of caffeine-induced c-fos mRNA expression in mouse brain. *Brain Res.* 501: 307-314.

Natthanson, J.A. (1977). Cyclic nucleotides and nervous system function. *Physiol. Rev.* 57: 157-256.

Nibuya, M., Morinobu, S., Duman, R.S. (1995). Regulation of BDNF and trkB mRNA in rat brain by chronic electroconvulsive seizure and antidepressant drug treatments. *J. Neurosci.* 15: 7539-7547.

Nibuya, M., Nestler, E.J., Duman, R.S. (1996). Chronic antidepressant administration increases the expression of cAMP response element binding protein (CREB) in rat hippocampus. *J. Neurosci*. 16: 2365-2372.

Ninan, P.T. (1999). The functional anatomy, neurochemistry, and pharmacology of anxiety. *J. Clin. Psychiatry* 60 (Suppl. 22): 12-17.

Ohl, F., Michaelis, T., Vollmannn-Honsdorf, G.K., Kirschbaum, C., Fuchs, E. (2000). Effect of chronic psychosocial stress and long-term cortisol treatment on hippocampus-mediated memory and hippocampal volume: a plot study in tree shrews. *Psychoneuroendocrinology* 25: 357-363.

Olivier, B., van Wijngaarden, I., Soudijn, W. (2000). 5-HT_3 receptor antagonists and anxiety; a preclinical and clinical review. *Eur. Neuropsychopharmacol.* 10: 77-95.

Ozawa, H., Saito, T., Takahata, N. (Eds.). (1998). Signal Transduction in Affective Disorders. Springer, Tokyo.

Pacher, P., Kohegyi, E., Kecskemeti, V., Furst, S. (2001). Current trends in the development of new antidepressants. *Curr. Med. Chem.* 8: 89-100.

Parker, K.J., Schatzberg, A.F., Lyons, D.M. (2003). Neuroendocrine aspects of hypercortisolism in major depression. *Horm. Behav.* 43: 60-66.

Pavlides, C., Watanabe, Y., Magarinos, A.M., McEwen, B.S. (1995). Opposing roles of type I and type II adrenal steroid receptors in hippocampal long-term potentiation. *Neuroscience* 68: 387-394.

Pham, K., Nacher, J., Hof, P.R., McEwen, B.S. (2003). Repeated restraintstress suppresses neurogenesis and induces biphasic PSA-NCAM expression in the adult rat dentate gyrus. *Eur. J. Neurosci.* 17: 879-886.

Pineyro, G., Blier, P.A. (1999). Autoregulation of serotonin neurons: role in antidepressant drug action. *Pharmacol. Rev.* 51: 533-591.

Plaisant, F., Dommergues, M.A., Spedding, M., Cecchelli, R., Brillaut, J., Kato, G., Munoz, C., Gressens, P. (2003). Neuroprotective properties of tianeptine : interactions with cytokines. *Neuropharmacology* 44 : 801-809.

Poldrack, R.A., Gabrieli, J.D. (1997). Functional anatomy of long-term memory. *J. Clin. Neurophysiol.* 14: 294-310.

Popoli, M., Gennarelli, M., Racagni, G. (2002). Modulation of synaptic plasticity by stress and antidepressants. *Bipolar Disord.* 4: 166-182.

Quitkin, F.M., Rabkin, J.G., Ross., D., McGrath, P.J. (1984). Duration of antidepressant drug treatment. What is an adequate trial? *Arch. Gen. Psychiatry* 41: 238-245.

Rang, H.P., Dale, M.M., Ritter, J.M. (1999). Pharmacology, 4th Edition, Churchill Livingstone, Edinburgh, pp. 483-538.

Reagan, L.P., Rosell, D.R., Wood, G.E., Spedding, M., Munoz, C., Rothstein, J., McEwen, B.S. (2004) Chronic restraint stress up-regulates GLT-1 mRNA and protein expression in the rat hippocampus: reversal by tianeptine. *Proc. Natl. Acad. Sci. USA* 101: 2197-2184.

Reyntjens, A., Gelders, Y.G., Hoppenbrouwers, M.L. (1986). Thymosthenic effects of ritanserin (R55667), a centrally acting serotonin S2 receptor blocker. *Drug Dev. Res.* 8: 205-211.

Richelson, E. (2001). Pharmacology of antidepressants. *Mayo Clin. Proc.* 76: 511-527.

Rocher, C., Spedding, M., Munoz, C., Jay, T.M. (2004). Acute stress-induced changes in hippocampal/prefrontal circuits in rats: effects of antidepressants. *Cerabral. Cortex* 14: 224-229.

Rogan, M.T., Staubli, U.V., LeDoux, J.E. (1997). Fear conditioning induces associative long-term potentiation in the amygdala. *Nature* 390: 604-607.

Roseboom, P.H., Klein, D.C. (1995). Norepinephrine stimulation of pineal cyclic AMP response element-binding protein phosphorylation: primary role of a beta-adrenergic receptor/cyclic AMP mechanism. *Mol. Pharmacol.* 47: 439-449.

Rossor, M.N. (1982). Neurotransmitters and CNS disease – Demantia. Lancet ii: 1200-1204.

Saarelainen, T., Hendolin, P., Lucas, G., Koponen, E., Sairanen, M., MacDonald, E., Agerman, K., Haapasalo, A., Nawa, H., Aloyz, R., Ernfors, P., Castrén, E. (2003). Activation of the TrkB neurotrophin receptor is induced by antidepressant drugs and is required for antidepressant-induced behavioral effects. *J. Neurosci.,* 23: 349-357.

Sagar, S.M., Sharp, F.R. (1993). Early response genes as markers of neuronal activity and growth factor action. *Adv. Neurol.* 59: 273-284.

Sah, D.W.Y., Ossipov, M.H., Porreca, F. (2003). Neuropathic factors as novel therapeutics for neuropathic pain. *Nature Reviews* 2: 460-472.

Sala, M., Perez, J., Soloff, P., di Nemi, S.U., Caverzasi, E., Soares, J.C., Brambilla, P. (2004). Stress and hippocampus abnormalities in psychiatric disorders. *Eur. Neuropsychopharmacol.* 14: 393-405.

Sapolsky, R.M., Uno, H., Rebert, C.S., Finch, C.E. (1990). Hippocampal damage associated with prolonged glucocorticoid exposure in primates. *J. Neurosci.* 10: 2897-2902.

Sapolsky, R.M. (2000). Glucocorticoids and hippocampal atrophy in neuropsychiatric disorders. *Arch. Gen. Psychiatry* 57: 925-935.

Savas, H.A., Herken, H., Yurekli, M., Uz, E., Tutkun, H., Zoroglu, S.S., Ozen, M.E., Cengiz, B, Akyol, O. (2002). Possible role of nitric oxide and adrenomedullin in bipolar affective disorder. *Neuropsychobiology* 45: 57-61.

Scaccianoce, S., Del Bianco, P., Caricasole, A., Nicoletta, F., Catalini, A. (2003). Relationship between learning, stress and hippocampal brain-derived neurotrophic factor. *Neuroscience* 121: 825-828.

Schaaf, M.J., De Kloet, E.R., Vreugdenhil, E. (2000). Corticosterone effects on BDNF expression in the hippocampus. Implications for memory formation. Stress 3: 201-208.

Schildkraut, J.J. (1965). The catecholamine hypothesis of affective disorders: a review of supporting evidence. *Am. J. Psychiatry* 122: 509-522.

Schmidt, H.D., Duman, R.S. (2007). The role of neurotrophic factors in adult hippocampal neurogenezis, antidepressant treatments and animal models of depressive-like behavior. *Behav. Pharmacol.* 18: 391-418.

Scott, B.W., Wojtowicz, J.M., Burnham, W.M. (2000). Neurogenezis in the dentate gyrus of the rat following electroconvulsive shock seizures. *Exp. Neurol.* 165: 231-236.

Selye, H. (1976). Forty years of stress research: principal remaining problems and misconceptions. *Can. Med. Assoc.* J 115: 53-56.

Sepinwall, J., Cook, L. (1980). Mechanisms of action of the benzodiazepines: *Behavioral aspect. Fed. Proc.* 39: 3024-3031.

Shamir, A., Agam, G., Belmaker, R.H. (2005). Neurogenesis and neuroprotection as new drug targets for bipolar disorder: a critical review. In: Den Boer, J,A,, George, M.S., ter Horst, G.J. (Eds.), Current and Future Developments in Psychopharmacology. Benecke NI, Amsterdam, pp. 217-229.

Sheline, Y.I. (2000). 3D MRI studies of neuroanatomic changes in unipolar major depression: the role of stress and medical comorbidity. *Biol. Psychiatry* 48: 791-800.

Sheline, Y.I., Gado, M.H., Kraemer, H.C. (2003). Untreated depression and hippocampal volume loss. *Am. J. Psychiatry* 160: 1516-1518.

Shirayama, Y., Chen, A.C., Nakagawa, S., Russel, R.S., Duman, R.S. (2002). Brain derived neurotrophic factor produces antidepressant effects in behavioral models of depression. *J. Neurosci.* 22: 3251-3261.

Shoval, G., Weizman, A. (2005). The possible role of neurotrophins in the pathogenesis and therapy of schizophrenia. *Eur. Neuropsychopharmacol.* 15: 319-329.

Shu, S.Y., Wu, Y.M., Bao, X.M., Leonard, B. (2003). Interactions among memory-related centers in the brain. *J. Neurosci. Res.* 71: 609-616.

Snyder, S.H. (1982). Neurotransmitters and CNS disease – Schizophrenia. *Lancet* ii: 970-973.

Snyder, S.H., Bredt, D.S. (1992). Biological roles of nitric oxide. *Sci. Am.* May: 68-77.

Sousa, N., Lukoyanov, N.V., Madeira, M.D., Almeida, O.F., Paula-Barbosa, M.M. (2000). Reorganization of the morphology of hippocampal neuritis and synapses after stress-induced damage correlates with behavioral improvement. *Neuroscience* 97: 253-266.

Squire, L.R. (1992). Memory and hippocampus: a synthesis from findings with rats, monkeys, and humans. *Psychol. Rev.* 99: 195-231.

Stahl, S.M. (1996). Essential Psychopharmacology. Cambridge University Press, Cambridge, pp. 1-47.

Stahl, S.M. (2000). Essential Psychopharmacology. Neuroscientific Basis and Practical Applications. Second Edition, Cambridge University Press, Cambridge.

Starkman, M.N., Giordani, B., Gebarski, S.S., Schteingart, D.E. (2003). Improvement in learning associated with increase in hippocampal formation volume. *Biol. Psychiat.* 53: 233-238.

Stein, L., Wise, D.C., Belluzi, J.D. (1975). Effects of benzodiazepines on central serotonergic mechanisms. *Adv. Biocehem. Psychopharmacol.* 10: 1-12.

Stein-Behrens, B.A., Lin, W.J., Sapolsky, R.M. (1994). Physiological elevations of glucocorticoids potentiate glutamate accumulation in the hippocampus. *J. Neurochem.* 63: 596-602.

Thome, J., Sakai, N., Shin, K., Steffen, C., Zhang, Y.J., Impey, S., Storm, D., Duman, R.S. (2000). cAMP response element-mediated gene transcription is upregulated by chronic antidepressant treatment. *J. Neurosci.* 20: 4030-4036.

Uno, H., Tarara, R., Else, J.G., Suleman, M.A., Sapolsky, R.M. (1989). Hippocampal damage associated with prolonged and fatal stress in primates. *J. Neurosci.* 9: 1705-1711.

Urenjak, J., Willliams, S.R., Gadian, D.G., Noble, M. (1993). Proton nuclear magnetic resonance spectroscopy unambiguously idendifies different neural cell types. *J. Neurosci.* 13: 981-989.

Uzbay, I.T., Çınar, M., Aytemir, M., Tuğlular, I. (1999). Analgesic effect of tianeptine in mice. *Life Sci.* 64: 1313-1319.

Uzbay, I.T., Oglesby, M.W. (2001). Nitric oxide and substance dependence. *Neurosci. Biobehav. Rev.* 25: 43-52.

Uzbay, I.T., Yüksel, N. (2002). Tianeptine in depression treatment. Journal of Clinical Psychiatry 5 (Suppl. 2): 10-17 (In Turkish).

Uzbay, I.T. (2004). Basics of Psychopharmacology and Experimental Technics. Çizgi Tıp Publishinghouse, Ankara, (In Turkish).

Uzbay, I.T., Çelik, T., Aydın, A., Kayir, H., Tokgöz, S., Bilgi, C. (2004) Effects of chronic ethanol administration and ethanol withdrawal on cyclic guanosine 3',5'-monophosphate (cGMP) levels in the rat brain. *Drug. Alcohol. Depend.* 74: 55-59.

Uzbay, T. (2005). Neuroplasticity and Depression. Çizgi Tıp Publishinghouse, Ankara, (in Turkish).

Uzbay, I.T. (2008). Tianeptine: Potential influences on neuroplasticity and novel pharmacological effects. *Prog Neuro-Psychopharmacol. Biol. Psychiat.* 32: 915-924.

Vallejo, M. (1994). Transcriptional control of gene expression by cAMP-response element binding proteins. *J. Neuroendocrinol.* 6: 587-596.

van der Hart, M.G., Czéh, B., de Biurrun, G., Michaelis, T., Watanabe, T., Natt, O., Frahm, J., Fuchs, E. (2002). Substance P receptor antagonist and clomipramine prevent stress-induced alterations in cerebral metabolites, cytogenesis in the dentate gyrus and hippocampal volume. *Mol. Psychiatry* 7: 933-941.

van Prag, H., Schinder, A.F., Christie, B.R., Toni, N., Palmer, T.D., Gage, F.H. (2002). Functional neurogenesis in the adult hippocampus. *Nature* 415: 1030-1034.

van Prag, H.M. (1982a). The significance of biological factors in the diagnosis of depressions: I. Biochemical variables. *Comp. Psychiatry* 23: 124-135.

van Prag, H.M. (1982b). Depression, suicide and metabolism of serotonin in the brain. *J. Affect. Dis.* 4: 275-290.

Vaswani, M., Linda, F.K., Ramesh, S. (2003). Role of serotonin reuptake inhibitors in psychiatric disorders: a comprehensive review. *Prog. Neuro-Psychopharmacol. Biol. Psychiat.* 27: 85-102.

Venero, C., Borrel, J. (1999). Rapid glucocorticoid effects on excitatory amino acid levels in the hippocampus: a microdialysis study in freely moving rats. *Eur. J. Neurosci.* 11: 2465-2473.

Vogel, G. (2000). New brain cells prompt new theory of depression. Science 290: 258-259.

Vollmann-Honsdorf, G.K., Flügge, G., Fuchs, E. (1997). Chronic psychosocial stress does not affect the number of pyramidal neurons in tree shrew hippocampus. *Neurosci. Lett.* 233: 121-124.

Vouimba, R.M., Munoz, C., Diamond, D.M. (2003). Influence of the antidepressant tianeptine and stress on the expression of synaptic plasticity in the hippocampus and amygdala. *Soc. Neurosci.* 376.6.

Waintraub, L., Septien, L., Azoulay, P. (2000). Efficacy and safety of tianeptine in major depression: evidence from a 3-month controlled clinical trial versus paroxetine. *Eur. Neuropsychopharmacol.*, 10 (Suppl. 2): S51.

Watanabe, Y., Gould, E., Daniels, D.C., Cameron, H., McEwen, B.S. (1992). Tianeptine attenuates stress-induced morphological changes in the hippocampus. *Eur. J. Pharmacol.* 222: 157-162.

Wegener, G., Volke, V., Harvey, B.H., Rosenberg, R. (2003). Local, but not systemic, administration of serotonergic antidepressants decreases hippocampal nitric oxide synthase activity. *Brain Res.* 959: 128-134.

Wilde, M.I., Benfield, P. (1995). Tianeptine. A review of its pharmacodynamic and pharmacokinetic properties, and therapeutic efficacy in depression and coexisting anxiety and depression. *Drugs* 49: 411-439.

Willner, P. (1985). Depression. *A Psychobiological. Synthesis*, New York,Wiley.

Wittenberg, G.M., Tsien, J.Z. (2002) An emerging molecular and cellular framework for memory processing by the hippocampus. *Trends Neurosci.* 25: 501-505.

Woolley, C.S., Gould, E., McEwen, B.S. (1990). Exposure to excess glucocorticoids alters dendritic morphology of adult hippocampal pyramidal neurons. *Brain Res.* 531: 225-231.

Yanik, M., Vural, H., Kocyigit, A., Tutkun, H., Zoroglu, S.S., Herken, H., Savas, H.A., Koylu, A., Akyol, O. (2003) Is the arginine-nitric oxide pathway involved in the pathogenesis of schizophrenia? *Neuropsychobiology* 47: 61-65.

Yaniv, D., Vouimba, R.M., Diamond, D.M., Richter-Levin, G. (2003a). Simultaneous induction of long-term potentiation in the hippocampus and the amygdala by entorhinal cortex activation: mechanistic and temporal profiles. *Neuroscience* 120: 1125-1135.

Yaniv, D., Vouimba, R.M., Diamond, D.M., Richter-Levin, G. (2003b). Effects of novel versus repeated mild stressful experiences on long-term potentiation induced simultaneously in the amygdala and hippocampus in freely behaving rats. *Ann NY Acad. Sci.* 985: 556-557.

Yin, Q., Kemp, G.J., Yu, L.G., Wagstaff, S.C., Frostick, S.P. (2001a). Expression of Schwann cell-specific proteins and low-molecular-weight neurofilament protein during regeneration of sciatic nerve treated with neurotrophin-4. *Neuroscience* 105: 779-783.

Yin, Q., Kemp, G.J., Yu, L.G., Wagstaff, S.C., Frostick, S.P. (2001b). Neurotrophin-4 delivered by fibrin glue promotes peripheral nerve regeneration. *Muscle Nerve* 24: 345-351.

Yocca, F.D. (1990). Novel Anxiolytic Agents: Actions on Specific Subtypes of Central 5-HT Receptors, Current and Future Trends in Anticonvulsant, Anxiety and Stroke Therapy, BS Meldrum, M Williams (Eds.), Wiley-Liss, New York, pp. 145-167.

Zethof, T.J., Van der Heyden, J.A., Tolboom, J.T., Olivier, B. (1995). Stress-induced hyperthermia as a putative anxiety model. Eur J Pharmacol 294: 125-135.

Zoladz, P.R., Park, C.R., Munoz, C., Fleshner, M., Diamond, D.M. (2008). Tianeptine: An antidepressant with memory-protective properties. *Current Neuropharmacology* 6: 311-321.

Zoroglu, S.S., Herken, H., Yurekli, M., Uz, E., Tutkun, H., Savas, H.A., Bagci, C., Ozen, M.E., Cengiz, B., Cakmak, E.A., Dogru, M.I., Akyol, O. (2002). The possible pathophysiological role of plasma nitric oxide and adrenomedullin in schizophrenia. *J. Psychiatr. Res.* 36: 309-315.

Zoroglu, S.S., Yurekli, M., Meram, I., Sogut, S., Tutkun, H., Yetkin, O., Sivasli, E., Savas, H.A., Yanik, M., Herken, H., Akyol, O. (2003). Pathophysiological role of nitric oxide and adrenomedullin in autism. *Cell Biochem. Funct.* 21: 55-60.

In: Antidepressants: Types, Efficiency …
Editor: Jayden T. Van Leeuwen, pp.67-89

ISBN 978-1-61668-581-2

Chapter 2

ANTIDEPRESSANT THERAPY AND THE RISK OF SUICIDE AMONG PATIENTS WITH MAJOR DEPRESSIVE DISORDERS

Maurizio Pompili[a,b], Gianluca Serafini[a], Marco Innamorati[a], Michele Battuello[a], Mariantonietta Milelli[a], Roberto Tatarelli[a], and David Lester[c]

[a.] Department of Neurosciences, Mental Health and Sensory Functions, Suicide Prevention Center Sant'Andrea Hospital, Sapienza University of Rome, Italy

[b.] McLean Hospital – Harvard Medical School, Belmont, MA, USA

[c.] The Richard Stockton College of New Jersey, Pomona, NJ, USA

ABSTRACT

The world-wide annual suicide rate currently averages approximately 13/100,000 (0.013%/year), with higher average rates for men than women in all but a few countries, very low rates in children, and relatively high rates in elderly men. Suicide rates vary markedly among regions of the world, countries, and locales, in part reflecting differences in case-identification and reporting procedures. Rates of attempted suicide average 20–30 times higher than rates of completed suicide in the general population, but are probably under-reported. A highly controversial question is whether antidepressant treatment modifies the risks of various aspects of "suicidality" among patients with major depressive disorders. Research on the relationship between pharmacotherapy and suicidal behavior was virtually unknown until a decade ago. A minority of ecological studies and most large clinical studies have found that decreases of suicide rates by region or time are correlated with higher rates of prescribing modern antidepressants. However, other studies and data from brief, randomized, controlled trials in patients with acute major depression have found increases for patients of some ages, particularly for the risk of suicide attempts, as well as increases in suicidal ideation in the young. Although other pharmacological treatments, such as clozapine and lithium, appear to have sound evidence for reducing the risk of attempted and completed suicide, in this paper we proposed to analyze the relationship between suicidality in depressed adults and only antidepressants.

INTRODUCTION

The world-wide annual suicide rate currently averages approximately 13/100,000 (0.013%/year), with higher average rates for men than women in all but a few countries, very low rates in children, and relatively high rates in elderly men (Goldsmith et al, 2002; APA, 2003; Simon and Hales, 2006; WHO, 2007). Suicide rates vary markedly among regions of the world, countries, and locales, in part reflecting differences in case-identification and reporting procedures (Diekstra, 1993; APA, 2003). Notably, suicide rates are extraordinarily high in Eastern Europe and relatively low in Latin America and Southern Europe. In the USA, annual suicide rates (per 100,000 people) are far higher in New Mexico (20.2) and other areas in the Southwest and the Intermountain West than on the East or West Coasts, with the lowest rates reported in Massachusetts and New York (6.5) and in the District of Columbia (6.0; Tondo et al, 2006). Internationally, the overall average suicide rate has been rising gradually over the past half-century, with increases reported in about half of reporting nations, mainly among men, and moderate decreases found in another half, including in Northern Europe and North America. These improvements could reflect improved diagnosis and treatment of mood disorders during the same era (Isacsson, 2000; Grunebaum et al, 2004; Tondo et al, 2006; Baldessarini et al, 2007b; WHO, 2007).

Estimated rates of attempted suicide are much less reliable than for completed suicides. Rates of attempted suicide average 20–30 times higher than rates of completed suicide in the general population, but are probably under-reported, and range widely in method and seriousness of intent (Tondo et al, 2003; Kessler et al, 2005). The ratio of attempts/suicides in clinical samples of mood-disorder patients is much lower, suggesting a greater lethality of suicidal behaviors (Baldessarini et al, 2006b). Most cases of suicide (81%–95%) in the general population involve psychiatric illnesses, nearly half of which (48.5%) are mood disorders (Roy, 2000).

In a study of men and women who attempted suicide and were evaluated in a medical emergency service (indicating, therefore, relatively serious attempts), the risk of completed suicide within five years was twice-higher among men than women (8.3% vs. 4.3%), as expected, and most occurred within a year of follow-up (Nordstrom et al, 1995). The ratio of attempts to subsequent suicides (A/S) also was half as great in men as in women (12:1 vs. 23:1), consistent with the greater lethality of suicide attempts in men. The risk of subsequent suicide was higher in men below the age of 35 versus above the age of 35 (9.7% vs. 7.0%), but higher in women older than this age than those below this age (6.0% vs. 2.5%). Accordingly, the relative risk among younger men was four-times higher than in younger women (9.7% versus 2.5%), whereas the relative risk in older men and women did not differ much (7.0% versus 6.0%), indicating that the lethality of suicidal behavior in women over age 35 approaches that of men of similar age.

In the last few years, there has been great interest in viewing the excess mortality associated with major mental illnesses as an important and plausible therapeutic target (Baldessarini and Jamison, 1999). Excessive mortality in mood, psychotic and substance-use disorders results from medical illnesses (2–3-times above the general population), particularly stress-sensitive disorders. Indeed, deaths associated with cardiovascular disorders probably account for the largest *number* of deaths among persons with mood disorders, as is the case in the general population.

However, the greatest source of the excess of mortality in patients with major mental illness is due to suicide, the rates of which in patients with mood disorders can exceed those in the general population by 20-fold, particularly in bipolar disorders and in severe, recurrent major depression, with lesser rates in psychotic, anxiety, or primary substance-use disorders (Harris and Barraclough, 1998; Tondo et al, 2003). Suicide rates are surprisingly high among persons diagnosed with anxiety disorders (Harris and Barraclough 1998; Khan et al. 2002), and severe anxiety may accompany suicidal behavior (Fawcett 2001), but evidence that anti-anxiety medications reduce suicidal risk in anxiety disorder patients is very limited (Khan et al, 2002).

The general risk factors for suicide include the presence of a major mood disorder with hopelessness, especially when co-occurring with alcohol or substance abuse (Tondo et al, 1999, 2003; Roy 2000; APA 2003). The risk is especially high among young, impulsive-aggressive and older unmarried men (APA 2003; Simon and Hales 2006). The risk of suicide in bipolar patients continues to be high, despite the introduction of a growing number of treatments with putative mood-stabilizing effects, reflecting the great difficulty in treating bipolar depressive and mixed manic-depressive states effectively. The unusually high risk of suicide among bipolar patients has been noted by several authors such as Tondo and Baldessarini (2007). They examined the medical records of nearly 3,000 outpatients with major mood disorders and found a substantially greater suicide risk among bipolar patients than in recurrent major depression patients. The risk of suicide among 843 bipolar I and II disorder patients was 150/100,000/year, or more than ten-times higher than in the general population, and three-times greater than among 1,983 patients diagnosed with recurrent major depressive disorder. These rates suggest that the risk of dying by suicide among bipolar disorder patients is nearly 10%, assuming potential risk-exposures of 60 years or more. More than one-third of all suicidal acts occurred within the first year from illness-onset, and more than half within the first five years of illness—indicating the need for early diagnosis and intervention in major mood disorders (Tondo and Baldessarini, 2007).

Surprisingly, approximately three-quarters of the high proportion of unresolved morbidity among bipolar disorder patients is depression (Judd et al, 2002; Post et al, 2003; Baldessarini et al, 2004; Joffe et al. 2004). This high level of residual depressive morbidity in treated bipolar patients no doubt encourages high rates of utilization of antidepressants in their treatment, even though such treatment is neither approved by regulatory bodies, nor well supported by available clinical research as either effective or safe in bipolar patients (Ghaemi et al, 2003; Baldessarini et al, 2007a). Furthermore, antidepressant treatments are associated in some patients with dysphoric-mixed-agitated or psychotic states that can increase suicidal risk (Koukopoulos and Koukopoulos, 1999; Akiskal et al, 2005; Maj et al, 2006).

The effects of treatments on suicidal risk have been a topic of growing research interest in recent years. Evidence that most modern psychiatric treatments reduce long-term suicide risks is very limited (Rose et al, 1985; Weinger, 2000; APA 2003; Oquendo et al, 2005; Simon and Hales, 2006).

In this chapter we will systematically review whether the use of antidepressants is associated with benefits in terms of completed or attempted suicide, whether the increasing use of SSRIs is associated with benefits in terms of decreased rates of suicide, and whether the use of antidepressant therapy is associated with increased rates of attempted or completed suicide, with the aim of generating evidence-based suggestions for daily clinical practice.

ANTIDEPRESSANTS

A highly controversial question is whether antidepressant treatment modifies the risk of various aspects of "suicidality" among patients with major depressive disorders (Baldessarini et al, 2005a, 2005b, 2006a; Mann et al, 2006; Healy, 2006; Klein, 2006; Moller, 2006), especially the selective serotonin reuptake inhibitors (SSRIs), which may cause worsening of suicidal thoughts in vulnerable people (Hall, 2006; Moller et al, 2008). In 2005, a systematic review of published randomized controlled trials comparing SSRIs with other active treatments or placebo found an almost 2-fold increase in the odds of fatal and nonfatal suicide acts among those exposed to SSRIs (Fergusson et al, 2005). No increase in risk was observed, however, when only fatal suicide acts were included. Another systematic review by Gunnell et al. (2005), which included both published and unpublished randomized controlled trials submitted by pharmaceutical companies to the safety review board of the Medicine and Healthcare Products Regulatory Agency, compared the use of SSRIs and placebo in adults with depression and other clinical conditions. This review showed no evidence of increased risk of completed suicide and only weak evidence of increased risk of self-harm. More recently, the US Food and Drug Administration (FDA) performed a meta-analysis of individual patient data from 372 randomized placebo-controlled trials of antidepressants with a total of nearly 100,000 patients (Laughren, 2005). This study reported that the incidence of reported suicidal behavior was strongly related to age. The risk associated with antidepressant use relative to placebo was increased among patients aged 25 or younger, but it was reduced among patients aged 65 or more. The risk among patients aged 25–64 years was neutral, but the risk was reduced when suicidal behavior and ideation were considered together (Laughren, 2006a, 2006b). Based on these findings, in May 2007 the FDA ordered that all antidepressant drugs carry an expanded black-box warning on their label that included information about increased risk of suicidal behavior in young adults aged 18–24 years (Leon, 2007; Barbui et al, 2008).

A controversial point of the FDA analysis is that the trials included were not primarily designed to measure suicidality (a composite outcome that includes suicide ideas, preparatory acts, suicide attempts and deaths by suicide) (Laughren, 2006a, 2006b). Of all suicidal events, less than 30% were serious suicide attempts or deaths. Additionally, considering that suicidality was self-reported rather than observed by others in most of the clinical trials, it is possible that antidepressant treatment, particularly in younger individuals, enhanced communication about suicidality, which may have allowed them to become more articulate and open about their thoughts and actions. Alternatively, antidepressant treatment might have enhanced communication about suicidality in all age groups, but increased attention to adverse effects might have led to enhanced detection of suicidality in younger individuals (Laughren, 2006a, 2006b). It is unlikely that individual randomized trials will be designed to primarily investigate the effect of antidepressant use on suicidality, and future systematic reviews of clinical trial data will not be able to overcome the limitations of the FDA analysis.

For children and adolescents, regulatory authorities in Europe, the UK, and the USA have issued warnings about the use of these agents. The European Medicines Agency (EMEA) has ruled that SSRIs and selective serotonin and norepinephrine reuptake inhibitors (SNRIs) should not be prescribed for depression for children and adolescents under the age of 18. The Committee for the Safety of Medicines in the UK has advised that the balance of risks and benefits for the treatment of depression in the pediatric population is unfavourable for paroxetine, citalopram, sertraline, venlafaxine, escitalopram, and mirtazapine. The regulatory authority in the USA requires a safety warning in bold text about suicide risk in package inserts for all antidepressant (AD) drugs.

In adults current evidence indicates no clear causal relationship between SSRIs and increased risk for suicide, although SSRIs may induce or worsen suicidal ideation and behavior during the early phases of treatment. In recent years, in order to shed light on this compelling issue, many different study designs have been employed, including randomized clinical trials, observational studies, case-control studies and ecological time-trend analyses.

Among adolescents, one study found that use of SSRIs significantly increased the risk of completed or attempted suicide (random-effect OR 1.92, 95% CI 1.51–2.44, I^2 0.0%) (Barbui et al, 2009). Among adults, SSRI use significantly decreased the risk of completed or attempted suicide (random-effect OR=0.57, 95%CI 0.47–0.70, I^2=52.5%). Among elderly people (aged 65 or more years), the use of SSRIs had a significant protective effect (random-effect OR=0.46, 95%CI 0.27–0.79, I^2=0.0%) (Barbui et al, 2009). Sensitivity analyses, which were performed to investigate the strength of the results, did not change these findings.

Among adults no individual antidepressant was significantly associated with completed or attempted suicide while among adolescents, exposure to paroxetine (random-effect OR=1.77, 95%CI 1.05–2.99, I^2=48.1%) and venlafaxine (random-effect OR=2.43, 95%CI 1.47–4.02, I2=0.0%) were significantly associated with increased risk (Olfson et al, 2006; Tiihonen et al, 2006).

Clearly the effect of age is critical (Barbui et al, 2009). Use of SSRIs decreased the risk of suicide by over 40% among adults and decreased the risk by over 50% among elderly people. However, among adolescents, use of SSRIs almost doubled the risk of suicide. These results are consistent with the main conclusion of the recent FDA meta-analysis of clinical trial data (Laughren, 2006). However, although the FDA reported a neutral effect of SSRIs (or a promoting effect among adults aged 18–25), Barbui et al. (2009) found a strong protective effect associated with SSRI treatment.

The large majority of studies on the effect of antidepressant therapy on the risk of suicide have a number of limitations. For example, observational studies have limited ability to adjust for baseline differences and are prone to bias and confounding. Additionally, among adolescents, SSRI treatment is often reserved for the very severe cases, and prescription of antidepressant drugs might have been triggered by suicidal ideation. Thus, the higher suicide rate might be confounded by severity, that is, adolescents who received SSRIs might have been more severely depressed (or more suicidal) than adolescents who did not receive SSRIs. In contrast, among adults SSRIs may be prescribed similarly in severe and less severe cases, and confounding might not have occurred. In some studies, confounding by the severity of the depression or suicidality was considered. For example, Olfson and colleagues (Olfson et al, 2006) limited their analysis to individuals who received inpatient treatment for depression, thereby ensuring a fairly comparable level of illness severity. In 2 other studies, comparability between groups was increased by the comparison of the risk of suicide during SSRI use with the risk during no antidepressant use in the same cohort (Rahme et al, 2008; Tiihonen et al, 2006).

Barbui et al (2009) concluded that it is not clear why the use of some antidepressants, such as paroxetine and venlafaxine, increases the risk of suicide more than others. Intriguingly, previous re-analyses of randomized studies, including the FDA study, reported similar differences between antidepressants (Cipriani et al, 2007; Barbui et al, 2008; Dubicka et al, 2007). Differences in long-term efficacy and safety should be confirmed in trials of head-to-head comparisons (Cipriani et al, in press). Such an evidence base would assist clinicians in making choices about optimal antidepressant treatment.

Data from observational studies should reassure doctors that prescribing SSRIs for patients with major depression is safe. However, children and adolescents should be followed very closely because of the possibility of increased risk of suicidal thoughts and suicidal acts. Paroxetine and venlafaxine should be avoided based on the evidence from randomized and observational studies that the risks might outweigh the benefits for most adolescents.

DATA FROM ECOLOGICAL STUDIES

The evidence that antidepressant treatment yields expected reductions in risk of suicides or attempts is controversial. It includes data from correlative or "ecological," pharmacoepidemiological studies that compare suicide rates by regions or years with concurrent rates of prescriptions for antidepressant drugs (Baldessarini et al, 2007b). In some Nordic countries and in the USA, the emergence of modern antidepressants over the past decade in current clinical practice was associated with generally moderate decreases in overall suicide rates, varying by sex and age groups (Isacsson, 2000; Grunebaum et al, 2004; Helgason et al, 2004; Gibbons et al, 2005, 2006; Ludwig and Marcotte, 2005; Henriksson and Isacsson, 2006; Søndergård et al, 2006c; Reseland et al, 2006; Baldessarini et al, 2007b). However, in the USA and some Nordic countries, similar trends regarding a reduction of suicide rates were also reported a decade before the introduction of fluoxetine, the first clinically successful modern antidepressant (Reseland et al, 2006; Baldessarini et al, 2007b).

In a recent review, Baldessarini et al. (2007) found that only nine of 29 ecological studies found significant inverse correlations between increased use of modern antidepressants and declining trends in suicide rates; another six found no relationships and 14 found correlations in some sex or age subgroups that were inconsistent across studies. Also, data from 78 reporting countries indicated that only about half (54%) experienced decreases in annual suicide rates between the 1950s (when antidepressants were not available) and the early 2000s (a decade after introduction of modern antidepressants) but a similar proportion (46%) reported increases. The distribution of decreases and increases in the suicide rates of nations between 1990 and the early 2000s was similar (Tondo and Baldessarini, 2006; WHO, 2007). Additionally, similar decreases and increases were reported in the separate regions of Western and Eastern Europe, Latin America and Asia. These data suggested the existence of a highly complex phenomenon which reflects the existence of many contributing factors.

It is possible that improvements in public health, changes in legal, cultural or social prohibitions against suicide, and improvements in identifying and reporting suicides might be associated with higher suicide rates despite the increased access to modern psychopharmacological treatment in the majority of countries. Socioeconomic factors may also contribute to the complex findings from the ecological studies as well as access to clinical services and social support. Also, all such correlational studies suffer from a fundamental inability to relate medication exposure or other specific factors causally to suicidal behavior at the level of individuals (Freedman, 2002). We may conclude that ecological studies cannot prove a direct, causal relationship between antidepressant treatment and reduced suicidal risk at the level of individual persons, and we need further research with less ambiguous methods.

Data from Cohort and Case-Control Studies

Other sources of data concerning antidepressants include large cohorts of depressed patients from general practice or health-maintenance organization data sources, and relatively large, case-control comparisons of subgroups varying in exposure to antidepressants. Such studies include over one-million, mainly clinically depressed subjects in 17 reports (Jick et al, 1995, 2004; Warshaw and Keller, 1996; Leon et al, 1999; Oquendo et al, 2002; Yerevanian et al, 2004; Angst et al, 2005; Barak et al, 2005; Didham et al, 2005; Martinez et al, 2005; Bauer et al, 2006; Juurlink et al, 2006; Olfson et al, 2006; Simon et al, 2006; Søndergård et al, 2006a, 2006b; Tiihonen et al, 2006). These studies have yielded inconsistent findings. Many (n=11) were designed to test for greater suicidal risks with SRI antidepressants compared to other agents or to non-treatment. Nine of these 11 studies did not find evidence of greater suicidal risk associated with antidepressant treatment, and a majority of other studies (4 out of the 6) found decreased or no difference in suicidal risk with more antidepressant treatment. A few of these studies found greater suicidal risk with more antidepressant treatment in general or, specifically, with the greater use of SSRIs and other modern antidepressants, in particular, small increases among adolescents (Olfson et al, 2006; Søndergård et al, 2006b), larger increases in elderly patients (Juurlink et al, 2006), as well as fewer completed suicides but more attempts (Tiihonen et al, 2006).

Data from these studies are severely compromised by the risk of "confounding by morbidity or by indication." For example medical treatments, in general, are more likely to be given to more severely ill patients at higher risk of suicide, and treatment with a low risk of toxic effects from acute overdosing (such as the SSRIs) are more likely to be selected clinically than more toxic agents (such as the tricyclic antidepressants) for patients at increased risk for suicide. The nonrandomized, clinically-selected treatment in such studies may severely distort the associations observed between greater suicidal risk and the use of some treatments.

Randomized Controlled Trials (RCTs)

RCTs should be the most reliable source of data on the effects of antidepressant treatment on suicidal risk. Individual trials are unlikely to include enough patients with identified suicidal acts to allow testing for treatment effects, especially since being acutely suicidal is usually a criterion for exclusion from such trials. However meta-analytic methods may yield substantial numbers of suicide attempts and even completed suicides. Rates of suicide attempts, and even of completed suicides, may be as high in controlled trials as in clinical samples of patients with major depressive disorder. Suicide rates taken from large meta-analyses of modern and older antidepressants or placebo (given similar rates with all treatments) averaged 862/100,000/year (Khan et al, 2000, 2003; Acharya et al, 2006), or 66-times above the average international general population rate of 13/100,000/year (WHO, 2007). In clinical samples of severely ill major depression patients, usually hospitalized patients, the standardized mortality ratio (SMR) for suicide compared to the general population was 20-fold higher (Harris and Barraclough, 1998), and among less severely ill, depressed patients this risk ratio may be about three-times higher (Bostwick and Pankratz, 2000). Such high observed rates of suicidal behaviors in RCTs reflect exaggeration arising from annualizing rates based on relatively brief exposure times (typically 8–12 weeks) in most trials in acute depression and early in the course of treatment.

There have been several recent reports based on pooling data on rates of suicides and attempts from large numbers of RCTs and subjects involving modern antidepressants, older standard agents, and placebo (Tollefson et al, 1994; Khan et al, 2000, 2003; Storosum et al, 2001; FDA, 2005; Gunnell et al, 2005; Fergusson et al, 2005a; Acharya et al, 2006; Baldessarini et al, 2006a; Hammad et al, 2006a,b; Laughren, 2006). With the exception of one report which found a significant excess of suicidal acts during treatment with SSRI antidepressants (Fergusson et al, 2005), other meta-analyses have found only minor differences in rates of suicidal behaviors between depressed patients treated with an SSRI, other antidepressants, or a placebo, overall tending toward an apparently greater risk with antidepressants. It was assumed that the trials included in the meta-analyses were well-randomized and with well-balanced exposures in both the drug and placebo arms throughout the duration of the trials.

In one meta-analysis, Baldessarini and colleagues (2006a) reported the overall pooled Rate Ratio (RR) and its 95% confidence interval (CI) is 1.42 (CI 1.10–1.85; z=2.65, p=0.008), compared to the null value of RR=1.0. One study (Fergusson et al, 2005) had a relatively large RR (3.52 [CI 1.43–8.69]). In addition, the computed, overall, pooled Risk Difference (RD) was 0.0015 [CI 0.00032–0.0027], or 0.15% [CI 0.03%–0.27%; z=2.49, p=0.013], indicating an estimated Number-Needed-to-Harm (NNH) of 667 [CI 373–3135]; without the Fergusson et al. (2005) study, NNH=1307 [CI 636–infinity], z=1.86, p=0.06. For completed suicide, RD=0.022% [CI 0.017%–0.060%; z=1.11, p=0.27], with an estimated NNH of 4651 [CI 1675–infinity]; for suicide attempts RD=0.163% [CI 0.014%–0.312%]; z=2.15, p=0.03), with a correspondingly NNH=613 [CI 321–6993]). Baldessarini et al. concluded that more than 600 depressed patients would have to be exposed to an antidepressant drug for approximately two months (or about 100 treated for a year), early in the course of an episode of acute major depressive disorder, when the suicidal risk is particularly high, to yield one excess suicide attempt, and over 4,500 depressed patients to yield one excess suicide over the number associated with untreated major depression.

In a large review, the American Food and Drug Administration (FDA) analyzed all available data from 386 controlled trials of modern antidepressant drugs involving 112,875 patients with major depressive or other disorders (Laughren, 2006). Most of the identified suicidal events involved suicidal ideation, but of uncertain clinical significance. Reported instances of suicides (0.013%) and attempts (0.198%) may be low due to the relatively brief exposure times, which averaged only two months. Among adult patients diagnosed with major depressive disorder, the observed suicide rate, based on estimated exposure-times averaging eight weeks, was 77/100,000/year, or only six-times above the general population rate of 13/100,000/year (WHO, 2007), compared to suicide rates of 862/100,000/year found in similar controlled trials of modern antidepressants, as already noted (Khan et al, 2000, 2003; Acharya et al, 2006). Initially, a slightly, but statistically nonsignificant, lower overall risk was found for new suicidal ideation and suicidal acts with antidepressants vs. placebo (OR=0.84, 95%CI 0.69–1.02) and, in addition, the decrease in the risk of completed and attempted suicide was age-associated and independent of treatment. A secondary analysis, based on stratifying by age-groups, suggested an increased risk of broadly defined "suicidality" (mainly ideation) with modern antidepressants versus placebo at younger ages, and possible beneficial effects in older patients. It is important to remember that the data are adapted from FDA analyses of spontaneous adverse-event reports and that most of the suicidal events pertain to ideation, whereas completed suicide and attempted suicide were rare.

These findings suggest an increased risk of presumably new suicidal ideation with SSRIs and other modern antidepressants over placebo among children, adolescents and young adults up to age 24 years, and these findings extended the initial impressions of a similar finding in meta-analyses involving children and adolescents by the UK drug regulatory agency (MHRA, 2004) and the FDA (FDA, 2005; Hammad et al, 2006b). In the initial FDA review of SSRI trials, data from some 4,400 depressed or anxious children and adolescents identified no suicides, but some self-injurious acts considered to be suicide attempts which resulted in a greater relative risk during treatment with SSRIs versus placebo (RR=1.90; 95%CI 1.00–3.63; FDA, 2005; Baldessarini et al, 2006a).

In conclusion, RCT data fail to support an expected overall reduction of risk of suicidal acts during treatment with antidepressants of all types and also suggest that the risk of suicide attempts and perhaps completed suicides may be greater during treatment with antidepressants of various types. However, many trials involving patients with depressive disorder found substantially larger reductions in average ratings of suicidal ideation with antidepressants of various types than with placebo (Beasley et al, 1991; Tollefson et al, 1994; Filteau et al, 1993; Pedersen, 2005; Acharya et al, 2006). Unfortunately, these trials reported subjective data, usually incidental, and based on post-hoc assessments of individual items on standard depression symptom-rating scales (Hamilton item 3 or Montgomery-Åsberg item 10).

RCTs have several limitations including potential unreliability of essentially incidental, passive reporting of suicidal thoughts or behaviors in most RCTs based on currently typical "adverse event reporting" systems. Additionally, the relatively short duration of most trials of treatments for acute depression may not provide an adequate evaluation of the effects of treatment on rare suicidal behaviors, comparable to the long-term trials available for clozapine, lithium and anticonvulsants. Another potential source of bias is that initial randomization in RCTs can break down during the conduct of trials. Premature, and potentially non-random, dropping out, usually a result of the lack of any perceived benefit or the emergence of intolerable side effects of the treatment, is routinely found in most RCTs. Observed rates of "suicidal events" are rarely corrected for the actual time of exposure of individual patients to specific treatments. Such correction for actual adverse event rates (events/persons/weeks) may be important if actual exposures are not closely matched across trial treatment arms, particularly when rare events such as completed and attempted suicides are involved (Baldessarini and Tondo, 2007c).

The FDA, after considering the findings from RCTs, demanded warnings about the possible increased of risk of suicidal ideation and perhaps behaviors during the treatment of juvenile and young adult patients with SSRIs and other modern antidepressants. The warnings carry the implication that special care is appropriate in the early treatment of young depressed patients (or any young patient) given an antidepressant (FDA, 2005). This recommendation limits the use of modern antidepressants in children, in addition to the fact that only fluoxetine is approved for juvenile major depression. This decision was based on at least four controlled trials (Tsapakis et al, 2007), one of which was a very large federally-funded trial with an unusually large separation of responses to the drug versus placebo (March et al, 2004). In 12 relatively large trials of SSRIs in juvenile patients with major depression, the relative rate of responding to the drug relative to the placebo (RR) averaged 1.23 (95%CI 1.14–1.33; $p<0.0001$) and in 14 much smaller trials of TCAs, the pooled RR of 1.15 (CI 0.98–1.34; $p=0.098$) was of similarly modest magnitude but statistically nonsignificant (Tsapakis et al, 2007).

The hypothesis about the possible worsening of suicidality in young antidepressant-treated patients implies that there are clinically developmental differences in affective and behavioral responses to antidepressants that require further study, especially with respect to the risks of actual suicidal behaviors.

Antidepressants and the Reduction of Suicide in Repeaters

Some research has focused on whether antidepressants are effective in reducing suicidality in repeaters. Data regarding this issue are scant. Considering the difficulties in studying the effects of treatments on rates of completed suicide, research has mainly focused on the evaluation of interventions following non-fatal suicidal behavior. Hawton and colleagues (2000), who systematically reviewed findings from all RCTs that examined the efficacy of treatments (problem-solving therapy, emergency contact card in addition to standard care, intensive aftercare plus outreach, dialectical behavioral therapy, and antidepressants) in patients who have deliberately harmed themselves, found a total of 23 clinical trials in which repetition of deliberate self-harm was reported as an outcome measure. Three studies compared antidepressant drugs with placebo. The pooled odds ratio for the three studies indicated no apparent benefit regarding repetition of deliberate self-harm for patients treated with mianserine, nomifensine or paroxetine. The paroxetine trial indicated that, among patients who had attempted suicide fewer than five times, 12 (36%) in the placebo group (N=33) and five (17%) in the paroxetine group (N = 30) made a subsequent suicide attempt, thereby generating the hypothesis that enhancing serotonergic function with an SSRI may reduce suicidal behavior at least in a subgroup of patients who had attempted suicide fewer than five times (Verkes et al, 1998).

Implications of the Increasing Prescribing of SSRIs on Suicide in Different Countries

In recent years, antidepressant prescribing has increased markedly in many developed countries, especially after the introduction of the SSRIs in the early 1990s. This might reflect the better recognition, treatment and prescribing for depression and an expected reduction in the rates of completed suicides as a consequence of this, but also because the newer antidepressants rarely result in lethal overdoses. The associations between antidepressants and suicide rates differ by country. In Italy, Barbui and colleagues described the impact of regulatory changes on antidepressant consumption in Italy from 1988 to 1996, examining whether the introduction of SSRIs was associated with changes in overall suicide rates (Barbui et al, 1999). From 1988 to 1996 the use of antidepressant rose from 1,843 to 2,814 units sold per 10,000 inhabitants. Data on suicide, available from 1988 to 1994, showed that, in the seven-year period during which SSRI use rose, male suicide rates increased from 9.8 to 10.2 per 100,000 inhabitants and females suicide rates declined from 3.9 to 3.2 per 100,000 inhabitants. The authors concluded that, in Italy, there was not any dramatic reduction in the overall suicide rates as a result of the increasing prescribing of SSRIs. Guaiana et al. (2005) investigated the impact of the increasing use of SSRIs and newer antidepressants on suicide rates, the proportion of completed suicides by poisoning with solid or liquid substances, admissions for depression and the proportion of admissions for depression that were first admissions. Their analysis revealed that, in Italy from 1983 to 2000, the use of tricyclic antidepressants remained stable and the use of SSRIs and newer agents dramatically increased. Suicide rates for males decreased from 1955 to 1974 and subsequently increased, reaching a peak in 1985 and then declining. In females, suicide rates remained substantially stable until 1978. A subsequent increase occurred up to 1985, followed by a steady decline. Suicide by poisoning dropped by nearly 50% from 1986 to 2000. Admissions to hospital for depression showed an erratic pattern, but no decline was observed. No change was observed in the rate of first admissions for depression. The analysis of long-term trends in suicide did not indicate that the increase in antidepressant prescribing was accompanied by a reduction in the suicide rate. Furthermore, in Italy, newer antidepressants had no impact on the total number of admissions for depression, nor on the proportion of all admissions that were first admissions.

Carlsten and colleagues (2001) carried out a time-series analysis using a two-slope model to compare suicide rates in Sweden before and after the introduction of the SSRIs. Antidepressant sales increased in men from 4.2 DDD/1,000 inhabitants/day during 1977-1979 to 21.8 in 1995-1997 and in women from 8.8 to 42.4 DDD/1,000 inhabitants/day between the same periods. A particularly rapid acceleration in antidepressant sales was observed during 1993-1996. In the two census periods suicide rates decreased in men by 30.9% and in women by 34.0%. The slope of suicide rates significantly changed after 1990, corresponding to 348 fewer suicides than expected during 1990-1997. This study showed a statistically significant change in the slope in suicide rates among men and women that coincided with the introduction of the SSRIs in Sweden but, as suggested by the same authors, the advent of these agents may explain only part of the declining suicide trend, since this trend started years before these drugs were introduced.

Isacsson (2000) found no correlation between suicide rates and alcohol consumption, or between suicide and unemployment, but the suicide rate decreased by 19% in parallel with the increased use of antidepressants in Sweden, Denmark, Norway and Finland. Moreover, in Sweden there was no demographic group with regard to age, gender or county in which the suicide rate decreased in the absence of an increased use of antidepressants. Isacsson concluded that the increased use of antidepressants agents appeared to be one of the contributing factors to the decrease in the suicide rate.

Hall and colleagues (2003) found that, in Australia between 1991 and 2000, the suicide rate markedly decreased in old men and women and increased in young adults especially young men, yielding a substantially stable total suicide rate. Exposure to antidepressants was higher for women than men in all age groups and increased markedly for both men and women, with the largest increases among older adults. A significant negative association was observed between antidepressants consumption and suicide in women but not in men. Among both men and women the largest declines in suicide occurred in the age groups with the highest exposure to antidepressants.

Ohberg and colleagues (1998) found that, in Finland from 1990 to 1995, the total suicide rate decreased from 30.3 per 100,000 inhabitants to 27.2. The total consumption of antidepressants drug more than doubled from 1990 to 1995. The authors concluded that the increased use of SSRIs in Finland coincided with a significant decline in suicide mortality. However, suicides using antidepressants showed an upward trend.

Rihmer reported that, in Hungary, the country with the one of the highest suicide rates in the world, the suicide rate steadily declined from 45.9 per 100,000 inhabitants in 1984 to 32.1 in 1998 (Rihmer, 2001; Rihmer et al, 2000; Rihmer, 2003). This decrease occurred together with the implementation of a new system of psychiatric care in which the number of outpatient psychiatric departments increased from 95 in 1982 to 136 in 1998, the number of psychiatrists increased from 550 in 1986 to 850 in 1998, and the number of emergency telephone services increased from 5 to 28 during the same period. Antidepressant consumption, mainly SSRIs, rose from 1984 to 1998, an approximately fivefold increase. In the same period there was a sixfold increase in unemployment, a 25% rise in official estimates of alcoholism rates and a 21% increase in divorce. Rihmer concluded that suicide rates are affected by many factors and the association between improved pharmacotherapy for depression and decreased suicide mortality is not easily demonstrated.

Grunebaum and colleagues (2004) showed that, in the United States from 1985 to 1999, the decline in the national suicide rate appeared to be associated with a greater use of non-tricyclic antidepressants. Suicide rates were already declining before 1985 in the United States, especially in females (Levi et al, 2003a; Levi et al, 2003b). In an ecological analysis over counties in the USA, Gibbons and colleagues (2005) found that the overall association between antidepressant prescriptions and the suicide rate was not significant for prescriptions for SSRIs, but the prescription of other new-generation non-SSRI antidepressants (nefazodone hydrochloride, mirtazapine, bupropion hydrochloride, and venlafaxine hydrochloride) were associated with lower suicide rates (both within and between counties). However, this finding may reflect not only on the efficacy of SSRIs, but also better compliance and quality of mental health care and a low toxicity in the event of a suicide attempt by overdose. In the pediatric population, higher SSRI prescription rates were associated with lower suicide rates in children and adolescents (Gibbons et al, 2006). Similar findings were reported by Olfson and colleagues (2006) in an extensive analysis of prescription data in the USA.

In the UK, Gunnell and colleagues (2003) reported a time-series analysis revealing an increase in young male suicide in England and Wales in the last 30 years, in parallel with a rise in a number of risk factors for suicide in this age group. In people aged over 60 an association was found between increases in the gross domestic product, antidepressant prescribing and other measures of improved healthcare provision and a decline in suicide. In Northern Ireland, Kelly and colleagues (2003) replicated these findings, observing that, in the younger group, there was no association between antidepressant prescribing and suicide, while for the older group increased antidepressants prescribing was associated with a reduction in suicide rate over a period of 10 years. However, a subsequent analysis of UK data suggested that the decline in suicide rates preceded increases in prescribing. Moreover, rises in antidepressant prescribing did not consistently coincide with clear changes in suicide trends (Gunnell and Ashby, 2004). Also in England, Morgan et al. (2004) investigated mortality from suicide and suggested that the increased prescribing of antidepressants, a proxy measure of improved diagnosis and treatment of depression in primary care, was accompanied by lower suicide rates .

In Iceland sales of antidepressants increased from 1975 to 2000, but suicide rates fluctuated during 1950-2000 and did not show any definite trend (Helgason et al, 2004).

Finally, in Israel, prescribing of antidepressants, particularly of SSRIs, increased 2.6-fold between 1998 and 2002. An overall reduction in suicides, significant only in elderly men, was reported in association with this increased rate of antidepressant prescription (Barak and Aizenberg, 2006).

Adverse Effect of Antidepressants and Suicide Mortality

In 2004, two systematic reviews analysing the efficacy and safety data of antidepressants for children and adolescents were simultaneously published, one in the *British Medical Journal* (Jureidini et al, 2004) and the other in *Lancet* (Whittington et al, 2004). Jureidini and colleagues checked the quality of methods and reporting of published trials of antidepressants drugs in children and adolescents in a total of 477 patients from six randomized trials who were treated with paroxetine, fluoxetine, sertraline or venlafaxine and 464 treated with placebo. Of 42 reported outcome measures, only 14 showed a statistical advantage for antidepressant drugs. Claims for effectiveness were based entirely on ratings by doctors. Regarding adverse effects of treatment, the authors suggested that some adverse effects might be more frequent than the authors of these studies imply. For example, up to half of young patients experienced an “activation syndrome”, and self-injurious ideation was seen in 6% of patients (Herxheimer and Mintzes, 2004). However, this analysis did not investigate the relative frequency of this rare outcome. By contrast, Whittington and colleagues (2004) published a systematic review of published and unpublished clinical trial data that assessed the risk-benefit of antidepressant drugs with a specific focus on suicidal behavior. No increased risk of suicidal behavior was observed for fluoxetine in comparison with placebo (3.6% versus 3.8%), but an increased risk of suicidal ideation or attempting suicide was observed for paroxetine (3.7% versus 2.5%), sertraline (2.6% versus 1.2%), citalopram (7.1% versus 3.6%,) and venlafaxine (7.7% versus 0.6%).

Jick et al (1995) followed 172,598 people who had at least one prescription for one of 10 antidepressant drugs in general practice in the UK. This epidemiological study found that the risk of suicide was higher in people who received fluoxetine (19/10,000 person years, 95%CI 9/10,000 person years to 34/10,000 person years) than in those receiving dosulepine (dothiepin; relative risk [RR] of suicide *V* dosulepine 2.1, 95%CI 1.1-4.1). In a nested case-controlled subgroup analysis in people with no history of suicidal behavior or previous antidepressant prescription, the risk remained the same, although the confidence interval broadened to make the result non-significant (RR 2.1, 95%CI 0.6=7.9). However, this study did not report the eventual association between the adverse events in patients taking antidepressants and the risk of suicide.

Jick and colleagues (2004) carried out a matched case-control study of more than 2,500 patients using the UK General practice Research Database and reported that the risk of suicidal behavior after starting antidepressant treatment was similar among users of amitriptyline, fluoxetine, and paroxetine compared with the risk among users of dothiepin. The risk of suicidal behavior was similar in patients taking SSRIs and tricyclics, but dothiepin might not be a useful comparison antidepressant for countries where this agent has never been licensed, such as Italy and USA (Barbui, 2004).

To replicate this finding, Jick et al (2004) used amitriptyline as a reference compound, and the OR (with 95%CI) for non-fatal suicidal behaviors among users of the other 3 antidepressants were 1.21 (0.80-1.83) for dothiepin, 1.40 (0.92-2.13) for fluoxetine and 1.55 (0.99-2.43) for paroxetine. A borderline value for paroxetine in comparison with amitriptyline emerged in this post-hoc analysis, leaving the possibility of an increased risk of non-fatal suicidal behaviors in users of this agent.

The potential empirical link between antidepressant treatment and suicide attempts was investigated by Valuck and colleagues (2004) who investigated 24,000 adolescents using a community sample of managed-care enrolees in USA. Crude suicide attempt rates ranged from 0.0% to 2.3% by index treatment group. Treatment with SSRIs (hazard ratio 1.59, 95% CI 0.89, 2.82), other antidepressant drugs (hazard ratio 1.03, 95%CI 0.43-2.44) or multiple antidepressants (hazard ratio 1.43, 95%CI 0.70-2.89) resulted in no significant increased risk of a suicide attempt. In contrast with these data, Martinez and colleagues (2005) analysed the risk of non-fatal self-harm and suicide in 146,095 patients with a new diagnosis of depression who were prescribed SSRIs or tricyclics. SSRI users in comparison with tricyclic users were not at increased risk of suicide or non-fatal self-harm. However, in patients aged 18 or less, weak evidence suggested a higher risk of non-fatal self-harm in those prescribed SSRIs (OR 1.59, 95%CI 1.01-2.50). Søndergård and colleagues (2006b) investigated the association between SSRIs and suicide in children and adolescents in Denmark and observed a statistically nonsignificant increased rate of suicides associated with SSRI use (RR 4.47, 95%CI 0.95-20.96).

Simon et al. (2006) identified more than 65,000 individuals with more than 82,000 episodes of antidepressant treatment. The risk of suicide during the acute-phase treatment was one in 3,000 treatment episodes and the risk of serious suicide attempt was one in 1,000. The data did not indicate a significant increase in risk of suicide or serious suicide attempt after starting treatment with newer antidepressants.

Isacsson et al. (2005) analyzed the presence of different antidepressants in the forensic toxicological screening of 14,857 suicides compared with those in 26,422 cases of deaths by accident or natural causes in Sweden from 1992 to 2000. In the toxicological screening, antidepressants were detected in 3,096 (20%) of the 14,857 cases of suicide investigated and a total of 3,411 antidepressants in these individuals. Of these, 48% were SSRIs, whereas the number of detections in the 26,422 controls was 1,538. SSRIs were under-represented compared with other antidepressants (OR 0.83, 99%CI 0.77-0.90). The differences within the SSRIs were insignificant, with the exception of fluvoxamine. The OR for the tricyclics as a class (including maprotiline) was 1.01 (99%CI 0.90-1.14), but it was higher for the class of moclobemide, mianserin, mirtazapine, reboxetine and venlafaxine (OR 1.78, 99%CI 1.46-2.16). In 52 cases of suicide in those aged less than 15 years, seven were positive for antidepressants (clomipramine, imipramine, maprotiline, trimipramine, mianserin and venlafaxine), but no SSRIs were detected. In 326 cases of suicide in the 15 to 19 year-old group, there were 13 cases which were positive for antidepressants (amitriptyline, clomipramine, trimipramine, citalopram, fluoxetine, sertraline and mirtazapine), and SSRIs had lower RR in suicides compared with non-SSRIs. The authors concluded that the hypothesis that treatment of depressed individuals with SSRIs leads to an increased risk of suicide was not supported by this analysis of the total suicidal outcome of the nationwide use of SSRIs in Sweden over a period of 9 years.

In a nationwide cohort study in Finland, Tiihonen et al. (2006) studied the association between the risk of suicide, attempted suicide, and overall mortality associated with antidepressant use, calculating the RR of completed suicides, suicide attempts leading to hospitalisation and overall mortality during tricyclic, SSRI and SNRI treatment versus no antidepressant use, after adjusting for possible confounders. In the entire cohort, fluoxetine use (RR 0.52, 95%CI 0.30-0.93) was associated with a lower risk of suicide and venlafaxine (RR 1.61, 95%CI 1.01-2.57) with a higher risk. Among suicidal subjects who had ever used antidepressants, the current use of any antidepressants was associated with a markedly increased risk of attempted suicide and with a markedly decreased risk of completed suicide and death.

The relationship between venlafaxine use and suicidality was investigated by Rubino and colleagues (2007) who found that patients prescribed venlafaxine were more likely to commit or attempt suicide compared with patients prescribed citalopram, fluoxetine and dothiepin, but adjustment for a number of possible confounders substantially reduced the excess risk. Finally, Juurlink and colleagues (2006) explored the relationship between the initiation of therapy with the SSRIs and completed suicide in older patients. During the first month of therapy, SSRI use was associated with a nearly fivefold higher risk of completed suicide over the other antidepressants (adjusted odds ratio 4.8, 95%CI 1.9-12.2). The risk was independent of a recent diagnosis of depression or the receipt of psychiatric care, and suicides of a violent nature were more common during SSRI therapy. However, the absolute risk of suicide was low, suggesting perhaps that an idiosyncratic response to these agents may induce suicide only in a vulnerable subgroup of patients.

Conclusion

Research on the possible relationship between pharmacotherapy and suicidal behavior was virtually unknown until a decade ago. An initial case series and several reports indicated that a minority of depressed patients experience adverse behavioral and emotional responses to treatment with various types of antidepressant drugs, including SSRIs (Teicher et al, 1990; Mann et al, 2006; Pompili et al, 2005). A minority of ecological studies have reported minor decreases of suicide rates by region or time correlated with higher rates of prescribing modern antidepressants, but such correlations are probably influenced by many factors associated with access to clinical care. Most large clinical studies indicate decreased suicidal risk with antidepressant treatment, but some find increases for patients in some age groups. However, these studies often have confounding variables such as an association between antidepressant treatment and more severe depression and, thus, greater suicidal risk. Data pooled from relatively brief, randomized, controlled trials in patients with acute major depression suggest an increase in the risk of suicide attempts, as well as increases in suicidal ideation in the young, but decreases in young and elderly adults. These data, taken together, suggested that antidepressants do not always have a beneficial effect on the risk of suicidal behaviors, but they may reduce suicidal ideation and other depressive symptoms. Peculiar responses emerging early in the course of antidepressant treatment require particularly close clinical follow-up in order to identify the suicidal risk. When this kind of risk is assessed, treatment must be appropriately modified, for example, changing antidepressant medication, adding sedating, antipsychotic or mood-stabilizing treatments, and providing additional individual support.

We conclude that antidepressant treatment appears to reduce suicidal ideation in depressed adults, but only pharmacological treatments such as clozapine (Hennen and Baldessarini, 2005) and lithium (Ahrens et al, 2001; Baldessarini et al, 2006b) have sound evidence for reducing the risk of completed and attempted suicide. "Suicidality" may not be a useful single therapeutic target. There may be a differential pharmacology for particular types of suicidality. One crucial target in order to reduce the risk of suicide may be limiting aggression and impulsivity in individuals at risk for suicide (Baldessarini et al, 2006b), and antipsychotic and mood-stabilizing agents rather than antidepressant drugs have these properties.

References

Acharya N, Rosen AS, Polzer JP, D'Souza DN, Perahia DG, Cavazzoni PA, Baldessarini RJ. Duloxetine: meta-analyses of suicidal behaviors and ideation in clinical trials for major depressive disorder. *J. Clin. Psychopharmacol.* 2006; 26: 587–594.

Akiskal HS, Benazzi F, Perugi G, Rihmer Z. Agitated "unipolar" depression re-conceptualized as a depressive mixed state: implications for the antidepressant-suicide controversy. *J. Affect. Disord.* 2005; 85: 245–258.

American Psychiatric Association (APA). Practice guideline for the assessment and treatment of patients with suicidal behaviors. *Am. J. Psychiatry.* 2003; 160 (11 Suppl): 1–60.

Angst J. Angst F, Gerber-Werder R, Gamma A. Suicide in 406 mood-disorder patients with and without long-term medication: a 40–44 years follow-up. *Arch. Suicide Res.* 2005; 9: 279–300.

Ahrens B, Müller-Oerlinghausen B. Does lithium exert an independent antisuicidal effect? *Pharmacopsychiatry* 2001; 34: 132–136.

Baldessarini RJ, Jamison KR: Effects of medical interventions on suicidal behavior: Summary and conclusions. *J. Clin. Psychiatry* 1999; 60 (Suppl. 2): 117–122.

Baldessarini RJ, Salvatore P, Tohen M, Khalsa HMK, Hennen J, González-Pinto A, Baethge C, Tohen M. Morbidity from onset in first-episode bipolar I disorder patients: The International-300 study. *Neuropsychopharmacology*. 2004; 29 (Suppl 1): S88.

Baldessarini RJ, Tarazi FI. Drug therapy of depression and anxiety disorders, psychosis and mania. Chapts. 17 and 18 in Brunton LL, Lazo JS, Parker KL, editors: Goodman and Gilman's Goodman and Gilman's The Pharmacological Basis of Therapeutics, eleventh edition. New York: McGraw-Hill Press, 2005a, pp 429–500.

Baldessarini RJ, Pompili M, Tondo L, Tsapakis E, Soldani F, Faedda GL, Hennen J: Antidepressants and suicidal behavior: Are we hurting or helping? *Clin. Neuropsychiatry*. 2005b; 2: 73–75.

Baldessarini RJ, Pompili M, Tondo L: Suicidal risk in antidepressant trials. *Arch. Gen. Psychiatry*. 2006a; 63: 246–248.

Baldessarini RJ, Tondo L, Davis P, Pompili M, Goodwin FK, Hennen J: Decreased suicidal risk during long-term lithium treatment: meta-analysis. *Bipolar Disord.* 2006b; 8: 625–639.

Baldessarini RJ, Leahy L, Arcona S, Gause D, Zhang W, Hennen J: Prescribing patterns of psychotropic medicines in the United States for patients diagnosed with bipolar disorders. *Psychiatr. Serv.* 2007a; 58: 85–91.

Baldessarini RJ, Tondo L, Strombom I, Dominguez S, Fawcett J, Oquendo M, Licinio J, Valuck R, Tollesfon G, Tohen M: Analysis of ecological studies of relationships between antidepressant utilization and suicidal risk. Harvard Rev. Psychiatry. 2007b; in revision.

Baldessarini RJ, Tondo L. Psychopharmacology for Suicide Prevention in Suicide in Psichiatric Disorders, Tatarelli R, Pompili M, Girardi P. Nova Science Publischers Inc. 2007c.

Barak Y, Aizenberg D: Association between antidepressant prescribing and suicide in Israel. *Int. Clin. Psychopharmacol.* 2006; 21(5):281-284

Barak Y, Olmer A, Aizenberg D. Antidepressants reduce the risk of suicide among elderly depressed patients. *Neuropsychopharmacology*. 2005; 31: 178–181.

Barbui C, Campomori A, D'Avanzo B, Negri E, Garattini S: Antidepressant drug use in Italy since the introduction of SSRIs: national trends, regional differences and impact on suicide rates. *Soc. Psychiatry Psychiatr. Epidemiol.* 1999; 34(3):152-156

Barbui C, Esposito E, Cipriani A. Selective serotonin reuptake inhibitors and risk of suicide: a systematic review of observational studies. CMAJ 2009; 180(3): 291–297.

Barbui C, Furukawa TA, Cipriani A. Effectiveness of paroxetine in the treatment of acute major depression in adults: a systematic re-examination of published and unpublished data from randomized trials. *CMAJ* 2008;178:296-305.

Barbui C: Antidepressants and the risk of suicidal behaviors. JAMA. 2004; 292(23):2833

Bauer MS, Wisniewski SR, Marangell LB, Chessick CA, Allen MH, Dennehy EB, Miklowitz DJ, Thase ME, Sachs GS. Are antidepressants associated with new-onset suicidality in bipolar disorder? A prospective study of participants in the Systematic Treatment Enhancement Program for Bipolar Disorder (STEP-BP). *J. Clin. Psychiatry*. 2006; 67: 48–55.

Beasley CM Jr, Dornseif BE, Bosomworth JC, Sayler ME, Rampey AH Jr, Heilgenstein JH, Thompson VL, Murphy DJ, Masica CN. Fluoxetine and suicide: a meta-analysis of controlled trials of treatment for depression. *BMJ*. 1991; 303: 685–692.

Bostwick JM, Pankratz VS. Affective disorders and suicide risk: a reexamination. *Am. J. Psychiatry*. 2000; 157: 1925–1932.

Carlsten A, Waern M, Ekedahl A, Ranstam J: Antidepressant medication and suicide in Sweden. *Pharmacoepidemiol. Drug Saf.* 2001; 10(6):525-530

Cipriani A, Furukawa T, Salanti G, et al. Comparative efficacy and acceptability of 12 new generation antidepressants: a multiple treatments meta-analysis. *Lancet*. In press.

Cipriani A, Geddes J, Barbui C: Venlafaxine for major depression: more evidence that risks outweigh benefits for most patients? *BMJ*. 2007; 334: 215-216.

Didham RC, McConnell DW, Blair HJ, et al. Suicide and self-harm following prescription of SSRIs and other antidepressants: confounding by indication. *Br. J. Clin. Pharmacol.* 2005;60:519-25.

Diekstra RFW. Epidemiology of suicide and parasuicide. *Acta Psychiatr. Scand.* 1993; 371 (Suppl): 9–20.

Dubicka B, Wilkinson P. Evidence-based treatment of adolescent major depression. *Evid. Based Ment. Health* 2007;10:100-2.

FDA (US Food and Drug Administration). Antidepressant use in children, adolescents, and adults. Available at: http://www.fda.gov/cder/drug/antidepressants. 2005. Accessed 22 June 2006.

Fergusson D, Doucette S, Glass KC, Shapiro S, Healy D, Hebert P, Hutton B. Association between suicide attempts and selective serotonin reuptake inhibitors: systematic review of randomized controlled trials. *BMJ*. 2005; 330: 396–402.

Filteau M-J, Lapierre YD, Bakish D, Blanchard A. Reduction in suicidal ideation with SSRIs: Review of 459 depressed patients. *J. Psychiatry Neurosci.* 1993; 18: 114–118.

Freedman DA. The Ecological Fallacy. Accessible at <http://www.stat.berkeley.edu/~census/ecofall.txt>. 2002. Accessed 10 January 2007.

Ghaemi SN, Hsu DJ, Soldani F, Goodwin FK. Antidepressants in bipolar disorder: the case for caution. *Bipolar Disord.* 2003; 5: 421–433.

Gibbons RD, Hur K, Bhaumik DK, Mann JJ. The relationship between antidepressant medication use and rate of suicide. *Arch. Gen. Psychiatry*. 2005; 62: 165–172.

Gibbons RD, Hur K, Bhaumik DK, Mann JJ. The relationship between antidepressant prescription rates and rate of early adolescent suicide. *Am. J. Psychiatry.* 2006; 163: 1898–1904.

Goldsmith SK, Pellmar TC, Kleinman AM, Bunney WE, editors. Reducing Suicide. Washington, DC: Institute of Medicine of the US National Academies of Science, 2002.

Grunebaum MF, Ellis SP, Li S, Oquendo MA, Mann JJ. Antidepressants and suicide risk in the United States, 1985–1999. *J. Clin. Psychiatry*. 2004; 65: 1456–1462.

Guaiana G, Andretta M, Corbari L, Mirandola M, Sorio A, D'Avanzo B, Barbui C: Antidepressant drug consumption and public health indicators in Italy, 1955 to 2000. *J. Clin. Psychiatry*. 2005; 66(6):750-755

Gunnell D, Ashby D: Antidepressants and suicide: what is the balance of benefit and harm. *BMJ.* 2004; 329(7456):34-38

Gunnell D, Middleton N, Whitley E, Dorling D, Frankel S: Why are suicide rates rising in young men but falling in the elderly?-- a time-series analysis of trends in England and Wales 1950-1998. *Soc. Sci. Med.* 2003; 57(4):595-611

Gunnell D, Saperia J, Ashby D. Selective serotonin reuptake inhibitors (SRIs) and suicide in adults: meta-analysis of drug company data from placebo controlled, randomized controlled trials **submitted to the MHRA's safety** review. *BMJ.* 2005; 330: 385–388.

Hall WD, Mant A, Mitchell PB, Rendle VA, Hickie IB, McManus P: Association between antidepressant prescribing and suicide in Australia, 1991-2000: trend analysis. *BMJ.* 2003; 326(7397):1008

Hall WD. How have the SSRI antidepressants affected suicide risk? *Lancet* 2006;367:1959-62.

Hammad TA, Laughren T, Racoosin JA. Suicidality in pediatric patients treated with antidepressant drugs. *Arch. Gen. Psychiatry.* 2006b; 63: 332–339.

Hammad TA, Laughren TP, Racoosin JA. Suicide rates in short-term randomized controlled trials of newer antidepressants. J. Clin. Psychopharmacol. 2006a; 26: 203–207.

Harris EC, Barraclough B. Excess mortality of mental disorder. *Br. J. Psychiatry.* 1998; 173: 11–53.

Hawton K, Townsend E, Arensman E, Gunnell D, Hazell P, House A, Van HK: Psychosocial versus pharmacological treatments for deliberate self harm. *Cochrane Database Syst. Rev.* 2000;(2):CD001764

Healy D. Did regulators fail over selective serotonin reuptake inhibitors? *BMJ.* 2006; 333: 92–95.

Helgason T, Tómasson H, Zoëga T. Antidepressants and public health in Iceland: time series analysis of national data. *Br. J. Psychiatry.* 2004; 184: 157–162.

Hennen J, Baldessarini RJ. Suicidal risk during treatment with clozapine: a meta-analysis. *Schizophrenia Res.* 2005; 73: 139–145.

Henriksson S, Isacsson G. Increased antidepressant use and fewer suicides in Jamtland county, Sweden, after a primary care educational programme on the treatment of depression. *Acta Psychiatr. Scand.* 2006; 114: 159–167.

Herxheimer A, Mintzes B: Antidepressants and adverse effects in young patients: uncovering the evidence. *CMAJ.* 2004; 170(4):487-489

Isacsson G, Holmgren P, Ahlner J: Selective serotonin reuptake inhibitor antidepressants and the risk of suicide: a controlled forensic database study of 14,857 suicides. *Acta Psychiatr. Scand.* 2005; 111(4):286-290

Isacsson G. Suicide prevention–a medical breakthrough? *Acta Psychiatr. Scand.* 2000; 102: 113–117.

Jick H, Kaye JA, Jick SS: Antidepressants and the risk of suicidal behaviors. *JAMA.* 2004; 292(3):338-343

Jick SS, Dean AD, Jick H. Antidepressants and suicide. BMJ. 1995; 310(6974):215-218

Joffe RT, MacQueen GM, Marriott M, Trevor Young L. A prospective, longitudinal study of percentage of time spent ill in patients with bipolar I or bipolar II disorders. *Bipolar Disord.* 2004; 6: 62–66.

Judd LL, Akiskal HS, Schettler PJ, Endicott J, Maser J, Solomon DA, Leon AC, Rice JA, Keller MB. Rel The long-term natural history of the weekly symptomatic status of bipolar I disorder. *Arch. Gen. Psychiatry.* 2002; 59: 530–537.

Jureidini JN, Doecke CJ, Mansfield PR, Haby MM, Menkes DB, Tonkin AL: Efficacy and safety of antidepressants for children and adolescents. *BMJ.* 2004; 328(7444):879-883

Juurlink DN, Mamdani MM, Kopp A, Redelmeier DA. The risk of suicide with selective serotonin reuptake inhibitors in the elderly. *Am. J. Psychiatry.* 2006; 163: 813–821.

Kelly CB, Ansari T, Rafferty T, Stevenson M: Antidepressant prescribing and suicide rate in Northern Ireland. *Eur. Psychiatry.* 2003; 18(7):325-328

Kessler RC, Berglund P, Borges G, Nock M, Wang PS: Trends in suicide ideation, plans, gestures, and attempts in the United States, 1990-1992 to 2001–2003. *JAMA.* 2005; 293: 2487–2495.

Khan A, Khan S, Kolts R, Brown WA. Suicide rates in clinical trials with SRIs, other antidepressants, and placebo: analysis of FDA reports. *Am. J. Psychiatry.* 2003; 160: 790–792.

Khan A, Leventhal RM, Khan S, Brown WA. Suicide risk in patients with anxiety disorders: a meta-analysis of the FDA database. *J. Affect. Disord.* 2002; 68: 183–190.

Khan A, Warner HA, Brown WA. Symptom reduction and suicide risk in patients treated with placebo in antidepressant clinical trials: analysis of the FDA database. *Arch. Gen. Psychiatry.* 2000; 57: 311–317.

Klein DF. FDA post-marketing safety decisions. J. Clin. Psychiatry. 2006; 67: 1305–1306.

Koukopoulos A, Koukopoulos A. Agitated depression as a mixed state and the problem of melancholia. Psychiatr. *Clin. North Am.* 1999; 22: 547–564.

Laughren T. Memorandum: overview for the December 13 meeting of Psychopharmacologic Drugs Advisory Committee. Food and Drug Administration; 2006. Available http://www.pubmedcentral.nih.gov/redirect3.cgi?andandauth=0lEQVNTg2RrBBJrrWncXefu5rv4NoNAU3hxL5AMnandreftype=extlinkandarticleid=2630355andissueid=175825andjournalid=77andFROM=Article%7CCitationRefandTO=External%7CLink%7CURIandrenderingtype=normalandandwww.fda.gov/ohrms/dockets/ac/06/briefing/2006-4272b1-01-fda.pdf (accessed 2008 Dec. 23).

Laughren TP. Overview of a meeting of the Psychopharmacology Drug Advisory Committee (PDAC) [concerning suicidal risk in trials of antidepressant drugs in juvenile and adult patients]. Accessible at: <http://www.fda.gov/ohrms/dockets/ac/06/ briefing/2006-4272b1-index.htm>, 2006, pp 27ff. Accessed 26 December 2006.

Leon AC, Keller MB, Warshaw MG, Mueller TI, Solomon DA, Coryell W, Endicott J. A prospective study of fluoxetine treatment and suicidal behavior in affectively ill subjects. *Am. J. Psychiatry.* 1999; 156: 195–201.

Leon AC. The revised warning for antidepressants and suicidality: unveiling the black box of statistical analyses. *Am J Psychiatry* 2007;164:1786-9.

Ludwig J, Marcotte DE. Antidepressants, suicide, and drug regulation. *J. Policy Anal. Manage.* 2005; 24: 249–272.

Maj M, Pirozzi R, Magliano L, Fiorillo A, Bartoli L. Agitated "unipolar" major depression: prevalence, phenomenology, and outcome. *J. Clin. Psychiatry.* 2006; 67: 712–719.

Mann JJ, Emslie G, Baldessarini RJ, Beardslee W, Fawcett JA, Goodwin FK, Leon FK, Meltzer HY, Ryan ND, Shaffer D, Wagner KD. ACNP task force report on SRIs and suicidal behavior in youth. *Neuropsychopharmacology.* 2006; 31: 473–492.

March J, Silva S, Petrycki S, Curry J, Wells K, Fairbank J, Burns B, Domino M, McNulty S, Vitiello B, Severe J; Treatment for Adolescents With Depression Study (TADS) Team. Fluoxetine, cognitive-behavioral therapy, and their combination for adolescents with depression: Treatment for Adolescents With Depression Study (TADS) randomized controlled trial. *JAMA*. 2004; 292: 807–820.

Martinez C, Rietbrock S, Wise L, Ashby D, Chick J, Moseley J, Evans S, Gunnell D. Antidepressant treatment and the risk of fatal and non-fatal self harm in first episode depression: nested case-control study. *BMJ*. 2005; 330: 389–392.

MHRA (UK Medicines and Health Regulatory Agency). Selective serotonin reuptake inhibitor (SSRI) antidepressants: Committee on Safety of Medicines (CSM) working group findings: <http://www.mhra.gov.uk/news/2004/2004.htm>, 2004. Accessed 22 September 2005.

Moller HJ, Baldwin DS, Goodwin G, et al. Do SSRIs or antidepressants in general increase suicidality? WPA Section on Pharmacopsychiatry: consensus statement. *Eur Arch Psychiatry Clin Neurosci* 2008;258(Suppl 3):3-23.

Moller HJ. Evidence for beneficial effects of antidepressants on suicidality in depressive patients: systematic review. *Eur. Arch. Psychiatry Clin. Neurosci.* 2006; 256: 329–343.

Morgan OW, Griffiths C, Majeed A: Association between mortality from suicide in England and antidepressant prescribing: an ecological study. BMC Public Health. 2004; 463

Nordstrom P, Samuelsson M, Åsberg M. Survival analysis of suicide risk after attempted suicide. *Acta Psychiatr. Scand.* 1995; 91: 336–340.

Ohberg A, Vuori E, Klaukka T, Lonnqvist J: Antidepressants and suicide mortality. *J. Affect. Disord.* 1998; 50(2-3):225-233

Olfson M, Marcus SC, Shaffer D. Antidepressant drug therapy and suicide in severely depressed children and adults: Case-control study. *Arch. Gen. Psychiatry*. 2006; 63: 865–872.

Oquendo MA, Chaudhury SR, Mann JJ. Pharmacotherapy of suicidal behavior in bipolar disorder. *Arch. Suicide Res.* 2005; 9: 237–250.

Oquendo MA, Kamali M, Ellis SP, Grunebaum MF, Malone KM, Brodsky BS, Sackeim HA, Mann JJ. Adequacy of antidepressant treatment after discharge and the occurrence of suicidal acts in major depression: a prospective study. *Am. J. Psychiatry.* 2002; 159: 1746–1751.

Pedersen AG. Escitalopram and suicidality in adult depression and anxiety. *Int. Clin. Psychopharmacol.* 2005; 20: 139–143.

Pompili M, Tondo L, Baldessarini RJ: Suicidal risk emerging during antidepressant treatment: Recognition and intervention. *Clin. Neuropsychiatry* 2005; 2: 66–72.

Post RM, Denicoff KD, Leverich GS, Altshuler LL, Frye MA, Suppes TM, Rush AJ, Keck PE Jr, McElroy SL, Luckenbaugh DA, Pollio C, Kupka R, Nolen WA. Morbidity in 258 bipolar outpatients followed for 1 year with daily prospective ratings on the NIMH life chart method. *J. Clin. Psychiatry*. 2003; 64: 680–690.

Rahme E, Dasgupta K, Turecki G, et al. Risks of suicide and poisoning among elderly patients prescribed selective serotonin reuptake inhibitors: a retrospective cohort study. *J. Clin. Psychiatry* 2008;69:349-57.

Reseland S, Bray I, Gunnell D. Relationship between antidepressant sales and secular trends in suicide rates in the Nordic countries. Br. J. Psychiatry. 2006; 188: 354–358.

Rihmer Z, Appleby L, Rihmer A, Belso N: Decreasing suicide in Hungary. *Br. J. Psychiatry.* 2000; 17784

Rihmer Z: Can better recognition and treatment of depression reduce suicide rates? A brief review. *Eur. Psychiatry.* 2001; 16(7):406-409

Rihmer Z: Do SSRIs increase the risk of suicide among depressives even if they are taking only placebo? *Psychother. Psychosom.* 2003; 72(6):357-358

Rose RM, Burt RA, Clayton PJ. Consensus development conference statement: Electroconvulsive therapy. *JAMA.* 1985; 254: 2103–2108.

Roy A. Suicide. (2000) Chapt 29.1 in Sadock BJ, Sadock VA, editors: Kaplan and Sadock's Comprehensive Textbook of Psychaitry, seventh edition, vol 2. Philadelphia: Lippincott Willians and Wilkins, pp 2031–2040.

Rubino A, Roskell N, Tennis P, Mines D, Weich S, Andrews E: Risk of suicide during treatment with venlafaxine, citalopram, fluoxetine, and dothiepin: retrospective cohort study. *BMJ.* 2007; 334: 242-247.

Simon GE, Savarino J, Operskalski B, Wang PS: Suicide risk during antidepressant treatment. *Am. J. Psychiatry.* 2006b; 163(1):41-47

Simon RI, Hales RE, editors. Textbook of Suicide Assessment and Management, Washington, DC: American Psychiatric Press, 2006a.

Søndergård L, Kvist K, Andersen PK, Kessing LV. Do antidepressants prevent suicide? *Int. Clin. Psychopharmacol. 2006a*; 21: 211–218.

Søndergård L, Kvist K, Andersen PK, Kessing LV. Do antidepressants precipitate youth suicide?–a nationwide pharmacoepidemiological study. Eur. Child Adolesc. *Psychiatry.* 2006b; 15: 232–240.

Søndergård L, Kvist K, Lopez AG, Andersen PK, Kessing LV. Temporal changes in suicide rates for persons treated and not treated with antidepressants in Denmark during 1995–1999. *Acta Psychiatr. Scand.* 2006c; 114: 168–176.

Storosum JG, van Zwieten BJ, van den Brink W, Gersons BP, Broekmans AW: Suicide risk in placebo-controlled studies of major depression. *Am. J. Psychiatry.* 2001; 158: 1271–1275.

Teicher MH, Glod C, Cole JO. Emergence of intense suicidal preoccupation during fluoxetine treatment. *Am. J. Psychiatry* 1990; 147: 207–210.

Tiihonen J, Lonnqvist J, Wahlbeck K, Klaukka T, Tanskanen A, Haukka J. Antidepressants and the risk of suicide, attempted suicide, and overall mortality in a nationwide cohort. *Arch. Gen. Psychiatry.* 2006; 63: 1358–1367.

Tollefson GD, Rampey AH Jr, Beasley CM Jr, Enas GG, Potvin JH. Absence of a relationship between adverse events and suicidality during pharmacotherapy for depression. *J. Clin. Psychopharmacol.* 1994; 14: 163–169.

Tondo L, Albert M, Baldessarini RJ: Suicide rates in relation to health-care access in the United States. *J. Clin. Psychiatry.* 2006; 67: 517–523.

Tondo L, Baldessarini RJ, Hennen J, Minnai GP, Salis P, Scamonatti L, Masia M, Ghiani C, Mannu P: Suicide attempts in major affective disorder patients with comorbid substance use disorders. *J. Clin. Psychiatry.* 1999; 60 (Suppl 2): 63–69.

Tondo L, Baldessarini RJ. Suicidal risks among 2826 major affective disorder patients. *Acta Psychiatr. Scand.* 2007; in revision.

Tondo L, Baldessarini RJ. Trends in suicide rates: an international perspective (Abstract). *Ital. J. Psychopathol.* 2006; 12 (2: Suppl): 202–203.

Tondo L, Isacsson G, Baldessarini RJ: Suicide in bipolar disorder: Risk and prevention. *CNS Drugs.* 2003; 17: 491–511.

Tsapakis E, Soldani F, Tondo L, Baldessarini RJ: Efficacy of antidepressants in depressed children and adolescents: A meta-analysis. *Br. J. Psychiatry.* 2007; in revision.

Valuck RJ, Libby AM, Sills MR, Giese AA, Allen RR: Antidepressant treatment and risk of suicide attempt by adolescents with major depressive disorder: a propensity-adjusted retrospective cohort study. *CNS Drugs.* 2004; 18(15):1119-1132

Verkes RJ, van der Mast RC, Hengeveld MW, Tuyl JP, Zwinderman AH, Van Kempen GM: Reduction by paroxetine of suicidal behavior in patients with repeated suicide attempts but not major depression. *Am. J. Psychiatry.* 1998; 155(4):543-547

Warshaw MG, Keller MB. The relationship between fluoxetine use and suicidal behavior in 654 subjects with anxiety disorders. *J. Clin. Psychiatry.* 1996; 57: 158–166.

Weinger RD, editor. Practice of Electroconvulsive Therapy: Recommendations for Treatment, Training, and Privileging. A Task Force Report of the American Psychiatric Association, Second Edition. Washington, DC: American Psychiatric Press, 2000.

Whittington CJ, Kendall T, Fonagy P, Cottrell D, Cotgrove A, Boddington E: Selective serotonin reuptake inhibitors in childhood depression: systematic review of published versus unpublished data. *Lancet.* 2004; 363(9418):1341-1345

World Health Organization (WHO). International suicide rates. Accessible at www.who.int/mental_health/prevention/suicide/country_reports/en/index.html, 2007. Accessed 10 January 2007.

Yerevanian BI, Koek RJ, Feusner JD, et al. Antidepressants and suicidal behaviour in unipolar depression. *Acta Psychiatr. Scand.* 2004;110:452-8.

In: Antidepressants: Types, Efficiency ...
Editor: Jayden T. Van Leeuwen, pp.91-113
ISBN 978-1-61668-581-2

Chapter 3

MONITORING OF ANTIDEPRESSANT THERAPY BY USING HEART RATE VARIABILITY

Sven Suefke, Hasib Djonlagic, and Thomas Kibbel
Medizinische Klinik I, Universitaetsklinikum Schleswig-Holstein,
Campus Luebeck, Luebeck, Germany

ABSTRACT

The cardiac autonomic nervous system is typically impaired in patients with major depression and panic disorder. Furthermore, this unfavorable condition will be dose dependent intensified by antidepressant drugs. This increases the cardiovascular risk and can be currently and non-invasively estimated by analysis of heart rate variability (HRV). The reduction of HRV is less expressed by SSRI than by TCA. This is in accordance to better acceptance of SSRI as published in the literature. The parasympathetic determinated components of HRV are in therapeutic doses more impaired than the rather sympathetic determinated components. This reduction is dependent on plasma concentration.

Under doxepin in toxic doses, a level dependent suppression of sympathetic parts (LF power) is added overtopping the suppression of vagal parts (HF power). The minimum of HRV was at that time attained that is associated in the literature with greatest mortality. This can be exlained by cardiac depression as a result of a quinidine-like effect. But the also described supraventricular and ventricular arrhythmias occur more frequently with time delay and seem to be less associated with the absolute level of developed sympathetic predominance, but rather with the dynamic of the increasing sympathetic influence in first recovery. Our results show a good Spearman correlation of (1) incidence of all arrhythmias within 48 h vs. (2) LF/HF after 48h / LF/HF in HRV minimum if frequency components of spectral analysis (LF and HF Power) are transformed into logarithms before ($p<.001$).

The already published results in the literature give sufficient information that HRV influences are agent specific and this may be important for prognosis. Because also starting conditions of patients are differing from each other, (1) a determination of agent specific profile of HRV changes as well as (2) a determination of basic HRV values of treated patients are desirable. If both parameters are known, the therapy could be better monitored in the future.

1. Introduction - New Opportunities for Estimation of Cardiovascular Side Effects in Antidepressant Therapy

The broad clinical use of antidepressant drugs is especially problematic in the older but always used tricyclic antidepressants (TCA). These agents show a narrow therapeutic width and a complex spectrum of adverse effects. Therefore, individual therapy will become much difficult, and in overdose, accidently or in attempt of committing suicide, TCA are the leading cause for severe intoxication treated in the ICU [1].

Further is increasing evidence that depressive disorders *per se* are associated with cardiovascular impairments and that the actual function of autonomic nervous system has prognostic relevance in cardiologic [2] as well as in psychiatric diseases [3]. Addionally was shown that diminished modulation of sympathetic and parasympathetic activity is leading to an unstable and therefore vulnerable status of central influences on cardiac autonomic regulation [4]. Such changes were associated with a greater incidence of sudden cardiac death [5].

Regarding to outcome, also low heart rate variability (HRV) has shown to predict mortality in patients with recent myocardial infarction or with stable coronary disease [6]. This method serves as a noninvasive instrument for measuring heart-brain interactions and autonomic nervous system dynamics [7]. Until now it can be concluded that depressive disorders are associated with a diminished HRV *per se* [8,9]. Additional anticholinergic effects that occurred in TCA use [10,11] are attributed to greater incidence of arrhythmias and sudden cardiac death [12]. In contrast to TCA, influences on HRV are significantly less expressed by selective serotonin reuptake inhibitors (SSRI) [13]. Therefore is commonly suggested that SSRI would provide lower cardiovascular risk [14].

Regarding to justified assumption that HRV analysis will provide advantageous information in individualization of therapy and in risk stratification, the following comment is summarizing the evidence of the literature in the context of possible explanations. Further, some preliminary results are mentioned that may be important for future outlook and innovative development.

2. Side Effects of Antidepressant Drugs – Severe Impairment in Overdose

Psychotherapeutic drugs can no more be neglected in the therapy of psychiatric diseases. But in therapy of depressive disorders such as in therapy of panic disorders customary substances are used which are strongly differing in their chemical structure and their pharmacological profile [15]. Furthermore, the same agents took place in the co-medication of chronic pain syndromes, in the therapy of peripheral neuropathies and in the prophylaxis of megrim [16]. Thereby, the broad clinical use is explained. Problematic become therapy especially by the older but always used tricyclic antidepressants (TCA). Individual therapy will become much difficult because of arising of dizziness, lightheadedness, drowsiness, confusion, constipation, bladder problems, sexual problems, dry mouth, and/or blurred vision. Also cardiovascular complications may arise already in therapeutic doses.

Especially in overdose, such side effects are more serious. A typical pattern is brief excitement and restlessness, sometimes myoclonus, tonic-clonic seizures, or dystonia, followed by rapid development of coma, often with depressed respiration, hypoxia, depressed reflexes, hypothermia, and hypotension. Because TCA have relatively strong antimuscarinic potency, they may commonly induce tachycardia and life-threatening cardiac arrhythmias for several days. Therefore, TCA overdoses are leading to 50% of ICU admissions because of acute intoxication. Mortality amounts to 2-3% under intensive medical care [1] but may increase to 15% in severe intoxication [17]. But not all patients are ariving the hospital alive. Because cardiac toxicity and hypotension may become suddenly much difficult, TCA-intoxicated patients require an early and close medical supervision [18]. Comparatively, the use of the newer selective serotonin reuptake inhibitors (SSRI) is suggested to be safer [19].

3. Depression, Antidepressant Therapy and Autonomic Nervous System - Association with Cardiac Disorders

Although depressive disorders are typically associated with an incidence of cardiovascular impairments [8,9], it is not known whether joint pathophysiological dysregulations are reponsible for. Discussed are autonomic dysregulations and proinflammatory or coagulatory processes [20,21]. But there is increasing evidence that the actual function of autonomic nervous system has prognostic relevance in cardiologic as well as in psychiatric diseases. Thus, depressive disorders are associated with an impairment of autonomic tone by simultaneously existing sympathetic predominance [3]. Similar constellations after myocardial infarction are leading to increased mortality [2].

The disease dependent changes of vegetative function are further negative influenced because the agents used in therapy are additionally diminishing the autonomic nervous sytem [22]. This is chiefly relevant in classic TCA. Because these agents are exerting greater anticholinergic effects than SSRI it is commonly suggested that TCA also are providing a greater cardiovascular risk. This was shown e.g. by nortriptyline in comparison with paroxetine [23]. But the question whether SSRI should be generally preferred is not yet verified scientificly [8,24]. Common side effects of SSRI are sexual problems, headache, nausea, nervousness, insomnia and agitation. Moreover some sporadic case reports of cardiovascular side effects exist under SSRI [25].

With regard to development of cardiovascular complications many publications have shown that a strongly diminished modulation of sympathetic and parasympathetic activity is leading to an unstable and therefore vulnerable status of central influencing the cardiac autonomic regulation [4]. If the suppression is additionally dysbalanced, i.e. there is a sympathetic or vagal predominance, supraventricular or ventricular arrhythmias may develop more frequently, especially if those changes would appear abruptly [26,27]. Such changes are associated with a greater incidence of sudden cardiac death [5]. Further is reported that the level of sympathetic activity is connected with better or poorer outcome in dependence of its duration [28]. In another paper the level of vagal activity is responsible for the brain-derived anti-inflammatory response [29]. This could be extensively important for comorbidity [30].

4. Autonomic Nervous System, Heart Rate Variability (HRV) and Prognosis - Principles of HRV

The autonomic nervous system plays an integrating role in the maintenance of hemodynamic stability and secures for internal homeostase by regulating the cardiovascular, gastrointestinal, urogenital, exocrine/endocrine, and pupillomotoric functions. These vegetative modulations are central controlled by diverse reflex interactions. On the level of sinus node, sympathetic and parasympathetic nervous tone is modulating the intrinsic pacemaker of the heart. Clinical relevance of reduction of parasympathetic and increase of sympathetic nervous system activity is lowering the threshold for myocardial ischemia and ventricular arrhythmias. This increases sudden cardiac death in patients with coronary heart disease or heart failure [31,32]. Regarding to outcome, low HRV has shown to predict mortality in patients with recent myocardial infarction or with stable coronary disease [6].

The cardiac vegetative function could not be estimated by simple heart rate measurement because sympathicus and parasympathicus are counteracting. If the functional status of cardiac nervous systym should be defined differentially, nowadays the analysis of heart rate variability (HRV) is suitable because of good reliability and validity. This method serves as a noninvasive instrument for measuring heart-brain interactions and autonomic nervous system dynamics [7]. The results are not only reflecting the vegetative activity in general but also are able to differentiate between sympathetic and parasympathetic activation or desactivation, respectively (see Figure 1). In spectral analysis of HRV, the LF/HF ratio is an effecient mean for detecting of autonomic dysbalance. But we have to consider that parts of power spectrum do not obey linear rules. Therefore, the LF/HF ratio is problematic in defining the sympathovagal balance over the complete range of measured values.

5. Depression, Antidepressant Therapy and Heart Rate Variability - Synopsis of the Literature

Because safety of patients has become more important regarding to progress in technical medicine and decreased HRV may not the reason but a valid indicator of an elevated mortality, analysis of HRV is used for risk stratification in cardiology [33] and diabetology [34]. In contrast, HRV analysis is not introduced in routine monitoring of antidepressant therapy. Mainly single investigations [35,36] and less comparative studies were performed [37] until now. Reflections to plasma concentrations [38,39] or clinical correlates [40] are scarce. Further the results were received by distinct methodical variations.

But independently to methodical differences, until now it can be concluded that depressive disorders are associated with a diminished HRV *per se*. Especially, the high frequency components of power spectrum activity are impaired [22]. These additional anticholinergic effects that occurred in TCA use [10,11] are attributed to a greater incidence of arrhythmias and sudden cardiac death particularly in older patients [12]. In contrast, the reduction of autonomic function is significantly less expressed by SSRI [13].

Thus, not only a greater diminution in high frequent component of HRV was seen under nortriptyline than under paroxetine [14], but also a reduction in the middle part of spectral analysis that is more in accordance to a depressed sympathetic tone [41].

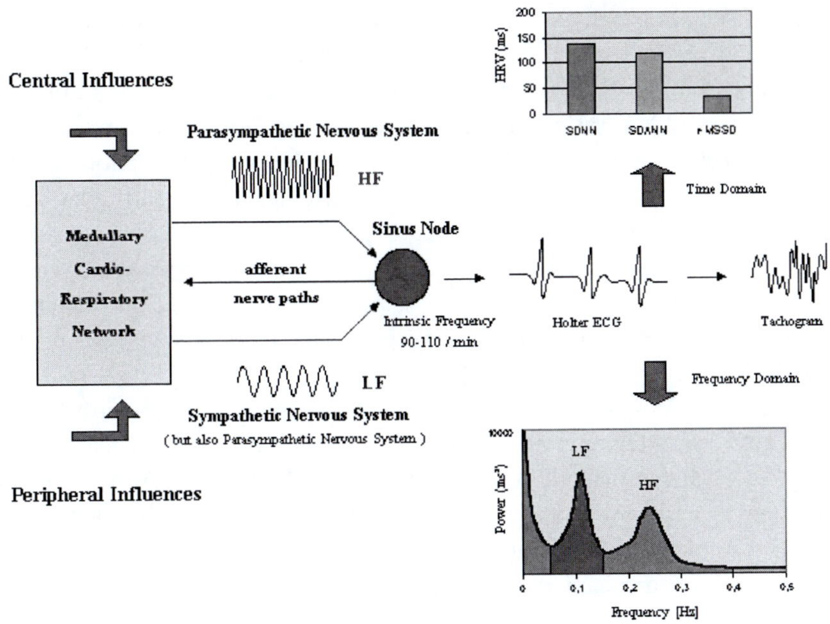

Figure 1. Influences on heart rate modulation in the sinus node.

Similarly, such signs of central sympathicolysis were seen under imipramine more than under mirtazepine [42].

Several studies in depressed patients have shown that all heart rate variability components will be deminished by TCA [43]. Conversely, no significant effects were seen in patients treated with SSRI [23]. Parallel to better acceptance of paroxetine [44] after 14 days significant changes in HRV were seen under amitriptyline and doxepin but not under paroxetine and fluvoxamine [37]. Similar holds for the comparison imipramine vs. fluoxamine [22]. Paroxetine normalized the HRV in patients with depression and anxiety disorders in contrast to TCA [45]. Venlafaxine as a combined serotonin-norepinephrine reuptake inhibitor showed a stronger HRV reduction than paroxetine, markedly of vagus describing parts [46]. Reboxetine as a selective norepinephrine reuptake inhibitor showed a significant decrease in absolute and relative low-frequency power and a significant decrease in the LF/HF ratio when patients with major depression were investigated [36]. But in healthy subjects, reboxetine revealed more reduction in HF Power [39]. Sertaline has positive effects on HRV but especially in the lower frequent components [47]. These differences may explain that the spectrum of side effects is dependent on the agent [48] and is further leading to different cardiotoxicity [49] and mortality [19]. The less influenced vagus in SSRI therapy is thought to be responsible for cardioprotection [14].

6. Intoxication with Antidepressant Drugs – Mechanisms of Cardiac Impairment

The alteration of many organ systems by TCA intoxication can be explained by the widespread working spectrum of those agents. In cases of less intoxication, the anticholinergic caused sinustachycardia is often the sole symptom. But in severe intoxication additionaly a strong cardiotoxicity occurred that is responsible for possibly fatal outcome [50,51]. Dependent from the dose of TCA, a quininine-like effect prevails in the membranes by inhibitioning the rapid Na^+ influx in the phase-0 depolarisation of the myocardium [52,53]. This causes myocardial conduction delays (seen on ECG as prolongation of PR and QRS duration), bradyarrhythmia and asystole, supraventricular and ventricular dysrhythmias, decreased cardiac output by decreased myocardial contractility, hypotension and therefore decreased coronary perfusion [53,54]. Further, TCA are inhibiting the cardiac rapidly activating delayed rectifier K^+ current (IKr) seen on ECG as QTc prolongation [55]. By inhibition of GABA-A receptor chloride uptake generalized convulsive seizures were seen in TCA overdose [56].

But the toxicity of TCA is not only due to these effects but also to antihistaminic effects, inhibition of neurotransmitter reuptake at central synaptic terminals, α_1-adrenergic blockade, and inhibition of central sympathetic reflexes [57]. The affinity of TCA on α_2-receptors is less expressed but may be relevant in toxic doses [58]. But autoreceptor interactions also reduce the synthesis of norepinephrine through the rate-limiting step at tyrosine hydroxylase [59]. These negative-feedback mechanisms are rapidely activated on TCA application but not on fluoxetine application [60].

Independently from direct TCA effects on α_1-receptors (blockade) and on myocardial contractility (depression), blood pressure may be tendentially elevated in the beginning because of an increased release of catecholamines. But in time course a lower blood pressure can be expected in the conception of an inadequate new synthesis of norepinephrine [61,62]. This later occurrence of diminished sympathetic activity may be also explained by an increased excitation of presynaptic α_2-receptors followed by prolonged resorption or redistribution phenomenons. Overall, the heart rate itself is less centrally reflectory modulated in the idea of total functional impairment and obtained a level that is reflecting the intrinsic frequency of sinus node. These complex and ultimately not completely understood findings as well as the partially contrary results on HRV in therapeutic doses induced us to further research on HRV in toxic plasma concentrations [63,64].

7. Changes of Heart Rate Variability in TCA Intoxication - Detailed Information on Doxepin

So far only reports are published that TCA in overdose can be detected [65] and that the severity of intoxication can be estimated by HRV analysis [38]. This is confirmed by our results. Moreover, by comparison of critical TCA vs. critical non-TCA intoxication (see Figure 2, **A**: f, 38 years, TCA intoxication with 2.5g trimipramine, .85mg/L plasma vs. **B** f, 31 years, mixed intoxication without special agent identification, Triage® test: TCA negative) could be shown (1) that heart rate in trimipramine intoxication has little changed within the first 24 h (narrow histogram as a sign of a widespread rigidity of frequency), (2) that the SDNN as a global HRV parameter is more reduced under trimipramine, and (3) that more cardiac arrhythmias occurred under trimipramine.

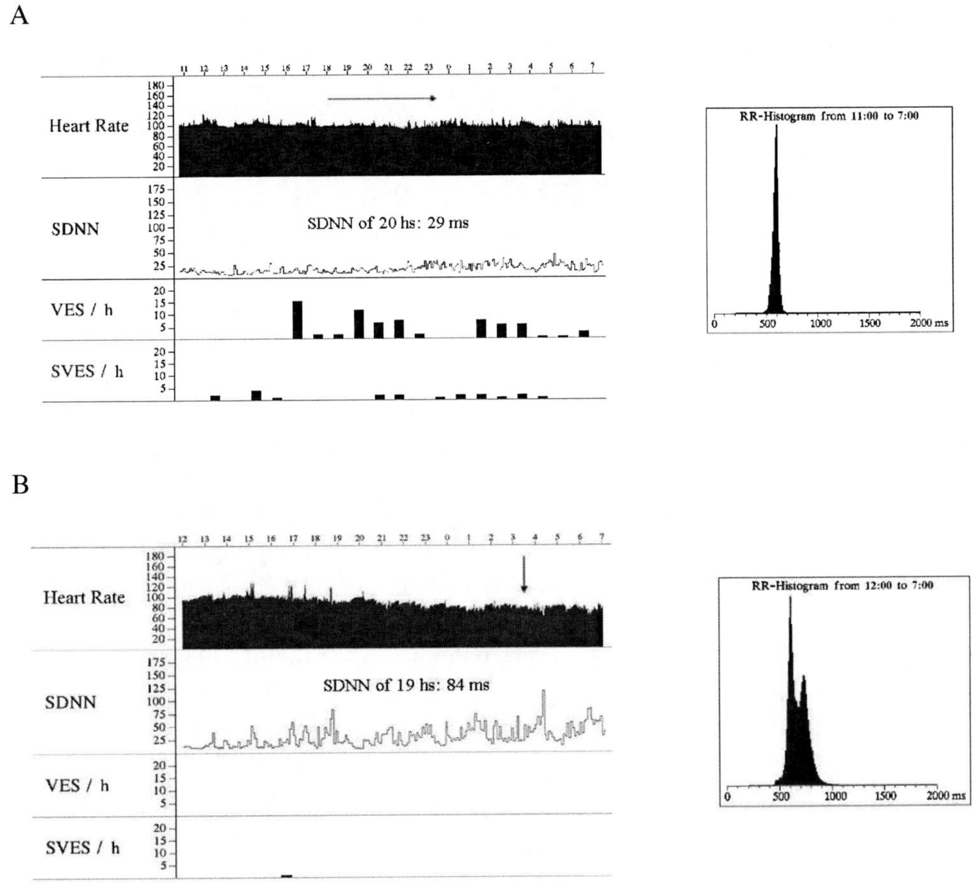

Figure 2. Comparison of two cases of critical drug intoxication (A: f, 38 years, TCA intoxication with 2.5g trimipramine, 0.85mg/L plasma vs. B f, 31 years, mixed intoxication on tablets without agent identification, [illegible])

Likewise, Waring et al. found a reduction of HRV in overdoses of antidepressive drugs in comparison to paracetamol intoxication [66]. This reduction revealed a *relative* increase of spectral HRV components that are more attributed to sympathetic activity (increase of LFnu). The possible coherence of changes in HRV and occurrence of cardiac arrhythmias is mentioned. But firstly, TCA intoxication (amitriptyline) amounts in the study only to 12.5%. Most evaluations (62.5%) are related to the group of SSRI which are reflecting less influences on HRV and certainly a lower potential for cardiovascular complications [67]. Secondly, in 19.4% of the cases also an intake of alcohol took part whereby a parasympathetic decrease can be explained by itself [68]. Thirdly, no graduation to severity of intoxication (plasma concentration, level of consciousness etc.) was performed. Because even the effects on receptors are different in dependence on individual antidepressant agent [69,70], we must also consider that the effects on autonomic function and therefore on HRV can be substance specificly different. An evaluation in general can only serve as a trend.

For not receiving of mixed results we restricted our investigation on pure doxepin intoxication [64], especially because clinical disorders are less severe under doxepin than under e.g. amitriptyline [19,71]. But only 10 patients could be included into the study because

TCA intoxication mostly occurred in suicidal intention and therefore much often mixed intoxication is present. By careful selection, we got 10 patients in that the effects could be mainly referred to doxepin overdoses with justification.

There is evidence that severe impairments of autonomic functions happened by doxepin in plasma concentrations with more than 500 mg/L due to its narrow therapeutic width [72]. In our performed investigation, the plasma concentration counts from 0.54 to 1.8 mg/L [64]. The reduction of HRV was dose dependent and the minimum of HRV was found in 5.4±2.2 h (2-9 h) after ICU admission, i.e. in that period of time that is mentioned to be associated with greatest risk when patients died within 24 h after admission [73]. At this moment HRV was reduced in all parts of frequency domain. On consideration of concentration dependent coherences, it can be concluded that parasympathetic parts are more reduced in moderate intoxication. But with increasing concentration are additionally more parts involved that are at least more attributed to sympathetic tone. This pattern was also seen under nortriptyline [41]. In accordance is published that higher concentrations of TCA greatly reduce or abolish the rate and force of beating in the presence of isoprenaline [74]. Furthermore, the data can be interpreted that doxepin in toxic doses works in the sense of a total blockade, i.e. as it can be expected by simultaneous application of atropin and a ß blocker [75]. Whether this holds true for all TCA must be confirmed.

According to HRV influences, the direct membrane stabilizing quinidine-like effect is evidently associated with a reduction of cardiac sympathetic activity and a reduction of LF Power [76,77]. Based on the complex profile of TCA effects, it is also possible that sympathetic activity may be reduced by an elevated serotonin level [78]. The importance of diminution of HRV in the LF Power band is underlined by some investigations that have shown that this is associated with an increased incidence of malignant arrhythmias [79-81]. But because the spectral LF component is sympathetic and parasympathetic influenced, the question is unanswered whether the mortality risk is more due to a total blockade or more due to a central sympatheticolysis. Also possible saturation effects must be considered [79].

Because the maximal occurrence of cardiac arrhythmias in our study is not connected with minimal HRV, the assumption is confirmed that highest risk for mortality should be more attributed to a direct myocardial depression than to arrhythmic events [82]. The reduction of myocardial contractility is depedent on ingested doses but works independently from effects on the cardiac conduction system [83]. Thus, widening of QRS complex and excessive prolongation of QTc interval are described [17] but their importance for risk stratification remains controversial [18,84].

8. Risk Of Higher Incidence of Arrhythmic Events in Doxepin Overdose – Differentiation of HRV Minimum and LF/HF Increase

The accumulated occurrence of tachyarrhythmias must be probably differentiated from the state of maximal autonomic impairment. This should be expected because in former studies arrhythmias in severe intoxication occurred in dependence on plasma levels more often and more aggravating [17] but also comparatively later [85]. Likewise in our investigation, the interval of preferred occurrence of arrhythmic events was not identical with the interval of measured HRV minimum in which most danger to life is suggested. Therefore we must assume that the reason for development of cardiovascular complications is clearly phase dependent. Also tachyarrhythmias can be dangerous but they are not prevailing in the beginning of therapy even when severest intoxication is concerned.

The initial condition of cardiac depression exists indepently from effects on the conduction system [83] and is associated with the tendency for bradycardia and asystole. These possibly fatal complications can be prevented by high therapeutical Na^+ levels [86] that certainly mainly led to the decrease of mortality in the last years if patients were early admitted to intensive care. But the mass of tachycardial arrhythmias certainly occur with some delay. In this, also their reduction as well as the reduction of conduction disturbences should be followed by an application of Na^+ [87]. The prolongation of arrhythmia incidence seems to be due to the profile of recovery of autonomic nervous system. That seems to be also dependent on plasma concentration because the in severe intoxication acutly more sympathetic depressed autonomic nervous system recovers better than the parasympathetic part. The retardation in normalization of vagal activity is leading to sympathetic predominance especially in severe intoxication. This could be the basis for later occurrence of tachycardial arrhythmias [5,63]. But there also reports that arrhythmogenesis will be more facilitated by change in the dynamics of R-R intervals rather than by the direction of change [26,88].

As is shown for example in Figure 3 (m, 37 years, intoxication with 6g doxepin, plasma concentration 1.7 mg/L, QTc 130% and QRS 135ms after 4h ICU stay), the autonomic function demonstrated by HRV analysis was still impaired after two days. In comparison to reference values of the Task Force [7] only values in %-dimension were found although we must consider that HRV in frequncy domain obeys notlinear rules and HRV impairment is *relatively* more expressed in low toxic state. Further, a sympathetic predominance (LF/HF: 9.14) has developed from the lowest level of autonomic nervous system function with vagal predominance (LF/HF: 0.11). On that basis (low HRV and change of sympathovagal balance) occurred many self-limitating arrhythmias in time course, but a clear relation of 1-hour LF/HF value and size of arrhythmias was not found. Because after 18 h QTc and QRS intervals had already widely normalized (QTc 116% and QRS 112 ms), it can be assumed that these parameters may have predictive value in the beginning of therapy, but they are certainly less responsible for the immediate development of tachycardial arrhythmias. Blood pressure has increased since the moment of maximal HRV suppression from 100/60 to 125/65 mmHg, and heart rate has decreased from 120 to 105/min.

9. Arrhythmic Events and Sympathovagal Balance - Correlation of Arrhythmic Incidence and LF/HF Increase

On the evidence from the literature might be considered that three sets of conditions contribute to the occurrence of arrhythmias in TCA treated patients: (1) deterioration of autonomic nervous system due to a chronic intense psychological state (2) myocardial electrical instability due to cardiac disease and/or medication, and (3) an acute triggering event like mental stress.

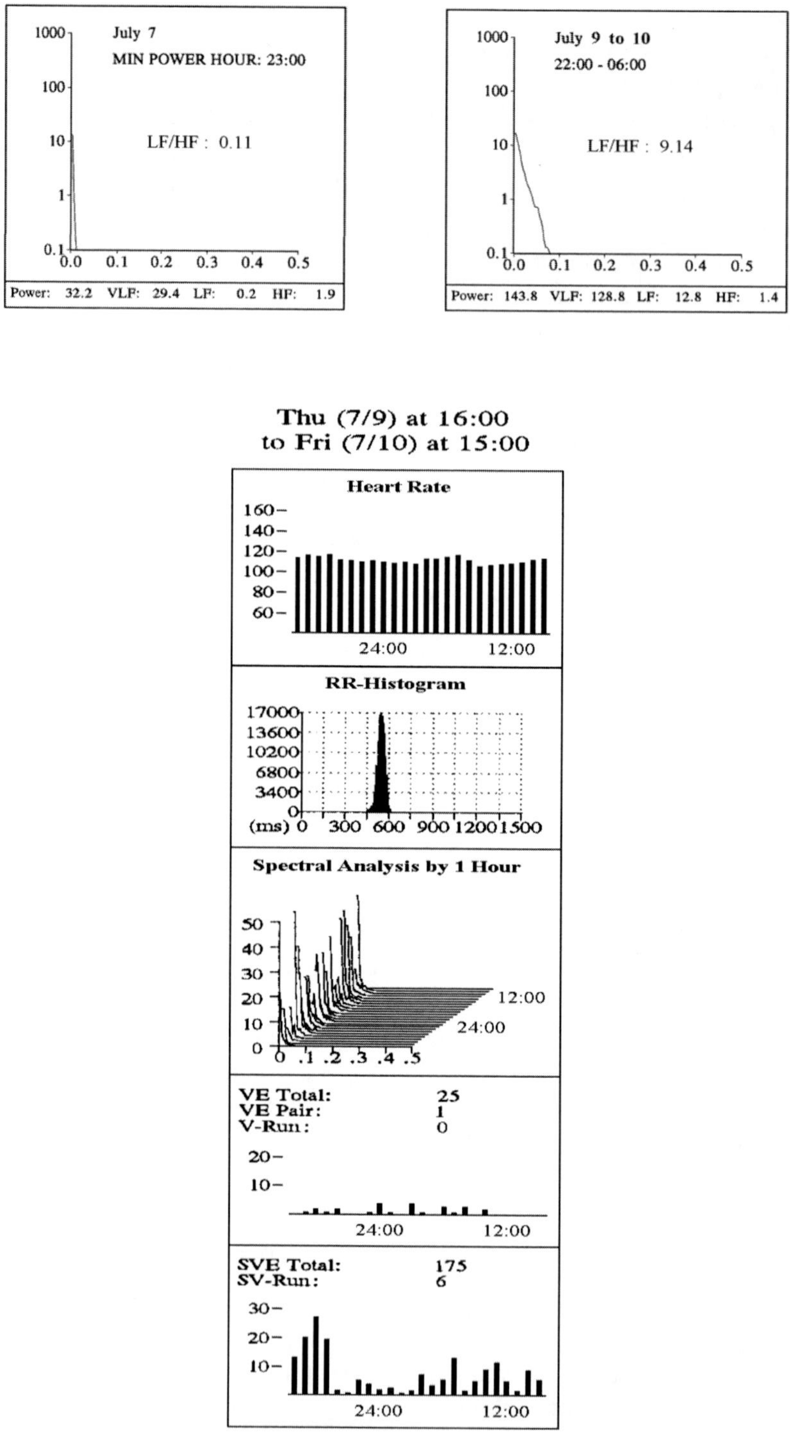

Figure 3. Development of self-limitating arrhythmias in low HRV and increased LF/HF ratio after two days related to ICU admission (m, 37 years, intoxication with 6g doxepin, plasma concentration 1.7 mg/L, QTc 130% and QRS 135ms after 4h ICU stay).

In this, patients with greatest changes in cardiac neural regulation demonstrated by decreased parasympathetic tone coupled with sympathetic predominance are thought to be at greatest risk for developing arrhythmias [45,89].

Related to our investigated patients [64], the subsequent evaluation of data revealed a similar but differentiated association between arrhythmia incidence and LF/HF ratio in the sense of an imaginable correlation (see Table 1). Based on our data of only 10 patients it can be assumed that the absolute level LF/HF ratio will not precisely predict the occurrence of arrhythmic events, but rather more the dynamics of change from relative vagal predominance (HRV minimum) to sympathetic predominance (48 h after ICU admission).

Table 1. Spearman Correlation of quantitity of arrhythmias with initial doxepin concentration, ECG parameters, and sympathovagal balance in HRV

1st Parameter	2nd Parameter	Spearman Correlation (r_S)	p
Supraventricular Arrhythmias (n/48h)	Initial Doxepin Concentration	.685	.029
Ventricular Arrhythmias (n/48h)	Initial Doxepin Concentration	.555	.096
All Arrhythmias (n/48h)	Initial Doxepin Concentration	.745	.013
All Arrhythmias (n/48h)	Initial QT_c Interval	.800	.005
All Arrhythmias (n/48h)	Initial QRS Interval	.506	>.1
All Arrhythmias (n/48h)	Total Power in HRV Minimum (=HRV Min)	-.333	>.1
All Arrhythmias (n/48h)	LF/HF in HRV Min	.559	.093
All Arrhythmias (n/48h)	LF/HF in Arrhythmia Maximum	.079	>.5
All Arrhythmias (n/48h)	LF/HF after 48h	.782	.008
All Arrhythmias (n/48h)	LF/HF after 48hs / LF/HF in HRV Min	.855	.002
Supraventricular Arrhythmias (n/48h)	LF/HF after 48hs / LF/HF in HRV Min	.806	.005
Ventricular Arrhythmias (n/48h)	LF/HF after 48hs / LF/HF in HRV Min	.781	.008
All Arrhythmias (n/48h)	logLF / logHF after 48hs / 1+logLF / 1+logHF in HRV Min	.952	<.001

These preliminary results could mean that not the sympathovagal balance itself may serve as a valid predictor for supraventricular and ventricular arrhythmias but rather the extent of autonomic counter action. That the evaluation of dynamics in relation to basic level may lead to better estimation is so far not surprising as the chosen difference is considering both the vulnerable substrate in the beginning (HRV minimum with vagal predominance) and the afterwards dysharmonic recovery (retarded normalization of vagal tone leading to sympathetic predominance). That the happened changes of HRV should be due to incidence of arrhythmias is in accordance with the results of Shusterman et al. [88]. But because of little patient size this result must be confirmed, especially the question whether raw data regarding to possible clinical relevance should be transformed into logarithms.

10. HRV Analysis in Time Course and Phase Dependent Side Effects – Changes of Blood Pressure and Heart Rate in Relation To HRV

The results of HRV analysis can well explain that a simple description of complications after TCA overdose may lead to controversial conclusions when there is no specification to period of time. Also is plausible that older depressive patients are markedly endangered because autonomic function is already reduced with growing age in general [11].

Table 2. Changes of blood pressure and heart rate from admission to 48h later in all 10 patients (.54 –1.8 mg /L doxepin in plasma) and correlation at HRV Minimum

	Admission	p	HRV Minimum	p	48 h
Systolic Blood Pressure [mmHg]	128 ± 14	.044	117 ± 13	.007	131 ± 13
Diastolic Blood Pressure [mmHg]	68 ± 8	>.1	65 ± 10	.066	74 ± 8
Heart Rate [1/min]	93 ± 15	>.1	97 ± 17	.069	88 ± 10

HRV Minimum		Spearman Correlation (r_S)	p
Systolic Blood Pressure	LF/HF	.641	.046
Systolic Blood Pressure	1+logLF / 1+log HF	.732	.016

Especially hypotension is a serious manifestation of TCA overdose. In this, several mechanisms as central or peripheral α-receptor blockade and depressed myocardial contractility by quinidinelike action may be involved [90,91]. Based on an α_1-adrenergic blockade typically orthostatic hypotension may arise [92]. But there are especially patients with sympathetic predominance and already existing vasoconstriction endangered that is relevant in heart failure [93]. This appearent discrepancy could be dissolved on our results. At least in doxepin intoxication the lowest systolic blood pressure was seen when HRV and LF/HF ratio were also most reduced [64]. A higher blood pressure was measured only in time course and not before sympathetic recovery took place (see Table 2). These findings are in accordance to former studies [94]. Simultaneuosly, heart rate after ICU admission stayed near assumed intrinsic frequency and decreased parallel to recovery of HRV.

11. Methodical Limitations of HRV - Partially Contrary Results Caused by the Lack of Consensus

Regarding to methods of HRV analysis it must be remembered that not only the evaluation of averaged 1-hour values based on 5-min intervals should be performed but also the illustration of genuine 5-min recordings in form of a trend (despite increased susceptibility to disturbances). Such illustration is important because the balance of sympathetic and vagal activity may change abruptly in conditions in that autonomic nervous system is severely impaired in general. Therefore, an averaging 1-hour value may mask the constellation which is responsible for triggering of arrhythmia. But unfortunately the more precise presentation of trend is not available by the used HRV software "Cardiovision" (MTM, Germany). Conversly, by using the system "Elatec" (ELA Medical, Germany) a trend presentation is possible, but instead of this, no online analysis is possible. Thus, an optimation of systems and a consensus in methods are necessary for achieving of valid and comparable results [67].

Further must be remarked that the already performed studies on HRV and antidepressants have focussed on different collectives, (1) healthy subjects [39,95], (2) major depressive disorder [42,47], and (3) panic disorder [96,97]. But we can assume with justification that in all groups of patients especially the tricyclic antidepressants are influencing the cardiac autonomic nervous system. Because these patients are certainly impaired by their diseases themselves, the therapy with antidepressants may increase the cardiac risk additionally [98]. For not discrediting the HRV analysis as a suitable method in risk stratification, a particular carefullness is necessary in valuation of received data. E.g. LF Power and LF (nu) Power should not simplified be used synonymously [66], because the LF Power describes the activity in absolute amount whereas the normalized LF Power offers relative information about the balance that is widely equivalent to LF/HF ratio. By this consideration, the findings of Waring et al. [66] are not in contrast to our results.

12. HRV Analysis in Antidepressant Therapy – Importance and Perspectives

Until now it can be assumed that results by HRV analysis may provide additional information in risk stratification of particularly endangered patients. There is much evidence that impairment of autonomic function is more pronounced in classic TCA than in newer SSRI. Especially the vagal parts are stronger diminished by TCA already in therapeutic doses. This is leading to sympathetic predominance that is probably responsible for elevating blood pressure and for greater incidence of arrhythmias. In overdose, this is added by a reduction of rather sympathetic activity describing components of HRV – at least in doxepin.

In life-threatening intoxication it may be important in practice that determination of plasma concentration is not always available or even not timely available. Therefore, it may be helpful that the status of autonomic function can be actually estimated by online HRV analysis. Until now, the usually determined ECG parameters like QTc and QRS duration are typically prolonged at admission, but they normalized widely within 48 h. In contrast, parameters of HRV remain always strongly reduced after 48 h. Further could be shown that the recovery of rather sympathetic components is preferred in comparison to vagal components. We can suggest that this change in sympathovagal balance is responsible for greater incidence of arrhythmias. Whether the therapy in intoxication should also lead to only little alteration, i.e. to an only slowly increase of LF/HF ratio, is in question and can only supposed until now. But our results are able to explain that the use of physostigmine or ß blockers can be problematic in the first phase of TCA intoxication [99]. But ß blockers may perhaps offer some advantages [13] in sympathetic predominance that can hold on for weeks when TCA are withdrawn [100].

Because the biochemical profiles of single TCA are differing from each other [101] it can be expected that the impairment of autonomic functions is not only existent between drug classes [37,39] but also in little extent within the single agent groups. What position selective norepinephrine reuptake inhibitors and combined serotonin-norepinephrine reuptake inhibitors are occupying in comparison to TCA and SSRI is not clear and must be investigated. Whereas in toxication with doxepin clear level dependent effects were found that seemed to be independent from individual basic status, it must be expected that the drug effect in therapeutic doses is more overwhelmed by inter- and intraindividual variances [11]. Consequently, the substance specific profile of effects will certainly only evident in relation to starting point because genetic predispositions [102] as well as specific factors like age, enviroment, and lifestyle [103] may contribute.

Based on this realization, new agents should be evaluated regarding to effects on autonomic nervous system in comparison to established drugs already before their permission. A nomination of a reference drug could be advantageous. If cardiac complications should be low as possible in patients treated with antidepressants, clinical studies should be accompanied by a Holter ECG – before and after permission as well. But for adequate analysis of HRV a detailled definition of procedure is needed [104]. In this, the recommendations of Task Force in 1996 [7] should be revised. Especially the reference values have to include age and gender specific influences [11,105]. Whether in studies as well as in therapy control position changes or mild standardized provocations should be addinionally performed can be discussed, if otherwise healthy patients are concerned [42,104].

Only after definition of commonly current regulations and in observance of reliable labor conditions, it can be expected that antidepressant therapy can be objectively valuated by HRV analysis. Further is possible that the use of HRV may yield useful information in therapy response [40,106]. But the results are not consistent and certainly dependent on the used drug. Nevertheless there should be no doubt that HRV measuring is revealing further evidence, this method is not established in therapy monitoring of psychiatric patients. Even in new permissions, e.g. in the combined serotonin-norepinephrine reuptake inhibitor dulexetine, no such data are published despite they can be easily and non-invasively recruited by Holter

ECG. In studies using PK-PD models, HRV analysis could lead to further knowledge [107]. But instead of demonstrating such causal coherences usually still profiles of side effects in comparison to placebo will be examined [108]. A determination to individual conditions before therapy is missed.

But HRV profiles are not only interesting in antidepressive drugs but also in other substances, markedly in antihypertensive and in antidiabetic drugs. This is surely important because patients that are treated with antidepressants are often multimorbid and need a polypharmaceutical treatment. Possibly mortality risk may further rise in such patients because many agents should express more or less influences on autonomic nervous system, e.g. by electrolyte disarrangement, pH change, increase of osmolarity or change in redox balance. A positive effect is known in ß blockers [109] and ACE inhibitors [110]. Impairing effects are also described but the extent should be underestimated because a major publication-bias must be assumed. Thus, a different but relevant drug induced reduction of cholinergic activity was recently shown by using a radioreceptor assay [111]. This means that we have not only to focus on drug induced prolongation of QT interval [112] but also on at least anticholinergic effects [113].

13. Conclusion – HRV for Non-Invasive Improvement of Antidepressant Monitoring

The severity of an antidepressiva overdose can be estimated by HRV measurement because acute changes of cardiac neurovegetative tone are important for prognosis. It can be assumed that parasympathetic components of HRV are more impaired in little doses of TCA than the sympathetic parts [100]. Under the conception that parasympathetic activity plays a guiding role in cardioprotection, an increased mortality in already coronary impaired patients is suggested [114]. Regarding to doxepin, with further increasing concentration also a reduction of more sympathetic defined parts took place. But in recovery, sympathetic HRV components normalized earlier. This change onto sympathetic predominance seems to be responsible for arrhythmia incidence.

The HRV analysis counts as a valid indicator for early detection of neurotoxic impairment. This method is non-invasive and therefore uncritical for the patient and can be principly unrestricted repeated. Because the data of HRV analysis are describing the actual constitution of autonomic nervous system, this method should be used for monitoring of therapy in the future [115]. Further reducing of fatal complications needs (1) determination of autonomic activity in the individual patient and (2) determination of the agent specific profile. If both conditions are known, the therapy can be sufficiently individualized and cardiac complications can be at least reduced.

References

[1] Arranto, C.A.; Mueller, C.; Hunziker, P.R.; Marsch, S.C. and Eriksson, U. (2003) Adverse cardiac events in ICU patients with presumptive antidepressant overdose. *Swiss Med. Wkly, 133,* 479-483

[2] Sandrone, G.; Mortara, A.; Torzillo, D.; La Rovere, M.T.; Malliani, A. and Lombardi, F. (1994) Effects of beta blockers (atenolol or metoprolol) on heart rate variability after acite myocardial infarction. *Am. J. Cardiol., 74,* 340-345

[3] Agelink, M.W.; Boz, C.; Ullrich, H. and Andrich, J. (2002) Relationship between major depession and heart rate variability. Clinical consequences and implications for antidepressive tratment. *Psychiatry Res., 15,* 130-149

[4] Hartikainen, J.E.; Malik, M.; Staunton, A.; Poloniecki, J. and Camm, A.J. (1996) Distinction between arrhythmic and nonarrhythmic death after acute myocardial infarction based on heart rate variability, signal-averaged electrocardiogram, ventricular arrhythmias and left ventricular ejection fraction. *J. Am. Coll Cardiol., 28,* 296-304

[5] Brembilla-Perrot, B.; Ross, M.; Jacquemin, L.; Beurrier, D. Houplon, P. and Danchin, N. (1997) Analysis of heart rate variability before and at the moment of cardiac death. *Arch. Mal. Cœur. Vaiss, 90,* 1477-1484

[6] Rich, M.W.; Saini, J.S.; Kleiger, R.E.; Carney, R.M.; teVelde, A. and Freedland, K.E. (1988) Correlation of heart rate variability with clinical and angiographic variables and late mortality after coronary angiography. *Am. J. Cardiol., 62,* 714-717

[7] Task Force of the European Society of Cardiology and the North American Society of Pacing and Electrophysiology (1996) Heart rate variability: standards of measurement, physiological interpretation and clinical use. *Circulation, 93,* 1043-1065

[8] Bounhoure, J.P.; Galinier, M.; Curnier, D.; Bousquet, M. and Bes, A. (2006) Influence of depression on the prognosis of cardiovascular diseases. *Bull. Acad. Natl. Med., 190,* 1723-1731

[9] Norra, C.; Skobel, E.C.; Arndt, M. and Schauerte, P. (2008) High impact of depression in heart failure: early diagnosis and treatment options. *Int. J. Cardiol., 125,* 220-231

[10] Mezzacappa, E.; Steingard, R.; Kindlon, D.; Saul, J.P. and Earls, F. (1998) Tricyclic antidepressants and cardiac autonomic control in children and adolescents. *J. Am. Acad. Child Adolesc. Psychiatry, 37,* 52-59

[11] Lehofer, M.; Moser, M.; Hoehn-Saric, R.; McLoad, D.; Hildebrandt, G.; Egner, S.; Steinbrenne, B.; Liebmann, P. and Zapotoczky, H.G. (1999) Influence of age on the parasympatholytic property of tricyclic antidepressants. *Psychiatry Res., 85,* 199-207

[12] Penttilä, J.; Scheinin, H. and Syvälahti, E. (2005) Measurement of anticholinergic effects of psychotropic drugs in humans. *Pharmacopsychiatry, 38,* 187-193

[13] Carney, R.M.; Freedland, K.E. and Veith R.C. (2005) Depression, the autonomic nervous system, and coronary heart disease. *Psychosom Med, 67 (Suppl 1),* S29-S33

[14] Yeragani, V.K.; Pesce, V.; Jayaraman, A. and Roose, S. (2002) Major depression with ischemic heart disease: effects of paroxetine and nortriptyline on long-term heart rate variability measures. *Biol. Psychiatry, 52,* 418-429

[15] Yildiz, A.; Gönül, A.S. and Tamam, L. (2002) Mechanisms of actions of antidepressants: Beyond the receptors. *Bull. Clin. Psychopharmacol., 12,* 194-200

[16] Glauser, J. (2000) Tricyclic antidepressant poisoning. *Cleve Clin J Med, 6,* 704-719

[17] Maitra, R.T.; Koniczek, K.H. and Cyran, J. (1999) Klinisches Erscheinungsbild und therapeutisches Management der schweren Intoxikation mit trizyklischen Antidepressiva. *Intensivmed, 36,* 462-466

[18] Boehnert, M.T.and Lovejoy, F.H. Jr. (1985). Value of the QRS duration versus the serum drug level in predicting seizures and ventricular arrhythmias after an acute overdose of tricyclic antidepressants. *N. Engl. J. Med., 313,* 474-479

[19] Buckley, N.A. and McManus, P.R. (2002) Fatal toxicity of serotoninergic and other antidepressant drugs: analysis of United Kingdom mortality data. *BMJ, 325,* 1332-1333

[20] Carney R.M.; Freedland, K.E.; Stein, P.K.; Miller, G.E.; Steinmeyer, B.; Rich, M.W. and Duntley, S.P. (2007) Heart rate variability and markers of inflammation and coagulation in depressed patients with coronary heart disease. *J. Psychosom. Res., 62,* 463-467

[21] Frasure-Smith, N.; Lespérance, F.; Irwin, M.R.; Talajic, M. and Pollock, B.G. The relationships among heart rate variability, inflammatory markers and depression in coronary heart disease patients. *Brain Behav. Immun.,* [online] 2009 Jul 25

[22] Volkers, A.C.; Tulen, J.H.; van den Broek, W.W.; Bruyn, J.A.; Passchier, J. and Pepplinkhuizen, L. (2004) Effects of imipramine, fluoxamine and depressive mood on autonomic cardiac functioning in major depressive order. *Pharmacopsychiatry, 37,* 18-25

[23] Roose, S.P.; Laghrissi-Thode, F.; Kennedy, J.S.; Nelson, J.C.; Bigger, J.T. Jr.; Pollock, B.G.; Gaffney, A.; Narayan, M.; Finkel, M.S.; McCafferty, J. and Gergel, I. (1998) Comparison of paroxetine and nortriptyline in depressed patients with ischemic heart disease. *JAMA, 279,* 287-291

[24] Guaiana, G.; Barbui, C. and Hotopf, M. (2007) Amitriptyline for depression. *Cochrane Database Syst. Rev.,* CD004186

[25] Erfurth, A.; Loew, M.; Dobmeier, P. and Wendler, G. (1998) EKG-Veränderungen nach Paroxetin. *Nervenarzt, 69,* 629-631

[26] Lombardi, F.; Tarricone, D.; Tundo, F.; Colombo, F.; Belletti, S. and Fiorentini, C. (2004) Autonomic nervous system and paroxysmal atrial fibrillation: a study based on the analysis of RR interval changes before, during and after paroxysmal atrial fibrillation. *Eur. Heart J., 25,* 1242-1248

[27] Fei, L.; Statters, D.J.; Hnatkova, K.; Poloniecki, J.; Malik, M. and Camm A.J. (1994) Change of autonomic influence on the heart immediately before the onset of spontaneous idiopathic ventricular tachycardia. *J. Am. Coll. Cardiol., 24,* 1515-1522

[28] Triposkiadis, F.; Karayannis, G.; Giamouzis, G.; Skoularigis, J.; Louridas, G. and Butler, J. (2009) The sympathetic nervous system in heart failure. Physiology, pathophysiology, and clinical implications. *J. Am. Coll. Cardiol., 54,* 1747-1762

[29] Pavlov, V.A.; Wang, H.; Czura, C.J.; Friedman, S.G. and Tracey, K.J. (2003) The cholinergic anti-inflammatory pathway: a missing link in neuroimmunomodulation. *Molecular Medicine, 9,* 125-134

[30] Haensel, A.; Mills, P.J.; Nelesen, R.A.; Ziegler, M.G. and Dimsdale, J.E. (2008) The relationship between heart rate variability and inflammatory markers in cardiovascular diseases. *Psychoneuroendocrinology, 33,* 1305-1312

[31] Schwartz, P.J. and Vanoli, E. (1981) Cardiac arrhythmias elicated by interaction between acute myocardial ischemia and sympathetic hyperactivity: a new experimental model for the study of antiarrhythmic drugs. *J. Cardiovac. Pharmacol., 3,* 1251-1259

[32] Behling, A.; Moraes, R.S.; Rohde, L.E.; Ferlin, E.L.; Nobrega, A.C. and Ribeiro, J.P. (2003) Cholinergic stimulation with pyridostigmine reduces ventricular arrythmia and enhances heart rate variability in heart failure. *Am. Heart J., 146,* 494-500

[33] La Rovere, M.T.; Pinna, G.D.; Hohnloser, S.H.; Marcus, F.I.; Mortara, A.; Nohara, R.; Bigger, J.T. Jr.; Camm, A.J. and Schwartz, P.J.; ATRAMI Investigators (2001) Baroreflex sensitivity and heart rate variability in the identification of patients at risk

for life-threatening arrhythmias: implications for clinical trials. *Circulation, 103,* 2072-2077

[34] Schroeder, E.B.; Chambless, L.E.; Liao, D.; Prineas, R.J.; Evans, G.W.; Rosamond, W.D. and Heiss, G. (2005) Diabetes, glucose, insulin, and heart rate variability: the Atherosclerosis Risk in Communities (ARIC) study. *Diabetes Care, 28,* 668-674

[35] Yeragani, V.K.; Jampala, V.C.; Sobelewski, E.; Kay, J. and Igel, G. (1999) Effects of paroxetine on heart period variability in patients with panic disorder: A dtudy on holter ECG records. *Neuropsychobiology, 40,* 124-128

[36] Agelink, M.W.; Ullrich, H.; Baumann, B.; Strum, S. and Majewski, T. (2002) Effects of reboxitine, a selective norepinephrine reuptake inhibitor, on sympathetic and parasympathetic outflow to the heart: preliminary data. *Psychopharmacololgy (Berl), 163,* 151-156

[37] Rechlin, T. (1994) The effects of amitriptyline, doxepin, fluoxamine, and paroxetine treatment on heart rate variability. *J. Clin. Psychopharmacol, 14,* 392-395

[38] Rechlin, T. (1995) Effects of psychopharmacologic therapy on heart rate variation. Nervenarzt, 66, 678-685

[39] Penttilä, J.; Syvälahti, E.; Hinkka, S.; Kuusela, T. and Scheinin, H. (2001) The effects of amitriptyline, citaprolam and reboxitine on autonomic nervous system. A randomised placebo-controlled study on healthy volunteers. *Psychopharmacology (Berl), 154,* 343-349

[40] Khaykin, Y.; Dorian, P.; Baker, B.; Shapiro, C.; Sandor, P.; Mironov, D.; Irvine, J. and Newman, D. (1998) Autonomic correlates of antidepressant treatment using heart rate variability analysis. *Can. J. Psychiatry, 43,* 183-186

[41] Veragani, V.K.; Srinivasan, K.; Pohl, R.; Berger, R.; Balon, R. and Ramesh, C. (1994) Effects of nortriptyline on heart rate variability in panic disorder patients: a preliminary study using power spectrum analysis of heart rate. *Neuropsychobiology, 29,* 1-7

[42] Tulen, J.H.; Bruijn, J.A.; de Man, K.J.; Pepplinkhuizen, L.; van den Meiracker, A.H. and Man in ´Veld, A.J. (1996) Cardiovascular variability in major depressive disorder and effects of imipramin or mirtazepine (Org 3770*). J. Clin. Psychopharmacol., 16,* 135-145

[43] Roose, S.P. (2003) Treatment of depression in patients with heart disease. *Biol. Psychiatry, 54,* 262-268

[44] Nelson, J.C.; Kennedy, J.S.; Pollock, B.G.; Laghrissi-Thode, F.; Narayan, M.; Nobler, M.S.; Robin, D.W.; Gergel, I.; McCafferty, J. and Roose, S. (1999) Treatment of major depression with nortriptyline and paroxetine in patients with ischemic heart disease. *Am. J. Psychiatry, 156,* 1024-1028

[45] Gorman, J.M. and Sloan, R.P. (2000) Heart rate variability in depressive and anxiety disorders. *Am. Heart J., 140,* S77-S83

[46] Davidson, J.; Watkins, L.; Owens, M.; Krulewicz, S.; Connor, K.; Carpenter, D.; Krishnan, R. and Nemeroff, C. (2005) Effects of paroxetine and venlafaxine XR on heart rate variability in depression. *J. Clin. Psychopharmacol., 25,* 480-484

[47] Glassman, A.H.; Bigger, J.T.; Gaffney, M. and van Zyl, L.T. (2007) Heart rate variability in acute coronary syndrome patients with major depression influence of sertaline and mood improvement. *Arch. Gen. Psychiatry, 64,* 1025-1031

[48] Alvarez, W. Jr. and Pickworth, K.K. (2003) Safety of antidepressant drugs in the patient with cardiac disease: a review of the literature. *Pharmacotherapy, 23,* 754-771

[49] Acosta, D.and Ramos, K. (1984) Cardiotoxicity of antidepressants in primary cultures of rat myocardial cells. *J. Toxicol. Environ. Health, 14,* 137-143

[50] Thorstrand, C. (1976) Clinical features in poisonings by tricyclic antidepressants with special reference to the ECG. *Acta Med. Scand., 199,* 337-344

[51] Goldberg RJ.; Capone, R.J. and Hunt, J.D. (1985) Cardiac complications following tricyclic antidepressant overdose. Issues for monitoring policy. *JAMA, 254,* 1772-1775

[52] Langou, R.A.; Van Dyke, C.; Tahan, S.R. and Cohen, L.S. (1980) Cardiovascular manifestations of tricyclic antidepressant overdose. *Am. Heart J., 100,* 458-464

[53] Shannon, M.; Merola, J. and Lovejoy, F.H. Jr. (1988) Hypotension in severe tricyclic antidepressant overdose. *Am. J. Emerg. Med., 6,* 439-442

[54] Pentel, P.R. and Benowitz, N.L. (1980) Tricyclic antidepressant poisoning: management of arrhythmias. *Med. Toxicol., 1,* 101-121

[55] Jo, S.H.; Youm, J.B.; Lee, C.O.; Earm, Y.E. and Ho, W.K. (2000) Blockade of the HERG human cardiac K^+ channel by the antidepressant drug amitriptyline. *Br. J. Pharmacol., 129,* 1474–1480

[56] Malatynska, E.; Knapp, R.J.; Ikeda, M. and Yamamura, H.I. (1988) Antidepressants and seizure-interactions at the GABA-receptor chloride-ionophore complex. *Life Sci., 43,* 303-307

[57] Weisman, R.S.; Howland, M.A.; Hoffman, R.S. and Cohen, H. (1994) Cyclic Antidepressants. In: Goldfrank, L.R.; Weisman, R.S.; Flomenbaum, N.E.; Howland, M.A.; Lewin, N.A. and Hoffman, R.S. (eds.) *Goldfrank´s Toxicologic Emergencies* (5th edn. , pp. 725-737). Norwalk (Connecticut): Appleton and Lange

[58] Schubert-Zsilavecz, M. and Stark, H. (2004) Wiederaufnahme-Hemmung an der Synapse als Wirkprinzip: Medizinische Chemie moderner Antidepressiva – Targets und Arzneistoffe. *Pharm. Unserer Zeit, 33,* 282–287

[59] Baldessarini R. (2001) Drugs and the treatment of psychiatric disorders. Depression and anxiety disorders. In: Hardman J, Limbird L, Goodman A (eds) Goodman and Gilman's. *The pharmacological basis of therapeutics* (10th edn., Chapter 19, pp. 447-483). New York: McGraw-Hill

[60] Huangfu, D.; Goodwin, W.B. and Guyenet, P.G. (1995) Sympatholytic effect of tricyclic antidepressants: site and mechanism of action inn anesthetized rats. *Am. J. Physiol., 268,* R1429-R1441

[61] Knudsen, K. and Abrahamsson, J. (1993) Effects of epinephrine and norepinephrine on hemodynamic parameters and arrhythmias during a continuous infusion of amitriptyline in rats. *J. Toxicol. Clin. Toxicol., 31,* 461-471

[62] Harrigan, R.A. and Brady, W.J. (1999) ECG abnormalities in tricyclic antidepressant ingestion. *Am. J. Emerg. Med., 17,* 387-393

[63] Djonlagic, I.; Djonlagic, H.; Kibbel, T.; Suefke, S. and Dodt, C. (2007) Heart rate reveals risk of arrhythmias after intoxication with a nidepressants. *Intesive Care Med., 33,* 200-202

[64] Suefke, S.; Djonlagic, H. and Kibbel, T. (2008) Continuous analysis of heart rate variability for examination of cardiac autonomic nervous system after doxepin intoxication. *Intensivmed, 45,* 121-131

[65] Rechlin, T. (1995) Decreased R-R variation: a criterium for overdosage of tricyclic psychotropic drugs. *Intensive Care Med, 21,* 598-601

[66] Waring, W.S.; Rhee, J.Y.; Bateman, D.N.; Leggett, G.E. and Jamie, H. (2008) Impaired heart rate variability and altered cardiac sympathovagal balance after antidepressant overdose. *Eur. J. Clin. Pharmacol., 64,* 1037-1041

[67] van Zyl, L.T.; Hasegawa, T. and Nagata, K. (2008) Effects of antidepressant treatment treatment on heart rate variability in major dpression: A quantitative review. *Biopsychosoc. Med., 2,* 12-21

[68] Suefke, S.; Fiedler, S.; Djonlagic, H. and Kibbel, T. (2009) Continuous analysis of heart rate variability for examination of cardiac autonomic nervous system after alcohol intoxication. *Med. Klin., 104,* 511-519

[69] Richelson, E. (1991) Biological basis of depression and therapeutic relevance. *J. Clin. Psychiatry, 52 (Suppl),* 4-10

[70] Broocks, A.; Junghanns, K.; Thiel, A.; Gleiter, C.H. and Bandelow, B. (2000) New antidepressive drugs in comparison with classical tricyclics. Mechanism of action and clinical evaluation. *Fortschr. Neurol. Psychiatr., 68,* 17-24

[71] Tobis, J.M. and Aronow, W.S. (1981) Cardiotoxicity of amitriptyline and doxepin. *Clin. Pharmacol. Ther., 29,* 359-364

[72] Preskorn, S.H. (1989) Tricyclic antidepressants: the whys and hows of therapeutic drug monitoring. *J. Clin. Psychiatry, 50 (Suppl),* 34-42

[73] Callaham, M. and Kassel, D. (1985) Epidemiology of fatal tricyclic antidepressant ingestion: implications for management. *Ann. Emerg. Med., 14,* 1-9

[74] Bradley, L. and Doggrell, S.A. (1983) Effects of amitriptyline, desipramine and mianserin on noradrenergic transmission in the rate isolated right ventricle. *J. Auton. Pharmacol., 3,* 287-295

[75] Akselrod, S.; Gordon, D.; Ubel, F.A.; Shannon, D.C.; Barger, A.C. and Cohen, R.J. (1981) Power spectrum analysis of heart rate fluctuation: A quantitative probe of beat to beat cardiovascular control. *Science, 213,* 220-222

[76] Lathers, C.M. and Roberts, J. (1985) Are sympathetic neural effects of digoxin and quinidine involved in their action of rhythm? *J. Cardiovasc. Pharmacol., 7,* 350-360

[77] Brembilla-Perrot, B.; Jacquemin, L. and Beurrier, D. (1997) Relationships between heart rate variability and antiarrhythmic effects of hydroquinidine. *Cardiovasc Drugs Ther, 11,* 493-498

[78] Baum, T. and Shropshire, A.T. (1975) Inhibition of efferent sympathetic nerve activity by 5-hydroxytryptophan and centrally administered 5-hydroxytryptamine. *Neuropharmacology, 14,* 227-233

[79] Shusterman, V.; Aysin, B.; Gottipathy, V.; Weiss, R.; Brode, S.; Schwartzman, D. and Anderson, K.P. (1998) Autonomic nervous system activity and the spontaneous initation of ventricular tachycardia. Electrophysiologic Study Versus Electrocardiograpic Monitoring (ESVEM) Trial. *J. Am. Coll. Cardiol., 32,* 1891-1899

[80] Lanza, G.A.; Cianflone, D.; Rebuzzi, A.G.; Angeloni, G.; Sestito, A.; Ciriello, G.; La Torre, G.; Crea, F. and Maseri, A.; Stratificazione Prognostica dell'Angina Instabile Study Investigators (2005) Prognostic value of ventricular arrhythmias and heart rate variability in patients with unstable angina. *Heart, 92,* 1055-1063

[81] Piccirillo, G.; Magrì, D.; di Carlo, S.; De Laurentis, T.; Torrini, A.; Matera, S.; Magnanti, M.; Bernardi, L.; Barillà, F.; Quaglione, R.; Ettorre, E. and Marigliano, V. (2006) Influence of cardiac-resynchronization therapy on heart rate and blood pressure variability: 1-year follow-up. *Eur. J. Heart Fail., 8,* 716-722

[82] Dziukas, L.J. and Vohra, J. (1991) Tricyclc antidepressant poisoning. *Med. J. Aust., 154,* 344-350

[83] Heard, K.; Cain, B.S.; Dart, R.C. and Cairns, C.B. (2001) Tricyclic antideprssants directly depress human myocardial mechanical function independent of effects on the conduction system. *Acad. Emerg. Med., 8,* 1122-1127

[84] Biggs, J.T.; Spiker, D.G.; Petit, J.M. and Ziegler, V.E. (1977) Tricyclic antidepressant overdose: incidence of symptoms. *JAMA, 238,* 135–138

[85] Noble, J. and Matthew, H. (1969) Acute poisoning by tricyclic antidepressants: Clinical features and management of 100 patients. *Clin. Toxicol., 2,* 403-421

[86] Crome, P. (1986) Poisoning due to tricyclic antidepressant overdosage. Clinical presentation and treatment. *Med. Toxicol., 1,* 2612-2685

[87] Nattel, S. and Mittleman, M. (1984) Treatment of ventricular tachyarrhythmias resulting from amitriptyline toxicity in dogs. *J. Pharmacol. Exp. Ther., 231,* 30-35

[88] Shusterman, V.; Aysin, B.; Weiss, R.; Brode, S.; Gottipaty, V.; Schwartzman, D. and Anderson, K.P. (2000) Dynamics of low-frequency oscillations preceding spontaneous ventricular tachycardia. *Am. Heart J., 139;* 126-133

[89] Walsh, B.T.; Giardina, E.G.; Sloan, R.P.; Greenhill, L. and Goldfein, J. (1994) Effects of desipramine on autonomic control of the heart. *J. Am. Acad. Child Adolesc. Psychiatry, 33,* 191-197

[90] Frommer, D.A.; Kulig, K.W.; Marx, J.A. and Rumack, B. (1987) Tricyclic antidepressant overdose. A review. *JAMA, 257,* 521-526

[91] Kerr, G.W.; McGuffie, A.C. and Wilkie, S. (2001) Tricyclic antidepressant overdose: a review. *Emerg. Med. J., 18,* 236-241

[92] Hegerl, U. and Möller, H.J. (1996) Nortriptylin: Stellenwert in der psychiatrischen Pharmakotherapie. *Psychopharmakotherapie, 3,* 13-27

[93] Fritze, J. (2002) Nicht-selektive Monoamin-Rückaufnahme-Inhibitoren (NSMRI), Unerwünschte Wirkungen, Kontraindikationen, Überdosierung, Intoxikation. In: Riederer P, Laux G, Pöldinger P (Hrsg.) *Neuro-Psychopharmaka, Band 3: Antidepressiva, Phasenprophylaktika und Stimmungsstabilisierer* (2. Aufl., S. 162-182) Wien, New York: Springer

[94] Pellinen, T.J.; Farkkila, M.; Heikkila, J. and Luomanmaki, K. (1987) Electrocardiographic and clinical features of tricyclic antidepressant intoxication. A survey of 88 cases and outlines of therapy. *Ann Clin Res, 19,* 12-17

[95] Pohl, R.; Balon, R.; Jayaraman, A.; Doll, R.G. and Yeragani, V. (2003) Effect of fluoxetine, pemoline, and placebo on heart rat period and QT variability in normal humans. *J. Psychosom. Res., 55,* 247-251

[96] Yeragani, V.K. and Rao, R. (2003) Effect of nortriptyline and paroxetine on measures of chaos of heart rate time series in patients with panic disorder. *J. Psychosom. Res., 55,* 507-513

[97] Garakani, A.; Martinez, J.M.; Aaronson, C.J.; Voustianiouk, A.; Kaufmann, H. and Gorman, J.M. (2009) Effect of medication and psychotherapy on heart rate variability in panic disorder. *Depress Anxiety, 26,* 251-258

[98] Davydov, D.M.; Shapiro, D.; Cook, I.A. and Goldstein, I. (2007) Baroreflex mechanisms in major depression. *Prog. Neuropschychopharmacol. Biol. Psychiatry, 31,* 164-177

[99] Bradberry, S.M.; Thanacoody, H.K.; Watt, B.E.; Thomas, S.H. and Vale, J.A. (2005) Management of the cardiovascular complications of tricyclicantidepressant poisoning: role of bicarbonate. *Toxicol. Rev., 24,* 195-204

[100] Rechlin, T. (2002) Heart rate analysis in patients with overdose of psychtropic central acting agents. *Intensiv- und Notfallbehandlung, 27,* 144-151

[101] Owens, M.J.; Morgan, W.N.; Plott, S.J. and Nereroff, C.B. (1997) Neurotransmitter receptor and transporter binding profile of antidepressants and their metabolites. *J. Pharmacol. Exp. Ther., 283,* 1305-1322

[102] Singh, JP.; Larson, M.G.; O'Donnell; C.J. and Levy, D. (2001) Genetic factors contribute to the variance in frequency domain measures of heart rate variability: *Auton. Neurosci., 20,* 122-126

[103] Faller, H. and Angermann, C.E. (2008) Depression in chronic heart failure: complication, risk factor or autonomous disease? *Internist 49:* 394-404

[104] Baumert, J.H.; Frey, A.W. and Adt, M. (1995) Analyse der Herzfrequenzvariabilität. *Anaesthesist, 44,* 677-686

[105] Stys, A. and Stys, T. (1998) Current clinical applications of heart rate variability. *Clin. Cardiol., 21,* 719-724

[106] Nahshoni, E.; Aizenberg, D.; Sigler, M.; Strasberg, B.; Zalsman, G.; Imbar, S.; Adler, E. and Weizman, A. (2004) Heart rate variability increases in elderly depressed patients who respond to electroconvulsive therapy. *J. Psychosom. Res., 56,* 89-94

[107] Scheinin, H.; Helminen, A.; Huhtala, S.; Grönroos, P.; Bosch, J.A.; Kuusela, T.; Kanto, J. and Kaila, T. (1999) Spectral analysis of heart rate variability as a quantitative measure of parasympatholytic effect – integrated pharmocokinetics and pharmacodynamics of three anticholinergic drugs. *Ther Drug Monit, 21,* 141-151

[108] Hudson J.I.; Wohlreich, M.M.; Kajdasz, D.K.; Mallinckrodt, C.H.; Watkin, J.G. and Martynov, O.V. (2005) Safety and tolerability of duloxetine in the treatment of major depressive disorder: analysis of pooled data from eight placebo-controlled clinical trials. *Hum. Psychopharmacol., 20,* 327-341

[109] Lurje, L.; Wennerblom, B.; Tygesen, H.; Karlsson, T. and Hjalmarson, A. (1997) Heart rate variability after acute myocardial infarction in patients treated with atenolol and metoprolol. *Int. J. Cardiol., 60,* 157-164

[110] Flapan, A.D.; Nolan, J.; Neilson, J.M. and Ewing, D.J. (1992) Effect of captopril on cardiac parasympathetic activity in chronic cardiac failure secondary to coronary artery disease. *Am. J. Cardiol., 69,* 532-535

[111] Chew, M.L.; Mulsant, B.H.; Pollock, B.G.; Lehman, M.E.; Greenspan, A.; Mahmoud, R.A.; Kirshner, M.A.; Sorisio, D.A.; Bies, R.R. and Gharabawi, G. (2008) Anticholinergic activity of 107 medications commonly used by older adults. *J. Am. Geriatr. Soc., 56,* 1333-1341

[112] Vieweg, W.V.R. and Wood, M.A. (2004) Tricyclic antidepressants, QT interval prolongation, and torsades de pointes. *Psychosomatics, 45,* 371-377

[113] Penttilä, J.; Kuusela, T. and Scheinin, H. (2005) Analysis of rapid heart rate variability in the assessment of anticholinergic drug effects in humans. *Eur. J. Clin. Pharmacol., 61,* 559-565

[114] Bhattacharyya, M.R.; Whitehead, D.L.; Rakhit, R. and Steptoe, A. (2008) Depressed mood, positive affect, and heart rate variability in patients with suspected coronary artery disease. *Pschychosom. Med., 70,* 1020-1027

[115] García-Gómez, R.G.; López-Jaramillo, P. and Tomaz, C. (2007) The role of played by the autoomic nervous system in the relation between depression and cardiovascular disease. *Rev. Neurol., 44,* 225-233

In: Antidepressants: Types, Efficiency …
Editor: Jayden T. Van Leeuwen, pp.115-133

ISBN 978-1-61668-581-2

Chapter 4

THE OVERLAP BETWEEN DEPRESSION AND SUICIDAL BEHAVIOUR: IMPLICATION FOR THE PREVENTATIVE EFFECT OF ANTIDEPRESSANT PHARMACOTHERAPY

Louise Brådvik[1] and Mats Berglund[2]

[1]Department of Psychiatry, Clinical Sciences, Lund University, Lund, Sweden
[2]Department of Clinical Alcohol Research, Health Sciences, Lund University, Malmö, Sweden

ABSTRACT

Retrospective diagnosis of suicide victims has revealed that about half of them have suffered from a depressive disorder. Treatment of depression with antidepressants would therefore be expected to prevent suicide but the role of antidepressant pharmacotherapy in the prevention of suicide has been difficult to evaluate.

Randomised double-blind placebo-controlled studies could be considered the best way of evaluating the effect on suicidal behaviour, but those studies have only been performed as secondary analyses examining the effect of pharmacotherapy on depressive symptoms. They have been performed on low-risk populations, and suicidal patients have been excluded for ethical reasons. Retrospective and pseudo-prospective case-control studies inherit the risk of confounders, as treatment was not randomised. Ecological studies of trends cannot investigate other factors related to a decrease in suicide rates. Descriptive studies on treatment before suicide may show low rates of treatment, but still do not prove that treatment would have been effective if given. Furthermore, complications of the prescription of antidepressants include non-compliance and risk of overdoses in suicidal people.

Apart from evaluating the possible effect of antidepressants in the prevention of suicide, certain questions need to be answered concerning the relationship between depression and suicide. Not all depressives suffer from an uncomplicated major depressive disorder. Sometimes depression is secondary to substance abuse and sometimes depression has melancholic or psychotic features. Furthermore, some investigators have postulated existence of a suicidal syndrome independent of depression, which may have implications for the efficacy of antidepressant pharmacotherapy on suicidal behaviour. Finally, a third way to investigate possible risk or benefit of antidepressants on non-fatal and fatal suicidal behaviour may be to identify certain risk groups for suicidal behaviour despite antidepressant pharmacotherapy.

Suicide and depression only partly overlap. Knowledge about this overlap may have implications for the role of antidepressant pharmacotherapy in the prevention of suicidal behaviour.

INTRODUCTION

Depression is a common disorder and a major health problem, and life-time risk of being affected by a depressive disorder is estimated at 22.5% for men and 30.7% for women [Mattisson et al. 2005]. The most feared complication is suicide. About a million people around the world commit suicide each year [who 2009]. Bearing in mind that many suicide victims are young, this represents the loss of many years of life. Antidepressant pharmacotherapy is the most commonly used treatment for depressive disorders. Suicide victims have often been undertreated so detection and treatment of depression is urgent in the work to prevent suicides.

The present review aims to describe aspects of the role of antidepressants in the prevention of suicide. The correlation between depression and suicide is discussed, as well as the efficacy of antidepressants, and finally the major studies on the preventative effect of antidepressants are summarised. A major issue is the impact of depressive sub-grouping of severe features and co-morbid substance use disorders. Antidepressants have an established effect on depressive symptoms, but there are certain limitations to be taken into consideration.

Detection and treatment with antidepressants should certainly be encouraged, but there are limitations in their efficacy. Therefore it is important to continue research in order to identify those who benefit from such treatment and those who do not.

This chapter will give some aspects of the limitations in efficacy of antidepressants as derived from literature, and which have to be taken into consideration in future research. Bipolar disorders are not included as the characteristics and treatment of this disorder differ from those of major depressive disorders.

RELATIONSHIP BETWEEN DEPRESSION AND SUICIDE

Depression Among Suicides

Mood disorder is the single diagnosis with the greatest impact on suicide. Reviews of psychological autopsies have revealed that about half of all completed suicides have been preceded by a depressive disorder. Lönnqvist [2000] reviewed studies involving 1,110 suicides and found that about half of the suicide victims suffered from a depressive disorder discovered in retrospective psychological autopsies. More recently Bertolote al. [2004] reviewed 31 studies involving 15,629 suicides and Arsenault et al. [2004] made a meta-analysis of 3,745 suicides. They found similar rates of mood disorders among the suicides, 44.4% and 43.2% respectively.

New studies appeared with similar findings. Chan et al. [2009] found that 27% of suicides had a current depression, and Fleischman et al. [2005] found 42.1% depressives among 895 young suicides.

Most studies do not distinguish between melancholic and/or psychotic features in the psychological autopsies. Prospective diagnostics in a sample of 66 suicides have shown that 29% of the suicide victims had suffered from major depressive disorders with melancholic and/or psychotic features while 15% had a major depressive disorder without severe features [Brådvik et al. 2009]. Consequently, even if severe depression with melancholic and/or psychotic features is a less common depressive diagnosis, these types predominate among accomplished suicides.This needs replication on a larger sample of suicides but may have implications for the work to prevent suicide.

Furthermore, co-morbidity between major depression and substance use disorders is common and important to take into consideration. Concurrent mood and substance-related disorders are commonly found in autopsies of accomplished suicides [Isometsä, 2001; Séguin et al., 2006].

In conclusion, there is general agreement that mood disorder is a leading diagnostic predecessor of suicide. However, diagnostic sub-grouping and co-morbid substance use disorders may have an impact on the risk of suicide.

Suicide Risk in Depression

Ideally, the life-time risk of suicide in people with mood disorders and other mental disorders would be calculated by following a cohort until all subjects were dead. To the best of our knowledge however, no adequately defined cohort of subjects with depressive disorder has yet been followed to its extinction. An early, often-cited review article involving a large number of follow-up studies of patients with a primary affective disorder has shown that an average of 15% eventually die from suicide [Guze and Robins, 1970] and a later review found a similar rate [Miles, 1977]. However, a computational modelling technique in a later review using the data in these previous studies estimated the final mortality in suicide at 6% [Inskip et al., 1998]. Furthermore, a calculation of the incidence of depression and suicide mortality based upon an entire sample of depressives showed an expected lifetime risk of 3.5% [Blair-West et al., 1997]. Another calculation was made on suicides in a British health district and found an even lower rate (2.4%) for any affective disorder [Boardman and Healy, 2001].

The discrepancy between older and more recent studies may be due to the fact that the older studies were performed on hospitalised patients, while the risk is much lower in the general population. The former are probably more severely depressed, as well as more suicidal (an indication for admission). The difference in suicide risk has been estimated in a retrospective longitudinal epidemiological study on a community sample of Icelanders born in the late nineteenth century. The sample was monitored until 1957, and the study revealed higher suicide rates in manic-depressive psychosis (including both major depressive disorders and bipolar disorders); 14% as compared to 1.7% in depressive neurosis [Helgason 1964]. Results in a more recent study of a community sample were similar, showing an increased risk of suicide in people with major depressive disorder with melancholic and/or psychotic features as compared with major depressive disorders without these features, 13.8% versus 3.7% [Brådvik et al., 2008].

Co-morbid substance use disorders have been found to increase the risk of suicide in major depressive disorder [Dumais et al., 2005; Sanchez and Le, 2001].

Finally, it should also be remembered that meta-analyses have concluded that almost all psychiatric disorders are related to an increased suicide risk, not only depression [Harris, 1997; Tidemalm et al., 2008].

In conclusion, the suicide risk in depressive disorders appears to be high, but is increased for severe depression with melancholic and/or psychotic features and also co-morbid substance use disorders.

The Suicidal Process in Depression

Suicidal Process

Depression is common among suicide victims, and depressive disorders inherit a high risk of suicide. Therefore, non-fatal and fatal suicidal behaviour has been seen as an ultimate consequence of depression.

The variation of suicide potential from more innocent to more dangerous behaviour has been postulated as the suicidal process [Beck et al., 1979; Beskow, 1979; Paykel et al., 1974; Zisook et al., 1994; Kessler, 1999]. It is used to describe the intra-individual process in reaction to a person's environment, starting with feelings of despair, then fleeting suicidal thoughts, and evolving through more concrete plans and suicide attempts, which are often recurrent and may show increasing levels of suicidal intent and lethality of methods used to completed suicide [van Heeringen et al., 2000].

However, some investigators have proposed that suicide completers are not on a continuum from suicidal ideation to completed suicide. Suicide attempts are heterogeneous and may represent more than one population of individuals with some overlap [Stengel et al., 1958; Maris, 1981; Linehan, 1986]. Suicide attempters and completers could be distinguished both epidemiologically and in terms of characteristics of the suicidal act. For instance, suicide attempters are more often young and female, while completers are more often male and older. Far from every suicide ideator goes on to make a suicide attempt, and most attempters never complete suicide.

Grant and Hasin [1997] examined the relationship between suicide ideation and major depression, alcohol dependence and major depression + alcohol dependence. They used data from 18,352 current drinkers from the National Longitudinal Alcohol Epidemiologic Survey. Suicide ideation in the previous year was present in 5.2% of the men and 6.9% of the women. In the group with alcohol dependence the suicide ideation rate was somewhat increased (men OR 2.2, and women OR 1.6). In the group with major depression the suicide ideation rate was strongly increased (men OR 13.6, women OR 10.9). There was no further increase in the co-morbid group alcohol dependence + major depression (men OR 9.9, women 9.0). Consequently, the major association is between suicide ideation and major depression.

The relationship between suicide attempt and major depression and alcohol use disorders + major depression was studied in 5,148 subjects with major depression in the National

Epidemiologic Survey on Alcohol and Related Conditions [Bolton et al., 2008] The rate of attempted suicide in the previous year in the major depression group was 17% in the male group and 17% in the female group. Corresponding figures in the alcohol use disorders + major depression group were 20% in the male group and 23% in the female group. The increase of suicide attempt in the co-morbid group was therefore small compared with the major depression group.

Consequently, suicide ideation is strongly associated with major depression, and the rate of ideation does not seem to increase in subjects with both major depression and substance use disorders. However, completed suicide is increased in subjects with major depression and substance use disorders. Other factors than suicide ideation are probably involved.

Suicidal Syndrome

Other investigators have proposed that suicidal behaviour may occur independent of depression. After the publication of Rouillon's investigation on maprotiline [Rouillon et al., 1989], it has been speculated that antidepressants may exert a different effect on depression and suicidal acts. It was found that maprotiline had a good effect on depressive symptoms, but it may also induce suicide attempts in some people. Furthermore, biological findings such as low 5-HIAA in cerebrospinal fluid (CSF) correlated with suicidal behaviour independent of type of psychiatric disorder, has led to a hypothesis of a suicidal syndrome [Åsberg, 1986]. Other authors tried to delineate this syndrome on a phenomenological level by describing core symptoms, such as hopelessness, etc. which appeared to be independent of illness [Ahrens and Linden, 1996; Ahrens et al., 2000]. Moreover, a stress-diathesis model has been proposed in which the risk of suicidal acts is determined not merely by a psychiatric illness (the stressor) but also by a diathesis, such as a tendency to experience more suicidal ideation and to be more likely to act on suicidal feeling [Mann et al., 1999]. In a study of the long-term course and treatment of severe depression, seriousness of suicide attempt appeared to be reduced in those with at least four weeks of antidepressant medication treatment [Brådvik and Berglund, 2006]. The suicide attempts at this point of treatment were actually interrupted by the attempter. This may be an indication that the urge to act on suicidal feelings was reduced but not extinguished when depression was relieved. Other investigators have found a non-significant tendency towards a reduced intention in suicide attempts during antidepressant pharmacotherapy [Leon et al., 1999].

Another factor which correlates with suicidal behaviour independent of diagnosis is "brittle and sensitive" personality. This factor is strongly related to suicide in male severe depression as well as alcoholism. [Berglund, 1984, Berglund and Nilsson, 1987; Brådvik and Berglund, 1993]. In addition, those alcoholics with "brittle and sensitive" personality who committed suicide did so during drinking, in contrast with other alcoholics [Berglund et al., 1987]. In the depressed sample three of the 16 future suicides with this diagnosis, but none of the controls, had made spontaneous reports that they were too cowardly to kill themselves [personal communication]. Some common mechanism could be present in alcoholism and depression in males.

This factor has a strong similarity with dependent personality disorder, as has been suggested by Bolton and co-workers [2008]. Dependent personality disorder was strongly related to a high rate of male attempted suicide in the NESARC study [Bolton et al., 2008]. It was the mental disorder most strongly correlated with suicide attempt among all Axis I and Axis II disorders with an almost four-fold increase in the probability of suicide attempt.

In conclusion, depressed feelings are related to suicidal behaviour, but there is disagreement whether there is a direct correlation or whether it is rather a stressor for a suicidal syndrome independent of depression. If suicidal behaviour is a final step of depression, treatment of depression will be expected to remove such behaviour. However, if there is suicidal syndrome independent of depression, you have may have to treat suicidal behaviour in itself apart from depression.

Treatment of Depression

The use of antidepressant pharmacotherapy is generally considered to be efficient in the relief of depressive symptoms. It is one of several treatment options, other examples being ECT [UK ECT Review group 2003], cognitive behavioural psychotherapy [Hollon et al., 2006], interpersonal psychotherapy [Luty et al., 2007], and short-time psycho-dynamic therapy [Driessen et al., 2009].

Efficacy of Antidepressant Pharmacotherapy

Though antidepressant pharmacotherapy is generally efficient, there are some important limitations in the efficacy of antidepressants, such as response rates, incomplete recovery and delay of effect or even initial worsening. Furthermore, non-compliance of treatment also limits the efficacy of antidepressant therapy [Demyttenaere et al., 2008; Nierenberg et al., 2008; Möller, 2008].

Placebo-controlled studies have shown that only about 70-80% of all depressed patients respond to antidepressant pharmacotherapy [Potter et al., 1991; Khan et al., 2000]. Furthermore, only a small group of patients with major depression are accepted for inclusion in randomised controlled studies. Blanco et al. [2008] used the NESARC database. They found that, among 3,119 subjects with major depression, 75.8% would be excluded in a randomised controlled study. Among 1,359 subjects who had been treated for major depression, 66.8% would be excluded, so the majority of patients with major depression would not be included in randomised studies. This is important for the evaluation of the effects of antidepressive treatment. In the Star*D real-life study, 2,876 patients were initially treated for 12 weeks with citalopram. Only 27.5% of the patients went into remission [Trivedi et al. 2008]. This figure is clearly much lower than those from the RCT studies.

Another limitation of efficacy is that some responders may still have a substantial degree of residual depressive symptoms. Several investigators have discussed incomplete recovery on antidepressant pharmacotherapy [Faravelli et al., 1986; Agosti et al., 1993; Fava, 1999; Fava et al., 2007]. Symptom reduction was for instance shown to be only 40.7% for investigational drugs in one meta-analytic study [Khan et al., 2000]. In a meta-analysis of randomised studies, only 46.4% receiving medication reached full remission [Cascalenda et al., 2002].

Non-response as well as residual symptoms are likely to limit the effect of antidepressant pharmacotherapy on suicidal behaviour.

Maintenance Treatment and Continuation Treatment

Most studies on the efficacy of antidepressant pharmacotherapy have been performed in the short-term acute phase. However, depression is often a recurrent disorder, and continuation treatment during the entire episode and maintenance treatment between the episodes are also important. A good effect in the prevention of new episodes has been shown, with better tolerability and compliance of new-generation antidepressants (imipramine versus paroxetine) [Claghorn and Feighner 1993].

Another indication of antidepressant pharmacotherapy is continuation treatment after ECT. This treatment is generally considered effective in the treatment of severe depression [Pagnin et al. 2004]. However, a frequent recurrence of depression after ECT has been shown in approximately 50% of cases, or even higher rates in for instance delusional depression [Bourgon and Kellner, 2000]. Continuation treatment with antidepressants has been shown to prevent relapse [Frank et al. 1990, Kay 1970, Wijkstra et al. 2000] or antidepressants in combination with Lithium [Sackheim et al. 2001, Kellner et al. 2006]. It has also been shown that depressed patients with pharmacotherapy treatment failure may benefit from the prophylactic effect of the same class of drug during maintenance therapy after response to ECT [van den Broek et al., 2006].

Risk of Suicide During Treatment

Another important issue to take into consideration is the possibility of an increased risk of suicide during antidepressant medication before the full effect is received.

It has been proposed that the relief of psychomotor retardation before the relief of depressive symptoms constitutes an increased risk of suicide [Benkert and Hippius, 1980; Feuerstein and Jackisch, 1986; Damluji and Ferguson, 1988].

Moreover, it is clinical practice to take precautions in prescribing antidepressants, as they may constitute a tool for suicide. The number of overdoses with antidepressants has been found to be around 4% of all suicides [Kelleher et al., 1992; Öhberg et al., 1996]. The frequency of lethal intoxication has been shown to be 8% among depressed suicides [Isacsson et al., 1994a, 1994b; Isometsä et al., 1994] or 3% among depressives with melancholic and/or psychotic features [Brådvik and Berglund, 2005]. Different studies showed that 20-30% of all deaths from overdose or poisoning were antidepressant-related [Obanunwa and Busuttil, 1994a, 1994b; Neeleman and Wessely, 1997; Shah et al., 2001]. A majority was associated with tricyclic antidepressants [Obanunwa and Busuttil, 1994a; Shah et al., 2001]. Other investigators found that 14% of all patients prescribed antidepressants used the drugs for their lethal overdose [Jick et al., 1995]. A risk of suicide during acute-phase antidepressant treatment has recently been estimated at approximately one in 3,000 treatment episodes, and risk of serious suicide attempt is approximately one in 1,000 [Simon et al. 2006].

Co-Morbid Substance Use Disorders and Major Depression

Nunes and Levin [2004] published a meta-analysis of treatment of depression in patients with alcohol or other drug dependence. They found 14 placebo-controlled studies including 848 subjects. The mean standardised effect size of antidepressant medication on outcome of depression was d=0.38. The effects of antidepressant medication on outcome of substance use were modulated by the effect on depression. Studies on treatment of depression with a standardised effect size of less than 0.50 showed no effect on substance use (d=0.07) while studies with a standardised effect size of more than 0.50 on depression had an effect size of d=0.56 on substance use. Consequently, effective antidepressive treatment of depression also had an important effect on outcome for substance use.

The Impact of Major Depression with Psychotic and Melancholic Features

The definition of melancholic and psychotic feature specifier of a major depressive disorder [APA, 1994] may indicate that they are on a continuum of the same disorder, a unitary view. Some investigators, however, have proclaimed that major depression and melancholia are two different disorders, a binary view [Parker and Hadzi-Pavlovic, 1996]. According to the latter study, psychomotor disturbances were regarded as the core symptom, while in the DSM IV the essential feature is loss of interest or pleasure in activities or a lack of reactivity to usually pleasurable stimuli. Likewise, psychotic features could be seen as a continuum of the melancholic entity or as a separate disease.

It has recently been proposed that the concept of melancholia or the doctrine of two depressions, non-melancholia and melancholia, should be restored [Fink et al., 2007; Fink and Taylor, 2007; Shorter, 2007; Coryell, 2007; Taylor and Fink, 2008].

According to a review, data on the differential efficacy of TCAs versus SSRIs and the newer antidepressants in severe depression appeared mixed, some concluded a better effect of TCA and others a similar effect, and the review also concluded that electroconvulsive therapy (ECT) may be indicated in severe psychotic depression and severe melancholic depression [Sonawalla and Fava, 2001]. A better efficacy of TCA and ECT in melancholia was found in a more recent review [Parker 2007]. In another recent review, the most consistent finding was poor response to placebo and relatively good response to antidepressants and ECT [Brown, 2007].

As mentioned earlier, major depressive disorders with melancholic or psychotic features inherit an increased risk of suicide and predominate over major depression almost two-fold amongst accomplished suicides. Therefore the identification and treatment of these conditions should be considered urgent in the effort to prevent suicide.

The Impact of Antidepressants on Suicidal Behaviour

There are great problems in the evaluation of the impact of treatment o suicidal behaviour, so all studies have limited evidence.

The ideal double-blind randomised placebo-controlled study on suicidal people could hardly be performed for ethical reasons and there would also be the difficulty of obtaining a large enough sample since suicide is such a rare event, even in a high-risk population. Randomised trials have therefore been performed only as secondary analyses. Retrospective and pseudo-prospective controlled studies are not randomised and may be confounded. The major problem of ecological studies is that causality cannot be inferred. There may be other factors that influence the increased use of antidepressants as well as the decreased suicide rates independently. Finally, early investigators found undertreatment of depression among suicide victims, indicating that treatment could prevent suicide. However, those studies were not controlled and could therefore not really prove a preventative effect had antidepressant therapy been given.

Undertreatment of Depression

Several studies on a general population have shown that only a minority of the depressed persons received adequate antidepressant therapy before suicide [Barraclough et al., 1974; Chynoweth et al., 1980]. Later studies included toxicological analyses and showed that 12-16% of the suicide victims were positive for antidepressants [Åsgård, 1990; Isacsson et al., 1994a, 1994b], including the finding that 4-6% of the depressives had taken lethal overdoses [Isacsson et al., 1994a, 1994b]. Nevertheless, other investigators found a high rate (55%) of antidepressant medication use in elderly depressed patients who had committed suicide, including 12% lethal overdoses [Waern et al. 1996].

Patients in psychiatric care are often treated as described in two studies [Schou and Weeke, 1988; Isometsä et al., 1994]. One of these showed that they were often adequately treated [Schou and Weeke, 1988], while the other found that most were inadequately treated [Isometsä et al., 1994].

Randomised Studies

Randomised double-blind placebo case-control studies have only been performed as secondary analyses of studies concerning the effect of pharmacotherapy on depressive symptoms. Those studies have been performed on low-risk populations and suicidal patients have been excluded for ethical reasons. One study even showed a higher rate of suicidal acts in patients treated with maprotiline [Rouillon et al., 1986]. Meta-analyses have failed to show a significant difference in favour of antidepressant medication [Tollefson et al., 1993; Montgomery et al., 1995; Mequies et al., 1998; Kahn et al., 2000; Khan et al,. 2003, Gunnell et al., 2005, Saperia et al., 2006]. A systematic review of randomised control trials documented an association between SSRI and suicide attempts but not an association with completed suicide [Fergusson et al. 2005]. Another meta-analysis showed that suicidality associated with use of antidepressants was strongly age-dependent, with a negative effect before 25 and a positive effect after 65 [Stone et al. 2009].

Controlled Studies

To the best of our knowledge, few case-control studies have been performed. Earlier studies could not show that antidepressant therapy had a preventative effect [Modestin and Schwarzenbach, 1992; Taiminen, 1993; Brådvik and Berglund, 2000]. One more recent study monitoring patients with affective disorders one year after discharge showed that treatment with antidepressant drugs at the censoring date were associated with a decrease in suicide risk [Høyer et al. 2009], while other investigators failed to show any difference in suicide rates between those who discontinued antidepressant treatment and those who did not [Erlangsen et al. 2009]. A longitudinal case-control study gave some evidence of lower suicide rates among patients treated with antidepressants [Angst et al., 2005].

Considering that ECT may be more efficient than antidepressant pharmacotherapy in severe depression [Sonawalla and Fava, 2001], but has a high risk of relapse [Bourgon and Kellner, 2000], continuation treatment with antidepressants may have a preventative effect on suicide in patients with a severe depression. However, little research focused on this possibility. In a seven-month double-blind trial of amitriptyline (n=59) and diazepam in ECT-treated patients (n=73) there were three suicides in the diazepam group but no suicides in the amitryptiline-group [Kay et al. 1970]. In a retrospective chart study comparing 34 patients receiving tricyclic antidepressants with 20 patients receiving lithium as continuation treatment after ECT, the patients were monitored for 6 months and there were no suicides in either group [Perry, Tsuang 1979]. None of these studies could give statistical evidence for a preventative effect of continuation treatment due to small sampling sizes. Another controlled study showed a significant difference in continuation treatment between suicides and controls [Brådvik and Berglund 2000], indicating a preventative effect of continuation treatment. A validation was made by comparing "suicides in treatment" (=those who were in treatment at suicide) with other "suicides not in treatment". "Suicides not in treatment" could be expected to resemble "suicides in treatment" more than non-suicides in depressive characteristics, and they showed similar rates of risk factors and similar age and sex distributions. There was a more common trend towards continuation treatment in the group that did not commit suicide at the time. In a later follow-up involving more suicide victims, the difference was significant [Brådvik and Berglund 2005].

Ecological Studies

Finally, there have been numerous ecological or population-based studies on correlational temporal trends in suicide rates and rates of usage of modern antidepressants including serotonin-reuptake inhibitors. A recent review yielded heterogeneous findings; only 8/19 found significant inverse correlations between rising sales of modern antidepressants in the 1990s and falling suicide rates not anticipated in the 1980s [Balderassini et al., 2007]. A steady decline in suicide rates has been recorded in the USA since records began in 1933 [Verberne, 2003]. It has been proposed that the general decline is connected to the introduction of ECT and antidepressants [O'Leary et al.]. However, on investigating a recent decline in suicide rates, it was found that people not receiving antidepressants also showed a decline as well, though to a lesser extent [Søndergård 2006]. One study provided evidence that decreasing suicide rates were associated with both increasing antidepressant sales and an increasing density of psychotherapists [Kapusta et al., 2009].

Induction of Suicidal Behaviour?

Apart from the difficulties in proving a preventative effect of antidepressants, some authors even proclaim an increased suicide risk when a patient is on medication, especially young adults [Healy, 2003; Healy and Whitaker, 2003]. A later comprehensive review concluded that there seems to be only a small amount of evidence from different research approaches that antidepressants, not only serotonin reuptake inhibitors (SSRIs), might induce, aggravate or increase the risk of suicidal ideation and suicide attempts, but no evidence for induction of accomplished suicide [Möller 2006].

A Summary of the Problem

There is an overlap between depression and suicide. Antidepressant pharmacotherapy is the most widely used treatment for depression, and its impact on suicidal behaviour is important to evaluate. Though antidepressants have a positive effect on depressive symptoms, there are several reasons *not* to believe that treatment with antidepressants is the only solution to the suicide problem.

Diagnostics matter. Depression is a major suicide precursor, but almost all psychiatric diagnoses are related to an increased risk of suicide. Furthermore, within the depression group co-morbidity with substance use disorders has to be taken into consideration. Another important consideration is the depressive subgroups, such as severe depression with melancholic and/or psychotic features. The latter has been shown to have an increased risk of suicide as compared to non-severe depression and predominates among completed suicides.

Antidepressants are not the only treatment available for depression. In cases of severe depression ECT may be more efficient. Continuation treatment with antidepressants is also needed to prevent relapse. This may be an important indication for use of antidepressants in the prevention of suicide, which has been mostly overlooked.

The efficacy of antidepressant pharmacotherapy has considerable limitations due to non-compliance, non-response and residual symptoms among responders. All of these shortcomings could be assumed to diminish the preventative effect on suicidal behaviour. The detection of antidepressants by autopsy of suicide victims is actually an indication of failure of preventative effect of antidepressants as well as an indication of undertreatment.

The possibility of lack of effect on suicidal feelings despite a positive effect on depression should not be overlooked.

The evaluation of the effect of antidepressants on suicidal behaviour is problematic.

For ethical reasons the ideal double-blind randomised control trial could never be performed on suicidal depressed individuals. Case-control studies have confounders.

Ecological studies inherit a risk of measuring coincidences instead of causal relationships.

The possibility that suicidal behaviour may even be induced by antidepressant therapy, especially among young people, is under debate but needs further exploration. In fact a major topic of future research would be not so much to discuss whether antidepressants are helpful or harmful but to continue research that aims to identify the people it benefits and those it does not.

Detection and treatment of depression with antidepressants remain an important clinical task, as well as improved diagnostics of co-morbid substance use disorders and severe depression with melancholic and/or psychotic features.

REFERENCES

Ahrens, B., and Linden, M. (1996). Is there a suicidality syndrome independent of specific major depressive disorder? Results of a split half multiple regression analysis. *Acta Psychiatrica Scandinavica, 94,* 79-86.

Ahrens, B., Linden, M., Zäske, H., and Berzewski, H. (2000). Suicidal behavior--symptom or disorder? *Comprehensive Psychiatry, 41(2 Suppl 1),* 116-121.

Agosti, V., Stewqart, J.W., Quitkin, F.M., and Ocepek-Welikson, K. (1993). How symptomatic do depressed patients remain after benefiting from medication treatment. *Comprehensive Psychiatry, 34,* 182-186.

American Psychiatric Association [APA]. (1994). *Diagnostic and Statistical Manual of Mental Disorders (DSM-IV)* (4th ed). Washington, DC: APA.

Angst, J., Angst, F., Gerber-Werder, R., Gamma, A. (2006). Suicide in 406 mood-disorder patients with and without long-term medication: a 40 to 44 years' follow-up. *Archives of Suicide Research 9,* 279-300.

Arsenault-Lapierre, G., Kim, C., and Turecki, G. (2004). Psychiatric diagnoses in 3275 suicides: a meta-analysis. *BMC Psychiatry, 4,* 37.

Åsberg, M., Nordström, P., and Träskman-Bendz, L. (1986). Cerebrospinal fluid studies in suicide. An overview. *Annals of the New York Academy of Sciences, 487*, 243-255.

Balasubramani, G.K., Fava, M., and STAR*D Study Team. (2006). Evaluation of outcomes with citalopram for depression using measurement-based care in STAR*D: implications for clinical practice. *American Journal of Psychiatry, 163(1),* 28-40.

Baldessarini, R.J., Tondo, L., Strombom, I.M., Dominguez, S., Fawcett, J., Licinio, J., Oquendo, M.A., Tollefson, G.D., Valuck, R.J., and Tohen, M. (2007.) Ecological studies of antidepressant treatment and suicidal risks. *Harvard Review of Psychiatry, 15(4),*133-145. Review.

Barraclough, B., Bunch, J., Nelson, B., and Sainsbury, P. (1974). A hundred cases of suicide: Clinical aspects. *British Journal of Psychiatry, 125,* 355-373.

Benkert, O., and Hippius, H. (1980). *Psychiatrische Pharmakotherapie.*(P. 35).Berlin Heidelberg New York: Springer.

Berglund, M. (1984). Suicide in alcoholism. A prospective study of 88 suicides. Part I: The multi-dimensional diagnosis at first admission. *Archives of General Psychiatry, 41,* 888-891.

Berglund, M., Krantz, P., and Lundqvist, G. (1987). Suicide in alcoholism. A prospective study of 55 cases with autopsy findings. *Acta Psychiatrica Scandinavica, 76,* 381-385.

Berglund, M., and Nilsson, K. (1987). Mortality in severe depression. A prospective study of 103 suicides. *Acta Psychiatrica Scandinavica, 76,* 372-380.

Bertolote, J.M., Fleischmann, A., De Leo, D., and Wasserman, D. (2004). Psychiatric diagnoses and suicide: revisiting the evidence. *Crisis, 25,* 147-155. Review.

Beskow, J. (1979). Suicide and mental disorder in Swedish men. *Acta Psychiatrica Scandinavica, Suppl. 277.*

Blair-West, G.W., Mellsop, G.W., and Eveson-Annan, M.L. (1997). Down-rating lifetime suicide risk in major depression. *Acta Psychiatrica Scandinavica, 95,* 259-263.

Blanco, C., Olfson, M., Goodwin, R.D., Ogburn, E., Liebowitz, M.R., Nunes, E.V., and Hasin, D.S. (2008). Generalizability of clinical trial results for major depression to community samples: results from the National Epidemiologic Survey on Alcohol and Related Conditions. *Journal of Clinical Psychiatry, 69(8),* 1276-80.

Boardman, A.P., and Healy, D. (2001). Modelling suicide risk in affective disorders. *European Psychiatry, 16,* 400-405.

Bolton, J.M., Belik, S., Enns, M.W., Cox, B.J., and Sareen, J (2008). Exploring the correlates of suicide attempts among individuals with major depressive disorder: Findings from the national epidemiologic survey on alcohol and related conditions. *Journal of Clinical Psychiatry, 69,* 1139-1149.

van den Broek, W.W., Birkenhäger, T.K., Mulder, P.G., Bruijn, J.A., and Moleman, P. (2006). Imipramine is effective in preventing relapse in electroconvulsive therapy-responsive depressed inpatients with prior pharmacotherapy treatment failure: a randomized, placebo-controlled trial. *Journal of Clinical Psychiatry, 67(2),* 263-268.

Brown, W.A. (2007). Treatment response in melancholia. *Acta Psychiatrica Scandinavica. Suppl., (433),* 125-129. Review

Brådvik, L., and Berglund, M. (1993). Risk factors for suicide in melancholia. A case record evaluation of 89 suicides and their controls. *Acta Psychiatrica Scandinavica, 87,* 306-311.

Brådvik, L., and Berglund, M. (2000). Treatment and suicide in severe depression. A case-control study on antidepressant therapy at last contact before suicide. *Journal of ECT, 16,* 399-408.

Brådvik, L., and Berglund, M. (2005). Suicide in severe depression related to treatment. Depressive characteristics and rate of antidepressant overdose. *European Archives of Psychiatry and Clinical Neuroscience, 255,* 245-250.

Brådvik, L., and Berglund, M. (2006). Long-term Treatment and Suicidal Behaviour in Severe Depression. ECT and Antidepressant Pharmacotherapy May Have Different Effects on the Occurrence and Seriousness of Suicide Attempts. *Depression and Anxiety, 23,* 34-41.

Brådvik, L., Mattisson, C., Bogren, M., and Nettelbladt, P. (2008). Long-term suicide risk of depression in the Lundby cohort 1947-1997 – severity and gender. *Acta Psychiatrica Scandinavica, 117(3),* 185-191 [Epub Jan 2008]

Brådvik, L., Mattisson, C., Bogren, M., and Nettelbladt, P. (2009). Mental disorders in suicide and undetermined death in the Lundby study. The contribution of severe depression and alcohol dependence. *Archives of Suicide Research.* In press.

Casacalenda, N., Perry, J.C., and Looper, K. (2002). Remission in major depressive disorder: a comparison of pharmacotherapy, psychotherapy, and control conditions. *American Journal of Psychiatry, 159(8),* 1354-1360. Review.

Chan, S.S., Chiu, H.F., Chen, E.Y., Chan, W.S., Wong, P.W., Chan, C.L., Law, Y.W., and Yip, P.S. (2009). Population-attributable risk of suicide conferred by axis I psychiatric diagnoses in a Hong Kong Chinese population. *Psychiatric Services, 60(8)*, 1135-1138.

Claghorn, J.L., and Feighner, J.P. (1993). A double-blind comparison of paroxetine with imipramine in the long-term treatment of depression. *Journal of Clinical Psychopharmacology, 103(6 Suppl 2),* 23S-27S.

Damluji, N.F., and Ferguson, J.M. (1988). Paradoxical worsening of depressive symptomatology caused by antidepressants. *Journal of Clinical Psychopharmacology, 8,* 347-349.

Demyttenaere, K., Adelin, A., Patrick, M., Walthère, D., Katrien de, B., and Michèle, S. (2008).

Six-month compliance with antidepressant medication in the treatment of major depressive disorder. *International Clinical Psychopharmacology, 23(1),* 36-42.

Driessen, E., Cuijpers, P., de Maat, S.C., Abbass, A.A., de Jonghe, F., and Dekker, J.J. (2009). The efficacy of short-term psychodynamic psychotherapy for depression: A meta-analysis. *Clinical Psychology Review,* Sep 3. [Epub ahead of print]

Dumais, A., Lesage, A.D., Alda, M., Rouleau, G., Dumont, M., Chawky, N., Roy, M., Mann, J.J., Benkelfat, C., and Turecki, G. (2005). Risk factors for suicide completion in major depression: a case-control study of impulsive and aggressive behaviors in men. *American Journal of Psychiatry, 162(11),* 2116-2124.

Erlangsen, A., Agerbo, E., Hawton, K., and Conwell, Y. (2009). Early discontinuation of antidepressant treatment and suicide risk among persons aged 50 and over: A population-based register study. *Journal of Affective Disorders, 119(1-3),* 194-199.

Faravelli, C., Ambonetti, A., Pallanti, S., and Pazzagli, A. (1986). Depressive relapses and incomplete recovery from index episode. *American Journal of Psychiatry 143,* 888-891.

Fava, G.A. (1999). Subclinical symptoms in mood disorders: pathophysiological and therapeutic implications. *Psychological Medicine, 29,* 47-61.

Fava, G.A., Ruini, C. and Belaise, C. (2007). The concept of recovery in major depression. *Psychological Medicine, 37(3),* 307-317. Review.

Fergusson, D., Doucette, S., Glass, K.C., Shapiro, S., Healy, D., Hebert, P., and Hutton, B. (2005).

Association between suicide attempts and selective serotonin reuptake inhibitors: systematic review of randomised controlled trials. *British Medical Journal, 330(7488),* 396. Review.

Feuerstein, T.J., and Jackisch, R. (1986). Why do some antidepressants promote suicide? *Psychopharmacology, 90,* 422.

Fink, M., Bolwig, T.G., Parker, G., and Shorter, E. (2007). Melancholia: restoration in psychiatric classification recommended. *Acta Psychiatrica Scandinavica, 115,* 89-92.

Fink, M., and Taylor, M.A. (2007). Resurrecting melancholia. *Acta Psychiatrica Scandinavica, 115 (Suppl. 433),* 14-20.

Fleischmann, A., Bertolote, J.M., Belfer, M., and Beautrais, A. (2005). Completed suicide and psychiatric diagnoses in young people: a critical examination of the evidence. *American Journal of Orthopsychiatry, 75(4),* 676-683.

Frank, E., Kupfer, D., Perel, J.M., Cornes, C., Jarrett, D.B., Mallinger, A.G., Thase, M.E., McEachran, A.B., and Grochocinski, V.J. (1990) Three-year outcome for maintenance therapies in recurrent depression. *Archives of General Psychiatry, 47,* 1093-1099.

Grant, B.F., and Hasin, D.S. (1997). Suicidal ideation among the United States drinking population: Results from the National longitudinal alcohol epidemiologic survey. *Journal of Studies on Alcohol, 60,* 422-429.

Gunnell, D., Saperia, J., and Ashby, D. (2005). Selective serotonin reuptake inhibitors (SSRIs) and suicide in adults: meta-analysis of drug company data from placebo controlled, randomised controlled trials submitted to the MHRA's safety review. *British Medical Journal, 330(7488),* 385.

Guze, S.B., and Robins, E. (1970). Suicide and primary affective disorders. *British Journal of Psychiatry, 117,* 37-438.

Harris, E.C., and Barraclough, B. (1997). Suicide as an outcome for mental disorders. A meta-analysis. *British Journal of Psychiatry, 170,* 205-228.

van Heeringen, K., Hawton, K., and Williams, J.M.G. (2000). Pathways to suicide: An integrative approach. In K. Hawton, and K. van Heeringen (Eds.), *The International Handbook of Suicide and Attempted Suicide.* (Pp. 223-234). Chichester: John Wiley and Sons Ltd.

Healy, D. (2003). Lines of evidence on the risks of suicide with selective serotonin reuptake inhibitors. *Psychotherapy and Psychosomatics, 72,* 71-79. Review.

Healy, D., and Whitaker, C. (2003). Antidepressants and suicide: risk-benefit conundrums. *Journal of Psychiatry and Neuroscience, 28,* 331-337. Review

Hollon, S.D., Stewart, M.O., Strunk, D. (2006). Enduring effects for cognitive behaviour therapy in the treatment of depression and anxiety. *Annual Review of Psychology,*
57, 285-315. Review

Høyer, E.H., Licht, R.W., and Mortensen, P.B. (2009). Risk factors of suicide in inpatients and recently discharged patients with affective disorders. A case-control study. *European Psychiatry, 24(5),* 317-321.

http://www.who.int/mental_health/prevention/suicide/suicideprevent/en/

Inskip, H.M., Harris, E.C., and Barraclough, B. (1998). Lifetime risk of suicide for affective disorder, alcoholism, and schizophrenia. *British Journal of Psychiatry, 172,* 35-37.

Isacsson, G., Bergman, U., and Rich, C.L. (1994a). Antidepressants, depression and suicide: an analysis of the San Diego study. *Journal of Affective Disorders, 32,* 277-286.

Isacsson, G., Holmgren, P., Wasserman, D., and Bergman, U. (1994b). Use of antidepressants among people committing suicide in Sweden. *British Medical Journal, 308,* 506-509.

Isometsä, E.T. (2001). Psychological autopsy studies--a review. *European Psychiatry, 16(7),* 379-385.

Isometsä, E.T., Aro, H.M., Henriksson, M.M., Heikinnen, M.E., and Lönnquist JK. (1994). Suicide in major depression in different treatment settings. *Journal of Clinical Psychiatry, 55,* 523-527.

Jick, H., Kaye, J.A., and Jick, S.S. (2004). Antidepressants and the risk of suicidal behaviours. *Journal of the American Medical Association, 292,* 379-381.

Jick, S.S., Dean, A.D., and Jick, H. (1995). Antidepressants and suicide. *British Medical Journal, 310,* 215-218.

Kapusta, N.D., Niederkrotenthaler, T., Etzersdorfer, E., Voracek, M., Dervic, K., Jandl-Jager, E., and Sonneck, G. (2009). Influence of psychotherapist density and antidepressant sales on suicide rates. *Acta Psychiatrica Scandinavica, 119,* 236-242.

Kay, D.W., Fahy, T., and Garside, R.F. (1970). A seven-month double-blind trial of amitryptiline and diazepam in ECT-treated depressed patients. *British Journal of Psychiatry, 117,* 667-671.

Kelleher, M.J., Daly, M., and Kelleher, M.J.A. (1992). The influence of Antidepressants in Overdose on the Increased Suicide Rate in Ireland Between 1971 and 1988. *British Journal of Psychiatry, 161,* 625-628.

Kessler, R.C., Borges, G., and Walters, E.E. (1999). Prevalence of and risk factors for lifetime suicide attempts in the national comorbidity survey. *Archives of General Psychiatry, 56,* 617-626.

Khan, A., Heather, A., Warner, M.A., and Brown, W.A. (2000). Symptom reduction and suicide risk in patients treated with placebo in antidepressant clinical trials. An analysis of the food and drug administration database. *Archives of General Psychiatry, 57,* 311-317.

Khan, A., Khan, S.R., Leventahl, R.M., and Brown, W.A. (2001). Symptom reduction and suicide risk in patients treated with placebo in antidepressant clinical trials: a replication analysis of the Food and Administration Database. *International Journal of Neuropsychopharmacology, 4,* 113-118.

Khan, A., Khan, S., Kolts, R., and Brown, W.A. (2003). Suicide rates in clinical trials of SSRIs, other antidepressants, and placebo: Analysis of FDA reports. *American Journal of Psychiatry, 160,* 790-792.

Leon, A.C., Keller, M.B., Warshaw, M.G., Mueller, T. I., Solomon, D.A., Coryell, W., and Endicott, J. (1999). Prospective study of fluoxetine treatment and suicidal behavior in affectively ill subjects. *American Journal of Psychiatry, 156,* 195-201.

Linehan, M.M. (1986). Suicidal people. One population or two? *Annals of the New York Academy of Sciences, 487,* 16-33.

Lönnquist, J.K. (2000). Psychiatric aspects of suicidal behaviour: depression. In K. Hawton, and K. van Heeringen (Eds.), *The International Handbook of Suicide and Attempted Suicide.* (Pp. 107-120). Chichester: John Wiley and Sons Ltd.

Luty SE, Carter JD, McKenzie JM, Rae AM, Frampton CM, Mulder RT, Joyce PR. (2007).Randomised controlled trial of interpersonal psychotherapy and cognitive-behavioural therapy for depression. *British Journal of Psychiatry, 190,* 496-502

Mann, J.J., Waternaux, C., Haas, G.L., and Malone, K.M. (1999).Toward a clinical model of suicidal behaviour in Psychiatric patients. *American Journal of Psychiatry*, 156, 181-189.Maris, R.A.W. *Pathways to Suicide.* Baltimore: The John Hopkins University Press; 1981.

Mattisson, C., Bogren, M., Nettelbladt, P., Munk-Jörgensen, P., Bhugra, D. (2005). First incidence depression in the Lundby Study: a comparison of the two time periods 1947-1972 and 1972-1997. *Journal of Affective Disorders, 87,* 151-60.

Mequies, L., Jasson, M., Soubrie, C., and Puech, A.J. (1998). Suicide prevention: the role of antidepressants. In M. Briley, and S. Montgomery (Eds.), *Antidepressant Therapy at the Dawn of the Third Millenium.* London: Martin Dunitz Ltd.

Miles, C.P. (1977). Conditions predisposing to suicide: a review. *Journal of Nervous and Mental Disease, 164,* 231-246.

Modestin, J., and Schwarzenbach, F. (1992). Effect of psychopharmacotherapy on suicide risk in discharged psychiatric in-patients. *Acta Psychiatrica Scandinavica, 85,* 173-175.

Möller, H.J. (2006). Is there evidence for negative effects of antidepressants on suicidality in depressive patients? A systematic review. *European Archives of Psychiatry and Clinical Neuroscience, 256(8),* 476-496.

Möller, H.J. (2008). Outcomes in major depressive disorder: the evolving concept of remission and its implications for treatment. *World Journal of Biological Psychiatry, 9(2),* 102-114. Review.

Montgomery, S.A., Dunner, D.L., and Dunbar, G.C. (1995). Reduction of suicidal thoughts with paroxetine in comparison with reference antidepressants and placebo. *European Neuropharmacology, 5,* 5-13.

Neeleman, J., and Wessely, S. (1997). Drugs taken in fatal and non-fatal self-poisoning: a study in South London. *Acta Psychiatrica Scandinavica, 95,* 283-287.

Nierenberg, A.A., Ostacher, M.J., Huffman, J.C., Ametrano, R.M., Fava, M., and Perlis, R.H. (2008). A brief review of antidepressant efficacy, effectiveness, indications, and usage for major depressive disorder. *Journal of Occupational and Environmental Medicine, 50(4),* 428-436.

Nunes, E.V., and Levin, F.R. (2004). Treatment of depression in patients with alcohol or other drug dependence: a meta-analysis. *Journal of the American Medical Association, 291(15),* 1887-1896.

Obafunwa, J.O., and Busttil, A. (1994a). Deaths from substance overdose in the Lothian and Border region of Scotland (1983-1991). *Human and Experimental Toxicology, 13,* 401-406.

Obafunwa, J.O., and Busttil, A. (1994b). A review of completed suicides in the Lothian and Border Region of Scotland (1987-1991). *Social Psychiatry and Psychiatric Epidemiology, 29,* 100-106.

Öhberg, A., Vuori, E., Ojanperä, I., and Lönnqvist, J. (1996). Alcohol and drugs in suicides. *British Journal of Psychiatry, 169(1),* 75-80.

O'Leary, D., Paykel, E., Todd, C., and Vardulaki, K. (2001). Suicide in primary affective disorders revisited: a systematic review by treatment era. *Journal of Clinical Psychiatry, 62(10),* 804-811. Review.

Pagnin, D., de Queiroz, V., Pini, S., and Cassano, G.B. (2004). Efficacy of ECT in depression: a meta-analytic review. *Journal of ECT, 20(1),* 13-20. Review

Parker, G., and Hadzi-Pavlovic, D. *Melancholia: A Disorder of Movement and Mood.* New York: Cambridge University Press; 1996.

Parker, G. (2007). Is the diagnosis of melancholia important in shaping clinical management? *Current Opinion in Psychiatry, 20,* 197-201.

Paykel, E.S., Myers, J.K., Lindenthal, J.J., and Tanner, J. (1974). Suicidal feelings in the general population: a prevalence study. *British Journal of Psychiatry, 124,* 460-69.

Perry, P., and Tsuang, M.T. (1979). Treatment of unipolar depression following electroconvulsive therapy. Relapse rate comparisons between lithium and tricyclic therapies following ECT. *Journal of Affective Disorders, 1,* 123-129.

Potter, W.Z., Rudorfer, M.V., and Manji, H. (1991). The Pharmacologic treatment of depression. *New England Journal of Medicine, 325,* 633-642.

Roullion, F., Phillips, R., Serruier, D., Ansaart, E., and Gérard, M.J. (1989). Rechutes de dépression unipolaire et efficacité de la maprotiline. [Recurrence of unipolar depression and efficacy of maprotiline.] *L'Encéphale, 15,* 527-534.

Sackeim, H.A., Haskett, R.F., Mulsant, B.H., Thase, M.E., Mann, J.J., Pettinati, H.M., Greenberg, R.M., Crowe, R.R., Cooper, T.B., and Prudic, J. (2001). Continuation pharmacotherapy in the prevention of relapse following electroconvulsive therapy: a randomized controlled trial.*Journal of American Medical Association, 285(10),* 1299-307.

Sanchez, L.E., and Le, L.T. (2001). Suicide in mood disorders. *Depression and Anxiety, 14(3),*177-182.

Saperia, J., Ashby, D., and Gunnell, D. (2006). Suicidal behaviour and SSRIs: updated meta-analysis. *British Medical Journal, 332(7555),* 1453.

Schou, M., and Weeke, A. (1988). Did manic-depressive patients who committed suicide receive prophylactic or continuation treatment at the time? *British Journal of Psychiatry, 153,* 324-327.

Simon, G.E., Savarino, J., Operskalski, B., and Wang, P.S. (2006). Suicide risk during antidepressant treatment. *American Journal of Psychiatry, 163(1),* 41-47.

Séguin, M., Lesage, A., Chawky, N., Guy, A., Daigle, F., Girard, G., and Turecki, G. (2006). Suicide cases in New Brunswick from April 2002 to May 2003: the importance of better recognizing substance and mood disorder comorbidity. *Canadian Journal of Psychiatry, 51(9),* 581-586.

Shah, R., Uren, Z., Baker, A., and Majeed, A. (2001). Deaths from antidepressants in England and Wales 1993-1997: analysis of a new national database. *Psychological Medicine, 31,* 203-210.

Sharma, V. (1999). Retrospective controlled study of in-patient ECT: does it prevent suicide? *Journal of Affective Disorders, 56,* 183-187.

Shorter, E. (2007). The doctrine of the two depressions in historical perspective. *Acta Psychiatrica Scandinavica, 115(Suppl. 433),* 5-13.

Sonawalla, S.B., and Fava, M. (2001). Severe depression: is there a best approach? *CNS Drugs, 15(10),* 765-776. Review.

Søndergård, L., Kvist, K., Lopez, A.G., Andersen, P.K., and Kessing, L.V. (2006). Temporal changes in suicide rates for persons treated and not treated with antidepressants in Denmark during 1995-1999. *Acta Psychiatrica Scandinavica, 114(3),* 168-176.

Stengel, E.N., Cook, N., and Kreeger, R.I. (1958). *Attempted Suicide.* Maudsley Monograph No. 4. London: Chapman and Hall.

Stone, M., Laughren, T., Jones, M.L., Levenson, M., Holland, P.C., Hughes, A., Hammad, T.A., Temple, R., and Rochester, G. (2009). Risk of suicidality in clinical trials of antidepressants in adults: analysis of proprietary data submitted to US Food and Drug Administration. *British Medical Journal, 339,* b2880. doi: 10.1136/bmj.b2880. Review.

Taiminen, T. (1993). Effect of psychopharmacotherapy on suicide risk in psychiatric in-patients. *Acta Psychiatrica Scandinavica, 87,* 45-47.

Taylor, M.A., and Fink, M. (2008). Restoring melancholia in the classification of mood disorders. *Journal of Affective Disorders, 105(1-3),* 1-14.

Tidemalm, D., Waern, M., Stefansson, C.G., Elofsson, S., and Runeson, B. (2008). Excess mortality in persons with severe mental disorder in Sweden: a cohort study of 12 103 individuals with and without contact with psychiatric services. *Clinical Practice and Epidemiology in Mental Health, 4,* 23.

Tollefson, G.D., Fawcett, J., Winokur, G., Beasley, C.M. Jr,, Potvin, J.H., Faries, D.E., Rampey, A.H. Jr., and Sayler, M.E. (1993).Evaluation of suicidality during pharmacologic treatment of mood and nonmood disorders. *Annals of Clinical Psychiatry, 5,* 209-224.

Trivedi, M.H., Rush, A.J., Wisniewski, S.R., Nierenberg, A.A., Warden, D., Ritz, L., Norquist, G., Howland, R.H., Lebowitz, B., McGrath, P.J., Shores-Wilson, K., Biggs, M.M., Balasubramani, G.K., and Fava, M., and STAR*D Study Team. (2006). Evaluation of outcomes with citalopram for depression using measurement-based care in STAR*D: implications for clinical practice. *American Journal of Psychiatry, 163(1),* 28-40.

UK ECT Review Group (2003). Efficacy and safety of electroconvulsive therapy in depressive disorders: a systematic review and meta-analysis. *Lancet, 361(9360),* 799-808. Review

Waern, M., Beskow, J., Runesson, B., and Skoog, I. (1996). High rate of antidepressant treatment in elderly people who commit suicide. *British Medical Journal, 313,* 1118.

Verberne, T.J. (2003). Antidepressant prescribing and suicide: Decline in suicide rate among older people predates 1991. *British Medical Journal, 327(7409),* 288.

Zisook, S., Goff, A., Sledge, P., and Shuchter, S.R. (1994). Reported suicidal behaviour and current suicidal ideation in a psychiatric out-patient clinic. *Annals of Clinical Psychiatry, 6,* 27-31.

In: Antidepressants: Types, Efficiency …
Editor: Jayden T. Van Leeuwen, pp.135-154
ISBN 978-1-61668-581-2

Chapter 5

SYNTHETIC INHIBITORS OF PROLYL ENDOPEPTIDASE EXHIBIT ANTIDEPRESSANT-LIKE EFFECTS IN RAT MODELS OF DEPRESSIVE SYNDROME AND ANXIETY-DEPRESSION STATE

N.A. Krupina [*,1]***, N.N. Khlebnikova*** [1]***, N.N. Zolotov*** [2]***,***
E.Yu Kushnareva [1]***, N.G. Bogdanova*** [1]***, and I.N. Orlova*** [1]

[1] Research Institute of General Pathology and Pathophysiology Russian Academy of Medical Sciences, Moscow, Russia

[2]Zakusov Research Institute of Pharmacology, Russian Academy of Medical Sciences, Moscow, Russia

ABSTRACT

Current theories of antidepressant action are substantially based on increasing the availability of the monoamine neurotransmitters. A new trend in antidepressant medication includes mechanisms connected with neuropeptides and peptide hormones lacking in side effects. Increasing evidence proves the involvement of neuropeptides in the development of depression and anxiety. However, there is a lack of data on the enzymes cleaving neuropeptides mediating depression and anxiety. Many neuropeptides involved in emotional responses are enriched in proline residues. The unique conformation of the prolyl bond protects peptides that contain proline residues from enzyme degradation. Thus, the enzymes cleaving prolyl bonds in neuropeptides are of particular interest.

Abnormal serum and plasma activities of the serine peptidases prolyl endopeptidase (EC 3.4.21.26) and dipeptidyl peptidase IV (EC 3.4.14.5) have been consistently observed in patients with mood disorders (Maes et al., 1994-2004). In our early experiments, synthetic inhibitors of PEP have been shown to have antidepressant-like activity in mice in a forced swimming test. We have found that the development of experimental dopamine deficit-dependent MPTP-induced depressive syndrome in rats is

[*] Corresponding author: Krupina NA. Email: krupina-na@yandex.ru.

accompanied by activation of PEP and DPPIV in the brain frontal cortex and in the striatum. Recently we have elaborated a new model of anxiety-depression state in rats exposed to irreversible synthetic inhibitor of DPPIV methionyl-2(S)-cyano-pyrrolidine in the early postnatal period. Adolescent and adult rats demonstrate increased anxiety, depression-related behavior in forced swimming test and anhedonia in sucrose preference test. Anxiety-depression state in males and females is associated with the increase of DPPIV/CD26 and PEP activity in frontal cortex, striatum, nucleus accumbens, hippocamp and hypothalamus in rat brain.

Competitive PEP inhibitor benzyloxycarbonyl-alanyl-proline promoted faster reduction of depression-like behavior in rats after MPTP withdrawal. Non-competitive PEP inhibitor benzyloxycarbonyl-methionyl-2(S)-cyano-pyrrolidine prevented the development of “behavioral despair” and disturbances in rhythmic organization of swimming behavior in forced swimming test both in rats with MPTP-induced depressive syndrome and in rats with DPPIV inhibitor-induced anxiety-depression state similar to NE/5-HT reuptake inhibitor imipramine.

The results obtained in two rat models of depression prove PEP inhibitors benzyloxycarbonyl-methionyl-2(S)-cyano-pyrrolidine and benzyloxycarbonyl-alanyl-proline to have antidepressant-like properties. Data afford grounds for a new approach to treatment strategy for depressive disorders based on modulation of PEP activity with synthetic inhibitors.

Introduction

Elucidation of the neurobiological basis of depression is rapidly increasing. Strong evidence exists for a preeminent role of the monoamine neurotransmitters, for overactivity of hypothalamic-pituitary-adrenal axis (HPA), for the role of peptide hormones, neuropeptides, proinflammatory cytokines and brain-derived growth factors [18, 23, 29, 40, 50, 60]. The function of G protein-coupled receptors and intracellular cascades initiated by the actions of neurotransmitters may also be altered in mental disorders, leading to downstream changes in neural function [9, 13, 74]. Recent works revealed the putative role of a depletion of omega-3 fatty acid levels and an imbalance between omega-3 and omega-6 polyunsaturated fatty acids in depressive patients [69].

Though great efforts are applied to overcome difficulties in recognizing affective disorders, thus far the genesis of these diseases remains elusive.

Search and studies of putative antidepressants, on the one hand, are based on known mechanisms, but, on the other hand, may reveal a new trend in understanding neurobiological mechanisms of the depression genesis. Despite reasonable attempts for revising the monoamine hypothesis [1], current theories of antidepressant action are substantially based on increasing the availability of the monoamine neurotransmitters [3], and no wonder monoamine pre-synaptic re-uptake inhibitors of serotonin, noradrenalin and dopamine are usually considered “first-line” antidepressants [30].

Among new future antidepressant targets including neurotrophic factors [71], components of the signal transduction pathways [79], omega-3 polyunsaturated fatty acids [76], much attention is paid to neuropeptides/peptide hormones and their receptors [6, 41] mediating therapeutic effect lacking in significant adverse effects. Modulation of monoaminergic transmission is the most likely mechanism by which neuropeptides may work in affective disorders. Many peptides and numerous regulatory neuropeptide signaling pathways are involved in pathophysiology of affective states [63]. Intervention at these molecular targets is expected to overcome the limitations of existing antidepressants. Substance P, neuropeptide Y, thyroliberin (TRH), corticoliberin (CRF), arginin-vasopressin, opioid peptides, oxytocin, galanin, are the most frequently nominated peptides for involving in the pathogenesis of affective disorders [5, 19, 38, 39, 60, 61, 64, 73]. These peptides are substrates for peptidases of different classes. Disturbances in peptides' processing may be due to the corresponding peptidases' abnormalities.

Our interest to proline-specific peptidases is founded on clinical and experimental data. Many neuropeptides involved in emotional responses are enriched in proline residues. The unique conformation of the prolyl bond protects peptides that contain proline residues against cleavage by non-specific proteases [15] giving rise to the search of the enzymes cleaving this bond [16]. Proline-specific peptidases belong to different classes.

Clinical data give evidence that at least two of the serine proline-specific peptidases probably play an important role in the development of depression and anxiety. Abnormal serum and plasma activities of the serine peptidases prolyl endopeptidase (PEP, EC 3.4.21.26, prolyl oligopeptidase) and dipeptidyl peptidase IV (DPPIV/CD26, EC 3.4.14.5) have been consistently observed in patients with mood disorders. In fact, numerous Maes' works demonstrated the association between the activities of proline-specific peptidases in plasma or serum and depressive and anxiety ratings in patients [43, 44]. Lowered serum DPPIV activity was associated with depressive symptoms [42, 44, 45]. As for PEP, the decrease of serum or plasma activity of PEP was observed in most cases [47, 48, 49, 81]. Antidepressant fluoxetine restored lowered plasma PEP activity to normal levels [46]. Maes and colleagues hypothesized that both proline-specific peptidases play a role in the pathophysiology of depression.

PEP and DPPIV are ubiquitously distributed in various tissues in mammals, including the brain [21, 58]. PEP is a predominantly cytosolic serine endopeptidase that hydrolyses peptide bonds on the carboxyl side of proline residue in peptides and proteins with a relatively small molecular weight [78]. Although PEP is associated with many functions [56, 57] its physiological role has remained unclear. Substrates for PEP include neuropeptides associated with various neurological and mental diseases (learning and memory, senescence, depression, anxiety, appetitive behavior and so on) suggesting a role for PEP in those processes [4, 11, 22].

DPPIV/CD26, also called adenosine deaminase binding protein, is put on the list of exopeptidases. It is a membrane-bound enzyme that cleaves the N-terminal dipeptides from regulatory peptides with a proline or an alanine residue in the second position from the amino end [2]. This peptidase is potentially involved in the regulation of functions of the immune, endocrine, and nervous systems [53, 66, 70, 80].

Recent experimental data in rodents with targeted inactivation of the gene of DPPIV testify for the implication of this enzyme in the pathophysiology of depression and anxiety. DPPIV-deficient mutant Japanese and German F344 rat substrains as compared with a wild-type-like F344 substrain from the U.S.A. demonstrated reduced stress-like responses in the open field, social interaction, and passive avoidance test as well as a reduced stress-induced analgesia [25]. CD26-/- (CD26-negative) mice resulting from targeted inactivation of the DPPIV gene demonstrated a decreased immobility in the forced swim and tail suspension tests that means a reduced depression-like behavior, higher horizontal and vertical activities in a motor activity test that means increased novelty-induced behavioral activation, no differences in anxiety as compared to controls in the black/white box and more head dips in the hole-board apparatus that, in the authors opinion, means increased curiosity [12]. Authors concluded that DPPIV inactivation in mice broadly leads to an antidepressant-like and hyperactive phenotype. At present DPPIV is considered a putative modulator of depression-related and anxiety-like behavior using neuropeptide Y [24] and substance P as substrates. Recently other substrates for DPPIV – opioid peptides and glucagon-like peptide-1 [53, 70] – also have been shown to take part in affective disorders [5, 14, 54].

Animal models in psychiatry are no doubt useful in understanding the neurobiological basis of mental diseases. Many (may be most) of behavioral scientists engaged in this problem now share the opinion that experimental modeling in psychiatry is one of the effective approaches to solving the problem and predicting successful treatment strategies [52, 65]. In early works, one of the co-authors of the present paper showed antidepressant effect for several synthetic dipeptide inhibitors of PEP (Z-AA-Pro-OH, where AA are the residues of amino acids Gly, Ala, Ile, and Pro) in Porsolt model of stress-induced depression (Porsolt forced swimming test) [82] in mice and revealed the modulation of dopaminergic function in brain in the presence of PEP inhibitors [59]. Given that, increased PEP activity in mice brain with experimental depression-like state is suggested.

Peptidase's activity in blood and brain may not coincide. Besides, the results in different experimental models are often distinct. We have used two other rat models of affective state in rodents to define PEP and DPPIV activity in brain structures.

The first model was elaborated in our previous investigations [31, 36, 62, 67]. Experimental depressive syndrome was induced in male Wistar rats by repeated systemic specific-for-dopamine-neurons proneurotoxin 1-methyl-4-phenyl-1,2,3,6-tetrahydropyridine (MPTP) administration. MPTP caused core symptoms of behavioral depression such as anhedonia, behavioral despair and low level of vital motivation and besides disturbances in rhythmic organization of swimming behavior. We consider MPTP-induced behavioral alterations in rats to be a model of dopamine deficiency-dependent depression-like syndrome in rats.

Using this model of depression-like behavior, we showed for the first time the increase of PEP and DPPIV activity in target structures of the central dopaminergic brain systems [35]. The development of MPTP-induced depressive syndrome in rats was accompanied by activation of PEP and DPPIV in the brain frontal cortex. PEP activity in the striatum also increased under the circumstances.

The second model has been recently elaborated in our studies. There is increasing recognition that many psychiatric disorders including depression and anxiety disturbances are neurodevelopmental in their origins [17, 20, 51]. Integrated data from human studies and from animal models point to a critical period for maturing neural circuits that mediate motivation and anxiety [7, 8, 20]. We have chosen the intervention in the DPPIV development at the first postnatal weeks when the peptidase activity is being increased [26]. Administration of original synthetic inhibitor of DPPIV methionyl-2(S)-cyano-pyrrolidine (Met-Prd-N) in Wistar rat pups of both genders increased anxiety in adolescent and adult experimental males and females in the elevated plus-maze, open field and in a battery of tests for evaluating anxiety-phobic states [33, 32]. Depression-related immobility behavior and index of depression indicating disturbances in rhythmic organization of swimming behavior in forced swimming test were higher in adult rats of both genders as compared with control. Adolescent and adult rats also presented anhedonia in sucrose preference test. The findings proved the development of long-term anxiety-depression-like state in rats exposed to the inhibitor of DPPIV in early postnatal period. Behavioral disturbances caused by postnatal modulation of peptidase activity are considered to be a new rat model of anxiety-depression-like state.

Anxiety-depression state in males and females postnatally exposed to the inhibitor of DPPIV was associated with the increase of DPPIV and PEP activity in frontal cortex, striatum, nucleus accumbens, hippocamp, and hypothalamus in rat brain [37].

The results obtained in two rat models of affective state indicate that proline-specific peptidases in the target structures of the brain dopaminergic system and in limbic structures are probably involved in the pathogenesis of depression and anxiety.

The aim of present investigation was to assess the effects of novel synthetic PEP inhibitors benzyloxycarbonyl-methionyl-2(S)-cyano-pyrrolidine (Z-Met-Prd-N) and benzyloxycarbonyl-alanyl-proline (Z-Ala-Pro) on behavioral deficits in two experimental models of depression-like behavior in rats - MPTP-induced depressive syndrome and anxiety-depression state induced by postnatal rat exposure to DPPIV inhibitor.

METHODS

All experiments were done in accordance with the Helsinki Declaration and with national and institutional guidelines. All animals were maintained under standard laboratory conditions and kept on a 12-h light-dark cycle with light onset at 7 a.m.

Model I. Experimental MPTP-induced depressive syndrome. Male Wistar rats ("Stolbovaya" nursery, Russia) were used weighing between 320-450 g at the time of the basic behavioral testing. The rats were kept individually in standard clear plastic cages (21 x 35 x 15 cm) on a 12-h light/dark cycle, with water and food available ad libitum during the experiments except the days when daily fluid intake and sucrose preference were assessed. All behavioral testing occurred between 10:00 and 17:00.

MPTP (synthesized at VV Zakusov Research Institute of Pharmacology, Russian Academy of Medical Sciences) was administered once a day intraperitoneally at a dose of 20 mg/kg for 14 days. Using that mild schedule of drug administration, we succeeded in minimizing extrapyramidal disorders and easier revealing emotional-behavioral disturbances in rats. Control rats were subjected to an equivolume (1 ml/kg) saline administration. We used several depression-related tests, which are thought to reflect different symptoms of depressive syndrome.

Sucrose preference test. Water and 10%-sucrose consumption were measured daily under free choice between water and sucrose solution through 3 weeks. Rats were kept in their home cages. Adaptation period to choice between sucrose solution and water lasted 4 days. Battles with sucrose solution and water were exchanged in places daily. Preference for sucrose over water was calculated as a relation of consumed 10%-sucrose solution (g) to daily fluid intake (water+sucrose, g) in percent. Decrease of preference for 10%-sucrose over water testified to anhedonia. Decrease in daily fluid intake testified to lowering drinking motivation.

Forced swimming test. Swimming behavior was assessed in modified forced swimming test based on classic method by Porsolt et al. [68]. Rats were placed in container with water at 25^0C for 10 min. The immobility time was assessed on drug administration and after drug withdrawal. Besides, the number of the shortest periods of immobility (less than 6 s) and total number of periods of active swimming were counted through the session. The relation of the number of the shortest periods of immobility to total number of periods of active swimming has been used as an indicator of disturbances in rhythmic organization of swimming behavior – so called index of depression (ID). Increase of immobility time testified to "behavioral despair", increase of ID – to the appearance of biorhythms' disturbances. Session 1 was conducted on the day 12 beginning from MPTP/saline administration, session 2 – on the day 12 of drugs withdrawal.

Repeated MPTP administration as a rule caused decrease of daily liquid consumption and lowering of preference for the 10%-sucrose over water, increase of immobility time and higher index of depression in forced swimming test. On the whole, MPTP-treated rats demonstrated a set of depressive-related symptoms that is an experimental depression-like syndrome.

Model II. Experimental anxiety-depression-like state induced by postnatal exposure to the inhibitor of DPPIV.

Pregnant females (from "Stolbovaya" nursery, Russia) weighing between 250-300 g were housed individually under standard conditions in the vivarium of the Institute of General Pathology and Pathophysiology (Moscow, Russia). Only male pups were used in present investigation.

Irreversible inhibitor of DPPIV Met-Prd-N [synthesized at VV Zakusov Research Institute of Pharmacology, Russian Academy of Medical Sciences, inhibitory constant with Gly-Pro-7-amine-4-cumarylamide as substrate is 2,7 nmol/l, does not decrease the activity of PEP, DPPII, DPPVIII, DPPI (catepsin C), tripsin, chimotripsin, prolidase] was administered in rat pups from postnatal day 5 to day 18 inclusive at a dose of 1 mg/kg, intraperitoneally. Pups from experimental and control groups were weighed daily before treatment and received either Met-Prd-N or vehicle in an equivolume (0.1 ml/10 g body weight) correspondingly. Makeup Met-Prd-N solution was used. Met-Prd-N was dissolved in 1-2 drops of TWEEN-80 and then diluted to the final concentration with saline.

Post weaning at postnatal day 30, rats were separated and grouped as necessary to produce experimental and control groups consisted of pups from 3-4 litters.

In this investigation rats were weighed weekly during 4 months after birth to consider any long-term effects on body weight gain (data not showen).

Depression-related behavior was evaluated in the *forced swimming test* in adult 2 (session 1) and 3 months-old rats (session 2) as described above.

Drugs. Two original PEP inhibitors were tested: non-competitive PEP inhibitor *Z-Met-Prd-N* and competitive PEP inhibitor *Z-Ala-Pro* (both synthesized at VV Zakusov Research Institute of Pharmacology, Russian Academy of Medical Sciences). In both models of depression-like state *imipramine* (NE/5-HT reuptake inhibitor, 10 mg/kg, dissolved in saline, i.p., «EGIS», Hungary) was used as a reference antidepressant.

In the model of MPTP-induced depressive syndrome *Z-Met-Prd-N* (1 mg/kg, i.p., inhibitory constant for PEP from subcortical structures with Z-Ala-Pro-7-amine-4-cumarylamide as substrate is 4.4 nmol/l, from cortex – 1.4 nmol/l) was administered daily, 30 min before MPTP injection, for 14 days (Figure1A). On day 15 rats from experimental and control groups were sacrificed and brain tissues were extracted for further biochemical analysis (data not shown in present paper). Just the same scheme was used for tricyclic antidepressant imipramine administration.

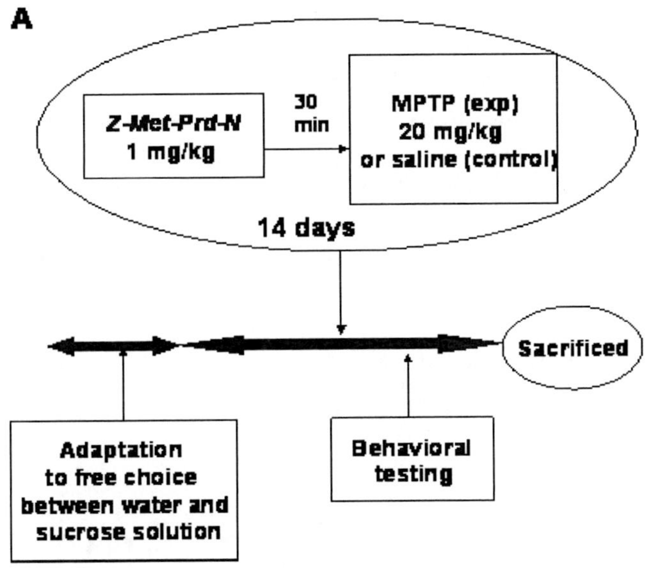

Figure 1A. Scheme of *Z-Met-Prd-N* study in rats with MPTP-induced depressive syndrome.

In the model of MPTP-induced depressive syndrome *Z-Ala-Pro-OH* (3 mg/kg, i.p., inhibitory constant for PEP from subcortical structures with Z-Ala-Pro-7-amine-4-cumarylamide as substrate is 20.0 μmol/l, from cortex – 90.0 μmol/l) was injected daily, 30 min before MPTP, from day 8 to day 14 inclusive. Observations were continued for two weeks after MPTP/saline withdrawal (Figure1B). Under both schemes, saline was injected in control rats instead of MPTP.

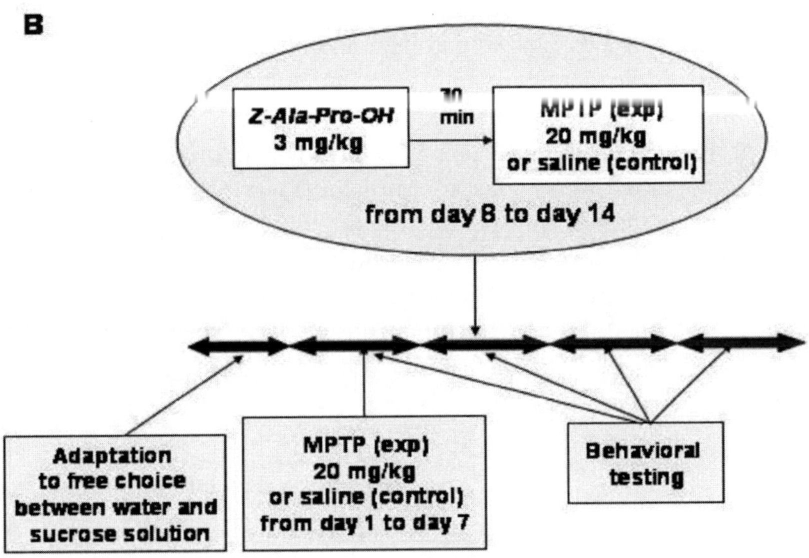

Figure 1B. Scheme of *Z-Ala-Pro* study in rats with MPTP-induced depressive syndrome.

In the rat model of DPPIV inhibitor-induced anxiety-depression-like state three pairs of groups were formed according to the results obtained in forced swimming session in 2-monthes-old rats. All experimental groups did not significantly differ in the immobility time and ID from each other. Values in experimental groups were significantly higher comparing to corresponding control groups. Rats of all experimental/control pairs were subjected to 10 days long drug injections: first pair – to PEP inhibitor *Z-Met-Prd-N* (2 mg/kg, i.p.) (Figure 2), second - to the injections of *imipramine*, third - to saline. All drugs and saline were injected in the same volume 1 ml/kg. Testing session was conducted one day after the last injection.

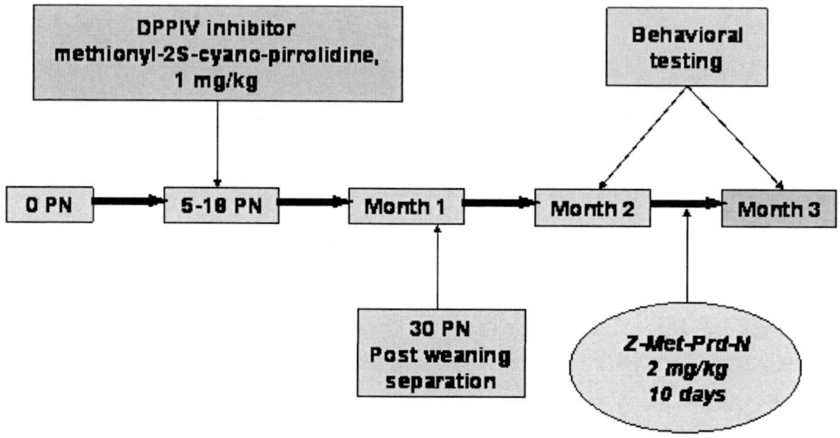

Figure 2. Scheme of *Z-Met-Prd-N* study in rats with DPPIV inhibitor-induced anxiety-depression state. PN – postnatal days. 0 – the day of birth.

Makeup solutions of PEP inhibitors were used. Z-Met-Prd-N and Z-Ala-Pro-OH were dissolved in 1-2 drops of TWEEN-80 and then diluted to the final concentration with saline. PEP inhibitors and vehicle were injected in the same volume 1 ml/kg.

Statistical analysis. Data are presented as groups mean (M)± standard error of the mean (SE). Data analyses were performed using STATISTICA software (Version 6.0). If normal distribution (Kolmogorov-Smirnov test for normality) was not rejected statistical significance of the results was determined with parametric single factor analysis of variance (ANOVA), single factor (drug exposure) repeated measures (days) ANOVA followed by individual comparisons by Newman-Keuls or Duncan tests, and Student T-test. If normal distribution was rejected, nonparametric single factor analysis of variance (Kruskall-Wallis ANOVA) followed by Mann–Whitney U-test, and Wilcoxon matched paired test were conducted. The α level was set at 0.05.

RESULTS

Model I. Experimental MPTP-Induced Depressive Syndrome

Z-Met-Prd-N. The effects of PEP inhibitor Z-Met-Prd-N on the MPTP-induced changes in the immobility time and ID are shown in Figure 3. In MPTP-treated rats immobility time

[H (3, N=40) = 8.090 p = 0.440] and ID [H (3, N=40) = 8.547 p = 0.036] were increased as compared to other groups that is “behavioral despair” and rhythmical disturbances in swimming behavior in the forced swimming test developed.

Z-Met-Prd-N prevented the increase of immobility time and ID in MPTP-treated rats likewise imipramine [27]. Imipramine, however, appeared to increase the immobility time in rats with a combination of Imipramine plus Saline (see Figure 3, upper row), but the effect did not reach the significance level [34]. Data may reflect side effects of imipramine.

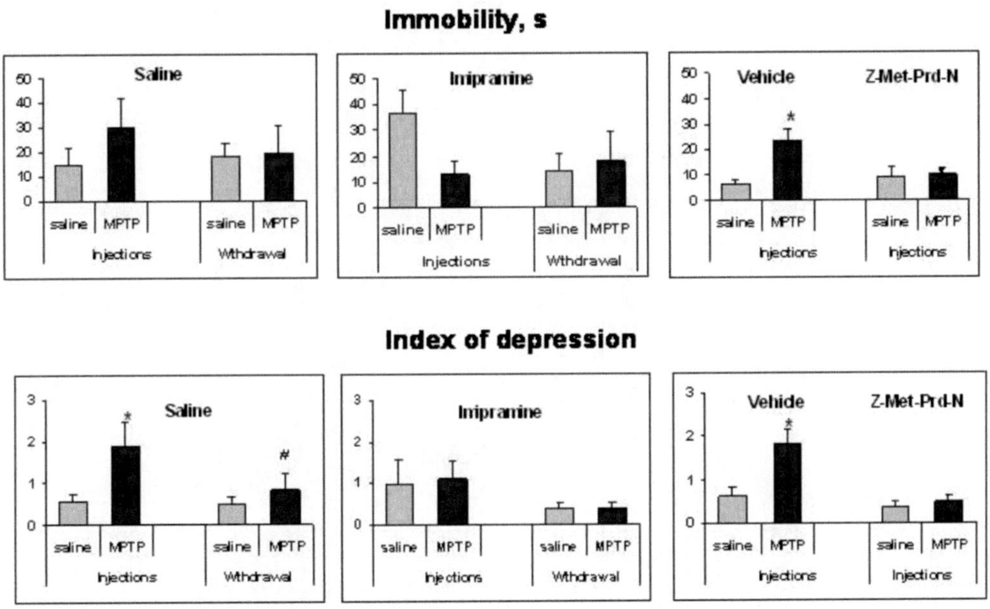

Figure 3. Immobility time (upper row) and index of depression (lower row) in rats with a combination of a Saline plus Saline (*N*=6), a combination of a Saline plus MPTP (*N*=7), a combination of an Imipramine 10 mg/kg plus Saline (*N*=[illegible]), a combination of an Imipramine 10 mg/kg plus MPTP (*N*=[illegible]), a combination of a Vehicle plus Saline (*N*=*12*), a combination of a Vehicle plus MPTP (*N*=*12*), a combination of Z-Met-Prd-N 1.0 mg/kg plus Saline (*N*=*8*), a combination of Z-Met-Prd-N 1.0 mg/kg plus MPTP (*N*=*8*) by the end of the period of drug administration and after withdrawal. Results are given as the mean ± S.E.M. *, significantly different from control; #, significantly different from a period of injections.

In MPTP-treated rats (a combination of a Vehicle plus MPTP) decrease in sucrose preference ($F_{(14, 154)} = 2.533$ $p = 0.003$) and daily fluid intake ($F_{(14, 154)} = 4.036$ $p = 0.000$) was observed that is anhedonia and decrease in drinking motivation appeared (Figure 4).

In rats with combinations of a Vehicle plus Saline and Z-Met-Prd-N plus Saline sucrose preference were not changed. As for fluid intake, it was not changed in rats with a combination of a Vehicle plus Saline but increased in rats with a combination of Z-Met-Prd-N plus Saline ($F_{(14, 84)} = 2.187$ $p = 0.015$).

In rats with a combination of Z-Met-Prd-N plus MPTP sucrose preference ($F_{(14, 98)} = 3.161$; $p = 0.000$) and daily fluid intake ($F_{(14, 98)} = 4.990$ $p = 0.000$) were decreased similar to rats with a combination of a Vehicle plus MPTP.

Thus, Z-Met-Prd-N had no effect on MPTP-induce anhedonia and the decrease in drinking motivation. Between groups comparison confirmed conclusion.

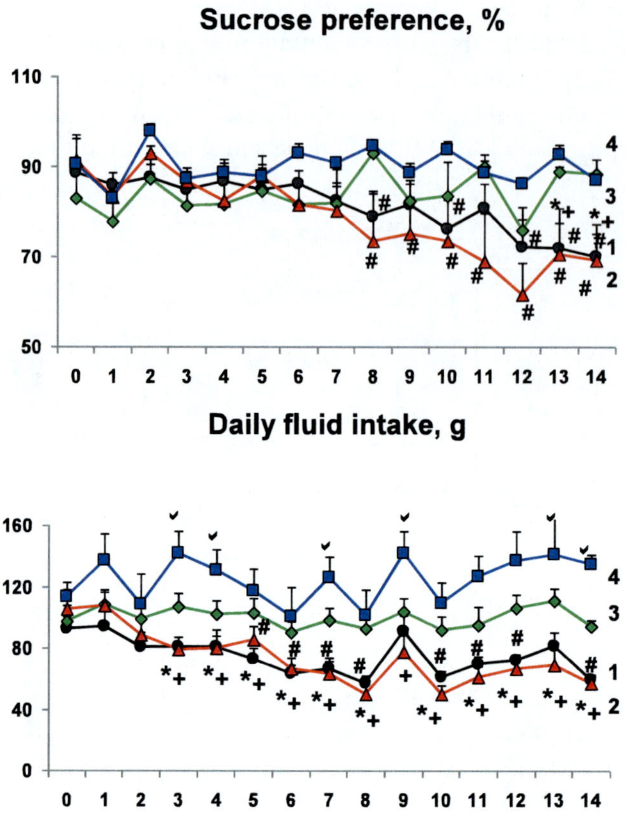

Figure 4. Sucrose preference and daily fluid intake in rats with a combination of a Vehicle plus MPTP (*N=12*) (curve 1, black), a combination of Z-Met-Prd-N 1.0 mg/kg plus MPTP (*N=8*) (curve 2, red), a combination of a Vehicle plus Saline (*N=12*) (curve 3,green), a combination of Z-Met-Prd-N 1.0 mg/kg plus Saline (*N=8*) (curve 4, blue) in the period of drug injection. 0 -14 – days of drug administration. Results are given as the mean ± S.E.M. *, significantly different for group 1 vs. group 3; +, significantly different for group 2 vs. group 4; ✔, significantly different for group 4 vs. group 3; #, significantly different from day 0 for groups 1 and 2.

Z-Ala-Pro-OH. In this series no significant changes in the immobility time and ID were revealed in rats with a combination of a Vehicle plus MPTP in the period of injection and after withdrawal (Figure 5). Nevertheless, the decrease in the values of immobility and ID after withdrawal was marked in all other groups.

In MPTP-treated rats (a combination of a Vehicle plus MPTP) decrease in the preference for the sucrose over water ($F_{(29, 174)} = 3.025$ $p = 0.000$) and in daily fluid intake ($F_{(29, 174)}=3.268$, $p=0.000$) was observed for two weeks of MPTP administration and two weeks after withdrawal. Data confirmed depressive symptoms in animals (Figure 6).

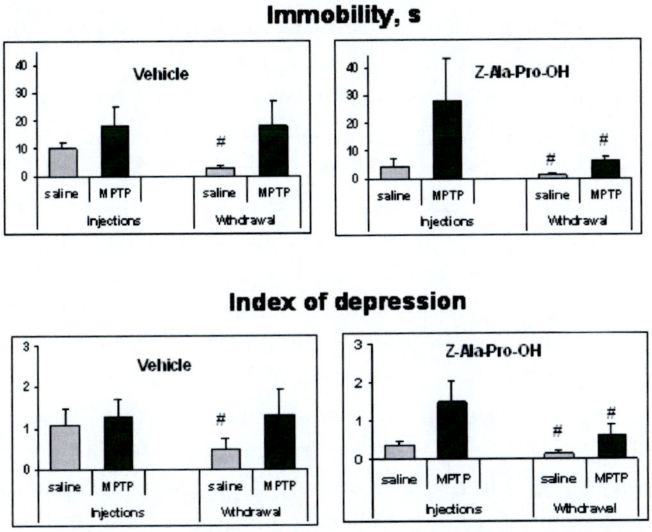

Figure 5. Immobility time (upper row) and index of depression (lower row) in rats with a combination of a Vehicle plus Saline (N=8), a combination of a Vehicle plus MPTP (N=8), a combination of Z-Ala-Pro-OH 3.0 mg/kg plus Saline (N=8), a combination of Z-Ala-Pro-OH 3.0 mg/kg plus MPTP (N=7) by the end of the period of drug administration and after withdrawal. Results are given as the mean ± S.E.M. #, significantly different from a period of injections.

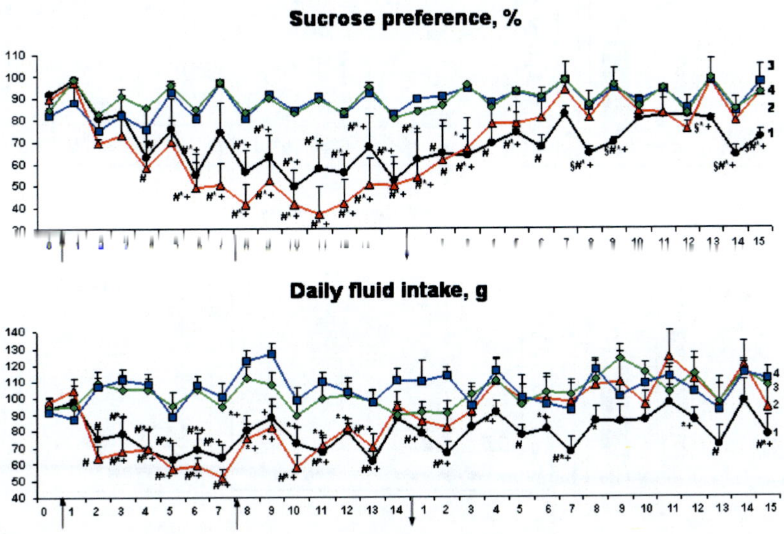

Figure 6. Sucrose preference and daily fluid intake in rats with a combination of a Vehicle plus MPTP (N=8) (curve 1, black), a combination of Z-Ala-Pro-OH 3.0 mg/kg plus MPTP (N=7) (curve 2, red), a combination of a Vehicle plus Saline (N=8) (curve 3, green), a combination of Z-Ala-Pro-OH 3.0 mg/kg plus Saline (N=8) (curve 4, blue). 0 – the day before drug administration; 1-7 – days of MPTP/saline administration without Z-Ala-Pro-OH/vehicle; 8-14 – days of MPTP/saline administration with Z-Ala-Pro-OH/vehicle; 1-15 – days after withdrawal. Arrows show changes in the schedule of the experiment. Results are given as the mean ± S.E.M. *, significantly different for group 1 and 2 vs. group 3; +, significantly different for group 1 and 2 vs. group 4; §, significantly different for group 1 vs. group 2; #, significantly different from day 0 for groups 1 and 3.

In rats with a combination of Z-Ala-Pro-OH plus MPTP decrease in sucrose preference ($F_{(29, 174)} = 5.376$, $p = 0.000$) and in daily fluid intake ($F_{(29, 174)} = 6.069$; $p = 0.000$) was observed in the period of drug administration however rapidly restored to normal after drug withdrawal [28].

In groups with a combination of a Vehicle plus Saline and Z-Ala-Pro-OH plus Saline no decrease in sucrose preference or daily fluid intake appeared. On the contrary, on some days increase in sucrose preference and fluid intake was revealed (correspondingly $F_{(29, 203)} = 18{,}335$ and $F_{(29, 203)} = 3{,}077$; $F_{(29, 203)} = 3{,}550$ and $F_{(29, 203)} = 3.220$ in all cases $p = 0.000$).

Between groups' analysis confirmed the difference in rats with a combination of a Vehicle plus MPTP and rats in other groups including the animals with a combination of Z-Ala-Pro-OH plus MPTP.

Model II. Experimental anxiety-depression-like state induced by postnatal exposure to the inhibitor of DPPIV. Z-Met-Prd-N likewise imipramine essentially decreased heighten ID and immobility time (Figure 7) in rats with anxiety-depression-like state induced by postnatal exposure to DPPIV inhibitor [32, 33]. Subchronic saline administration did not normalize rats' behavior in forced swimming test.

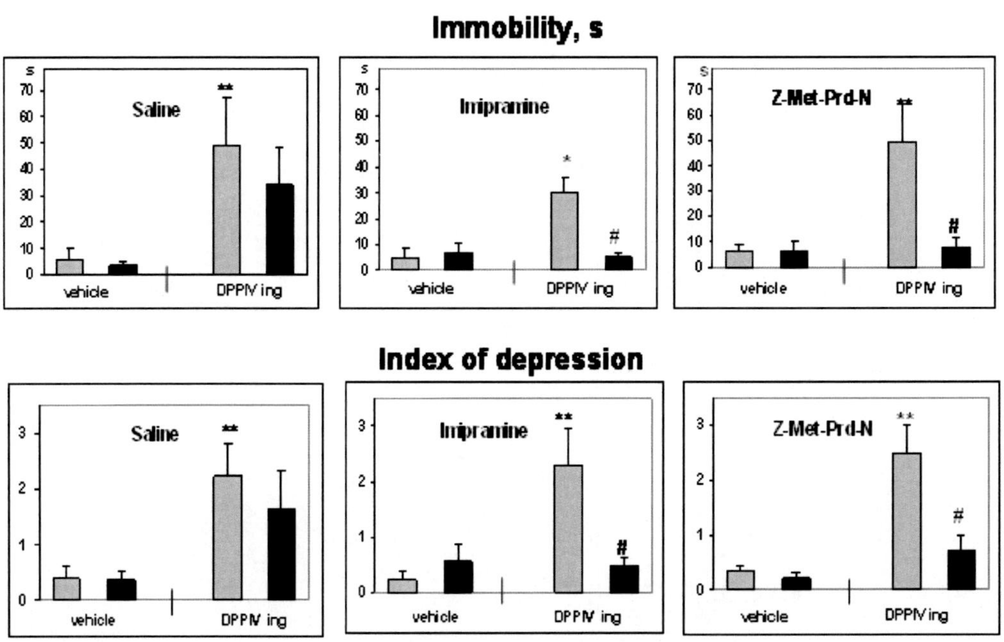

Figure 7. Immobility time (upper row) and index of depression (lower row) in rats with a combination of a Saline plus Vehicle (*N=8*), a combination of a Saline plus DPPIV inhibitor (*N=7*), a combination of an Imipramine 10 mg/kg plus Vehicle (*N=7*), a combination of an Imipramine 10 mg/kg plus DPPIV inhibitor (*N=6*), a combination of Z-Met-Prd-N 2.0 mg/kg plus Vehicle (*N=8*), a combination of Z-Met-Prd-N 2.0 mg/kg plus DPPIV inhibitor (*N=7*) before (grey columns) and just after (black columns) subchronic drug administration. Results are given as the mean ± S.E.M. *, significantly different from control (groups with Vehicle); #, significantly different from the same group before drug administration.

DISCUSSION

The main finding of the present study is that the novel synthetic inhibitors of PEP with different mechanism of the enzyme inhibiting action - Z-Met-Prd-N and Z-Ala-Pro-OH - prevent or suppress depression-like behavior. These effects were comparable to those observed with the reference antidepressant imipramine but lacking side effect on immobility time. Nevertheless, mild increase in daily fluid intake under subchronic administration of Z-Met-Prd-N was observed. This fact needs further investigation. Importantly that effective dose of Z-Met-Prd-N in DPPIV inhibitor-induced model of behavioral depression was of five lower as compared to imipramine.

In present investigation PEP inhibitors demonstrated antidepressant-like efficacy in two different rat models: first based on experimental dopamine deficient state, second – on the inhibition of DPPIV in early postnatal period. The last model is one of the newest models. Nevertheless, we have already obtained data testifying to the deficit of dopaminergic function in adult rats postnatally exposed to the inhibitor of DPPPIV (unpublished data). Given that, and consider the decrease in catecholaminergic function to be one of the accepted mechanisms in depression [60] we suppose that PEP inhibitors may realize their antidepressant-like effects, at least partly, by enhancing dopaminergic function in CNS in indirect way.

PEP distribution in CNS founded the opportunity to promote functions of some neurotransmitter systems - glutamatergic, GABAergic, and cholinergic neurotransmission systems [57] with altered activity in mood disorders [75] that interact with dopaminergic system [55]. Disturbances of neuropeptides that serve as PEP substrates may also contribute to the genesis of affective disorders [77]. If this is the case, PEP inhibitors may normalize neurotransmitter and peptides function followed by restoration of CNS activity.

Recent data elucidate putative molecular mechanisms of antidepressant-like effects of PEP inhibitors. Inhibition of PEP activity is reported to enhance phosphoinositide signaling and mood stabilizers may limit mood swings to depression by inhibiting PEP thus increasing phosphoinositide signalling [10, 56, 72]

Anyhow, it is clear that the mechanism of antidepressant-like action of PEP inhibitors is probably complex and in turn suggests the mechanisms of PEP involvement in pathophysiology of depression.

As for DPPIV, the fact that modulation of the enzyme's activity in early ontogenesis may cause persistent disturbances in behavior similar to anxiety-depression-like state gives the basis to suggest the role of DPPIV in triggering affective disorders.

In whole, the data testify to the involvement of proline-specific peptidases, particularly PEP, in the mechanisms of depression. Although the specific mechanisms underlying the role of these enzymes in mood disorders have yet to be clarified, it is clear that PEP inhibitors may be effective as antidepressants. Given our early results, increase activity of PEP in brain structures in animal models of depression-like behavior founded putative therapeutic efficacy of PEP inhibitors.

Conclusion

The results obtained in two rat models of depression-like behavior give the evidence to antidepressant-like properties in PEP inhibitors Z-Met-Prd-N and Z-Ala-Pro-OH. Our findings suggest a role for PEP and probably DPPIV in the pathophysiology of depression and give much promise for the development of new approaches to complex pathogenetic therapy of depressive disorders with PEP-modulating drugs.

References

[1] Aan het Rot M, Mathew SJ, Charney DS. Neurobiological mechanisms in major depressive disorder. *CMAJ* 2009;180(3) 305-313. doi:10.1503/cmaj.080697

[2] Aertgeerts K, Ye Sh, Shi L, Prasad SG, Witmer D, Chi E, Sang B-Ch, Wijnands RA, Webb DR, Swanson RV. N-linked glycosylation of dipeptidyl peptidase IV (CD26): Effects on enzyme activity, homodimer formation, and adenosine deaminase binding. *Protein Science* 2004;13:145-154. doi:10.1110/ps.03352504

[3] Artigas F, Nutt DJ, Shelton R. Mechanism of Action of Antidepressants. *Psychopharmacol Bull.* 2002; 36(Suppl 2):123-132.

[4] Bellemere G, Morain P, Vaudry H, Jegou S. Effect of S 17092, a novel prolyl endopeptidase inhibitor, on substance P and alpha-melanocyte-stimulating hormone breakdown in the rat brain. *J. Neurochem.* 2003;84(5):919-929. doi:10.1046/j.1471-4159.2003.01536.x

[5] Bodnar RJ. Endogenous Opiates and Behavior: 2006. *Peptides* 2007;28(12):2435–2513. doi:10.1016/j.peptides.2007.09.002.

[6] Brain SD, Cox HM. Neuropeptides and their receptors: innovative science providing novel therapeutic targets. *Brit. J. Pharmacol.* 2006;147:S202–S211. doi: 10.1038/sj.bjp.0706461.

[7] Card JP, Levitt P, Gluhovsky M, Rinaman L. Early experience modifies the postnatal assembly of autonomic emotional motor circuits in rats. *Neuroscience* 2005;25(40):9102–9111. doi:10.1523/JNEUROSCI.2345-05.2005

[8] Cassano P, Hidalgo A, Burgos V, Adris S, Argibay P. Hippocampal upregulation of the cyclooxygenase-2 gene following neonatal clomipramine treatment (a model of depression). *Pharmacogenomics* 2006;6(6):381-387. doi:10.1038/sj.tpj.6500385

[9] Catapano LA, Manji HK. G protein-coupled receptors in major psychiatric disorders. *Biochim Biophys Acta* 2007;1768(4):976–993. doi:10.1016/j.bbamem.2006.09.025

[10] Cheng L, Lumb M, Polgár L, Mudge AW. How can the mood stabilizer VPA limit both mania and depression? *Mol. Cell Neurosci.* 2005;29(2):155-161.

[11] Cunningham D.F., O'Connor B. Proline specific peptidases. *Biochim Biophys Acta* 1997;1343:160-186. doi:10.1016/S0167-4838(97)00134-9

[12] El Yacoubi M, Vaugeois JM, Marguet D, Sauze N, Guieu R, Costentin J, Fenouillet E Behavioral characterization of CD26 deficient mice in animal tests of anxiety and antidepressant-like activity. *Behav Brain Res* 2006;171(2):279-285. doi:10.1016/j.bbr.2006.04.003

[13] Feng P, Guan Z, Yang X, Fang J. Impairments of ERK signal transduction in the brain in a rat model of depression induced by neonatal exposure of clomipramine. *Brain Res* 2003;991(1-2):195-205. doi:10.1016/j.brainres.2003.08.018

[14] Filliol D., Ghozland S., Chluba J., Martin M, Matthes HW, Simonin F, Befort K, Gavériaux-Ruff C, Dierich A, LeMeur M, Valverde O, Maldonado R, Kieffer BL. Mice deficient for delta- and mu-opioid receptors exhibit opposing alterations of emotional responses. *Nat. Genet.* 2000;25:195–200. doi:10.1038/76061

[15] Fülöp V, Jones DT. Beta propellers: structural rigidity and functional diversity. *Curr Opin Struct Biol* 1999;9(6):715-721. doi:10.1016/S0959-440X(99)00035-4

[16] Fülöp V, Szeltner Z, Polgár L. Catalysis of serine oligopeptidases is controlled by a gating filter mechanism. *EMBO Rep* 2000;1(3):277–281. doi:10.1093/embo-reports/kvd048.

[17] Hansen HH, Sánchez C, Meier E. Neonatal administration of the selective serotonin reuptake inhibitor Lu 10–134-C increases forced swimming-induced immobility in adult rats: a putative animal model of depression? *Pharmacol. Exp. Ther.* 1997;283(3):1333-1341.

[18] Hauger RL, Risbrough V, Brauns O, Dautzenberg FM. Corticotropin releasing factor (CRF) receptor signaling in the central nervous system: new molecular targets. *CNS Neurol Disord Drug Targets* 2006; 5(4):453–479.

[19] Heilig M, Zachrisson O, Thorsell A, Ehnvall A, Mottagui-Tabar S, Sjögren M, Asberg M, Ekman R, Wahlestedt C, Agren H. Decreased cerebrospinal fluid neuropeptide Y (NPY) in patients with treatment refractory unipolar major depression: preliminary evidence for association with preproNPY gene polymorphism. *J Psychiatr Res* 2004;38(2):113-121. doi:10.1016/S0022-3956(03)00101-8

[20] Heim C, Plotsky PM, Nemeroff CB. Importance of studying the contributions of early adverse experience to neurobiological findings in depression. *Neuropsychopharmacology* 2004;29(4):641-648. doi:10.1038/sj.npp.1300397

[21] Irazusta J, Larrinaga G, González-Maeso J, Gil J, Meana JJ, Casis L. Distribution of prolyl endopeptidase activities in rat and human brain. *Neurochem Int* 2002;404:337-345.

[22] Irazusta J, Silveira PF, Gil J, Varona A, Casis L. Effects of hydrosaline treatments on prolyl endopeptidase activity in rat tissues. *Regul Pept* 2001;101(1-3):141-147. doi:10.1016/S0167-0115(01)00277-4

[23] Jolley SN, Elmore Sh, Barnard KE, Carr DB. Dysregulation of the hypothalamic-pituitary-adrenal axis in postpartum depression. *Biol Res Nurs* 2007; 8(3): 210-222.

[24] Karl T, Duffy L, Herzog H. Behavioural profile of a new mouse model for NPY deficiency. *Eur J Neurosci* 2008;28(1):173-180. doi:10.1111/j.1460-9568.2008.06306.

[25] Karl T, Hoffmann T, Pabst R, von Hörsten S. Extreme reduction of dipeptidyl peptidase IV activity in F344 rat substrains is associated with various behavioral differences. *Physiol Behav* 2003; 80(1):123-134. doi:10.1016/S0031-9384(03)00229-4

[26] Kato T, Hama T, Nagatsu T, Kuzuya H, Sakakibara S. Changes of X-prolyl dipeptidyl-aminopeptidase activity in developing rat brain. *Experientia* 1979;35(10):1329-1330.

[27] Khlebnikova NN, Krupina NA, Bogdanova NG, Zolotov NN, Kryzhanovskii GN. Effects of prolylendopeptidase inhibitor benzyloxycarbonyl-methionyl-2(S)-cyanopyrrolidine on experimental depressive syndrome development in rats. *Bull Exp Biol Med* 2009;147(1):26-30. doi: 10.1007/s10517-009-0458-6

[28] Khlebnikova NN, Krupina NA, Orlova IN, Bogdanova NG, Zolotov NN, Kryzhanovskii GN. Effect of a prolyl endopeptidase inhibitor benzyloxycarbonyl-alanyl-proline on the development of experimental depressive syndrome in rats. *Bull Exp Biol Med* 2009;147(3):291-295. doi: 10.1007/s10517-009-0494-2

[29] Kiecolt-Glaser JK, Belury MA, Porter K, Beversdorf DQ, Lemeshow S, Glaser R. Depressive symptoms, omega-6:omega-3 fatty acids, and inflammation in older adults. *Psychosom Med* 2007;69(3):217-224. doi: 10.1097/PSY.0b013e3180313a45

[30] Koenig AM, Thase ME. First-line pharmacotherapies for depression – what is the best choice? *Pol Arch Med Wewn* 2009;119(7-8):478-485.

[31] Krupina NA, Kryzhanovskiĭ GN. Insufficiency of nigrostriatal dopaminergic system as a disregulation mechanism of dopamine-dependent depression syndrome. *Zh Nevrol Psikhiatr Im S S Korsakova* 2003;103(4):42-47. [Russian]

[32] Krupina NA, Kushnareva EIu, Khlebnikova NN, Zolotov NN, Kryzhanovskiĭ GN. Experimental model of anxiety-depression state in rats exposed to inhibitor of dipeptidyl peptidase IV methionyl-2(S)-cyano-pyrrolidine in early postnatal period. *Zh Vyssh Nerv Deiat Im I P Pavlova* 2009;59(3):360-372. [Russian]

[33] Krupina NA, Kushnareva EY, Khlebnikova NN, Zolotov NN, Kryzhanovskii GN. Behavioral changes in rats induced by a dipeptidyl peptidase IV inhibitor methionyl-2(S)-cyanopyrrolidine: experimental model of anxiety-depression disorder. *Bull Exp Biol Med* 2009;147(3):285-290. doi: 10.1007/s10517-009-0493-3

[34] Krupina NA, Orlova IN, Kryzhanovskii GN. Effect of melipramine on the development of experimental depressive syndrome induced by systemic administration of 1-methyl-4-phenyl-1,2,3,6-tetrahydropyridine (MPTP). *Bull Exp Biol Med* 1995;120(2):805-808. doi: 10.1007/BF02445959

[35] Krupina NA, Zolotov NN, Bogdanova NG, Orlova IN, Khlebnikova NN, Kryzhanovskii GN. Activities of prolyl endopeptidase and dipeptidyl peptidase IV in brain structures of rats with dopamine deficiency-dependent MPTP-induced depressive syndrome. *Bull Exp Biol Med* 2006;142(5):554-556. doi: 10.1007/s10517-006-0416-5

[36] Kryzhanovskii GN., Krupina NA., Kucheryanu VG. A new model of the depressive syndrome induced by administration of 1-methyl-4-phenyl-1,2,3,6-tetrahydropyridine (MPTP) in rats. *Bull Exp Biol Med* 1995;119(2):116-119. doi: 10.1007/BF02445853

[37] Kushnareva E, Krupina N, Khlebnikova N, Zolotov N. Activities of prolyl endopeptidase and dipeptidyl peptidase iv in brain structures of rats with anxiety-depression state induced by postnatal administration of dipeptidyl peptidase iv inhibitor. New Research Abstract Book. XIV World Congress of Psychiatry. Sept 20-25, 2008. Prague. Czech Republic. Česká a slovenská psychiatrie. *J Czech and Slovak psychiatry* 2008;104(Suppl 1):30.

[38] Kuteeva E, Hokfelt T, Ogren SO. Behavioural characterisation of young adult transgenic mice overexpressing galanin under the PDGF-B promoter. *Regul Pept* 2005;125(1–3):67–78. doi:10.1016/j.regpep.2004.07.028

[39] Landgraf R. The involvement of the vasopressin system in stress-related disorders. *CNS Neurol Disord Drug Targets* 2006;5:167–179.

[40] Liu Y, Heiberg T, Reichelt Kl-L. Towards a possible aetiology for depressions? *Behav Brain Funct* 2007;3:47-53. doi:10.1186/1744-9081-3-47

[41] Madaan V, Wilson DR. Neuropeptides: relevance in treatment of depression and anxiety disorders. *Drug News Perspect* 2009;22(6):319-324. doi:10.1358/dnp.2009.22.6.1395255

[42] Maes M, Bonaccorso S, Marino V, Puzella A, Pasquini M, Biondi M, Artini M, Almerighi C, Meltzer H. Treatment with interferon-alpha (IFN alpha) of hepatitis C patients induces lower serum dipeptidyl peptidase IV activity, which is related to IFN alpha-induced depressive and anxiety symptoms and immune activation. *Mol. Psychiatry* 2001;6(4):475-480.

[43] Maes M, Bonaccorso S. Lower activities of serum peptidases predict higher depressive and anxiety levels following interferon-alpha-based immunotherapy in patients with hepatitis C. *Acta Psychiatr Scand* 2004;109(2):126-131. doi:10.1046/j.0001-690X.2003.00230.x

[44] Maes M, Capuron L, Ravaud A, Gualde N, Bosmans E, Egyed B, Dantzer R, Neveu PJ. Lowered serum dipeptidyl peptidase IV activity is associated with depressive symptoms and cytokine production in cancer patients receiving interleukin-2-based immunotherapy. *Neuropsychopharmacology* 2001;24(2):130-40. doi:10.1038/sj.npp.1395576

[45] Maes M, De Meester I, Verkerk R, De Medts P, Wauters A, Vanhoof G, Vandoolaeghe E, Neels H, Scharpé S. Lower serum dipeptidyl peptidase IV activity in treatment resistant major depression: relationships with immune-inflammatory markers. *Psychoneuroendocrinology* 1997;22(2):65-78. doi:10.1016/S0306-4530(96)00040-6

[46] Maes M, Goossens F, Scharpé S, Calabrese J, Desnyder R, Meltzer HY. Alterations in plasma prolyl endopeptidase activity in depression, mania, and schizophrenia: effects of antidepressants, mood stabilizers, and antipsychotic drugs. *Psychiatry Res* 1995,58(3):217-225. doi:10.1016/0165-1781(95)02698-V

[47] Maes M, Goossens F, Scharpé S, Meltzer HY, D'Hondt P, Cosyns P. Lower serum prolyl endopeptidase enzyme activity in major depression: further evidence that peptidases play a role in the pathophysiology of depression. *Biol Psychiatry* 1994;35(8):545-552. doi:10.1016/0006-3223(94)90101-5

[48] Maes M, Libbrecht I, Lin A, Goossens F, Ombelet W, Stevens K, Bosmans E, Altamura C, Cox J, de Jongh R, Scharpé S. Effects of pregnancy and delivery on serum prolyl endopeptidase (PEP) activity: alterations in serum PEP are related to increased anxiety in the early puerperium and to postpartum depression. *J Affect Disord* 2000;57(1-3):125-137. doi:10.1016/S0165-0327(99)00081-6

[49] Maes M, Lin AH, Bonaccorso S, Goossens F, Van Gastel A, Pioli R, Delmeire L, Scharpé S. Higher serum prolyl endopeptidase activity in patients with post-traumatic stress disorder. *J Affect Disord* 1999;53(1):27-34. doi:10.1016/S0165-0327(98)00086-X

[50] Maletic V, Robinson M, Oakes T, Iyengar S, Ball SG, Russell J. Neurobiology of depression: an integrated view of key findings. *Clin Pract* 2007;61(12):2030-2040. doi:10.1111/j.1742-1241.2007.01602.x

[51] Mathew SJ, Price RB, Charney DS. Recent advances in the neurobiology of anxiety disorders: implications for novel therapeutics. *Med Genet C Semin Med Genet* 2008;148(2):89-98. doi:10.1002/ajmg.c.30172

[52] McArthur R, Borsini F. Animal models of depression in drug discovery: a historical perspective. *Pharmacol Biochem Behav* 2006;84(3):436-452. doi:10.1016/j.pbb.2006.06.005

[53] Mentlein R. Dipeptidyl-peptidase IV (CD26)--role in the inactivation of regulatory peptides. *Regul Pept* 1999;85(1):9-24. doi:10.1016/S0167-0115(99)00089-0

[54] Möller C, Sommer W, Thorsell A, Rimondini R, Heilig M. Anxiogenic-like action of centrally administered glucagon-like peptide-1 in a punished drinking test // *Prog Neuropsychopharmacol Biol Psychiatry* 2002;26(1):119-122. doi:10.1016/S0278-5846(01)00223-8

[55] Mora F, Segoviaa G, del Arco A. Glutamate–dopamine–GABA interactions in the aging basal ganglia. *Brain Res Rev* 2008;58(2):340-353. doi:10.1016/j.brainresrev.2007.10.006

[56] Myöhänen TT, García-Horsman JA, Tenorio-Laranga J, Männistö PT. Issues about the physiological functions of prolyl oligopeptidase based on its discordant spatial association with substrates and inconsistencies among mRNA, protein levels, and enzymatic activity. *J Histochem Cytochem* 2009;57(9):831-848.

[57] Myöhänen TT, Venäläinen JI, Garcia-Horsman JA, Piltonen M, Männistö PT. Cellular and subcellular distribution of rat brain prolyl oligopeptidase and its association with specific neuronal neurotransmitters. *J Comp Neurol* 2008;507(5):1694–1708. doi:10.1002/cne.21642

[58] Myöhänen TT, Venäläinen JI, Tupala E, Garcia-Horsman JA, Miettinen R, Männistö PT Distribution of immunoreactive prolyl oligopeptidase in human and rat brain. *Neurochem Res* 2007;32(8):1365-1374. doi:10.1007/s11064-007- 9316-y

[59] Narkevich VB, Nazarova GA, Zolotov NN, Pozdnev VF, Raevskiĭ KS. Neuroleptic catalepsy in rats is accompanied by activation of brain prolyl endopeptidase and is eliminated by inhibitors of this enzyme. *Dokl Akad Nauk* 1994;339(5):691-693. [Russian].

[60] Nemeroff CB. Recent advances in the neurobiology of depression. *Psychopharmacol Bull* 2002;36(Suppl 2):6-23.

[61] Neumann ID, Krömer SA, Toschi N, Ebner K. Brain oxytocin inhibits the (re)activity of the hypothalamo-pituitary-adrenal axis in male rats: involvement of hypothalamic and limbic brain regions. *Regul Pept* 2000;96(1-2):31-38. doi:10.1016/S0167-0115(00)00197-X

[62] Pankova NB, Krupina NA, Orlova IN, Khlebnikova NN, Kryzhanovskii GN. Involvement of brain dopaminergic systems in the development of an MPTP-induced depressive state in rats. *Neurosci Behav Physiol* 2008;38(4):383-391. doi:10.1007/s11055-008-0055-6

[63] Paschos KA, Veletza S, Chatzaki E. Neuropeptide and sigma receptors as novel therapeutic targets for the pharmacotherapy of depression. *CNS Drugs* 2009;23(9):755-772. doi: 10.2165/11310830-000000000-00000

[64] Peteranderl C, Antonijevic IA, Steiger A, Murck H, Held K, Frieboes RM, Uhr M, Schaaf L. Nocturnal secretion of TSH and ACTH in male patients with depression and healthy controls. *J Psychiatr Res* 2002;36(3):189-196. doi:10.1016/S0022-3956(02)00004-3

[65] Phillips ML, Drevets WC, Rauch SL, Lane R. Neurobiology of emotion perception II: Implications for major psychiatric disorders. *Biol Psychiatry* 2003;54:515-528. doi:10.1016/S0006-3223(03)00171-9

[66] Polgar L. The prolyl oligopeptidase family. *Cell Mol Life Sci* 2002;59(2):349-362. doi: 10.1007/s00018-002-8427-5

[67] Popkova EV, Krupina NA, Kryzhanovskii GN, Orlova IN, Iordanskaya TE. Monoamine content in the rat brain structures with MPTP-induced depressive syndrome. *Bull Exp Biol Med.* 1999;127(1):19-23. doi: 10.1007/BF02432791

[68] Porsolt RD, Anton G, Blavet N, Jalfre M. Behavioural despair in rats: a new model sensitive to antidepressant treatments. *Eur J Pharmacol* 1978;47(4):379-391.

[69] Riemer S, Maes M, Christophe A, Rief W. Lowered omega-3 PUFAs are related to major depression, but not to somatization syndrome. *J Affect Disord* 2010;123(1-3):173-180. doi:10.1016/j.jad.2009.08.004

[70] Scharpé S, De Meester I, Verh K. Peptide truncation by dipeptidyl peptidase IV: a new pathway for drug discovery? *Verh K Acad. Geneeskd Belg*. 2001;63(1):5-32.

[71] Schmidt HD, Banasr M, Duman RS. Future antidepressant targets: neurotrophic factors and related signaling cascades. *Drug Discov Today Ther Strateg* 2008;5(3):151–156. doi:10.1016/j.ddstr.2008.10.003.

[72] Schulz I, Gerhartz B, Neubauer A, Holloschi A, Heiser U, Hafner M, Demuth HU. Modulation of inositol 1,4,5-triphosphate concentration by prolyl endopeptidase inhibition. *Eur J Biochem* 2002;269(23):813-820. doi:10.1046/j.1432-1033.2002.03297.x

[73] Sergeyev V, Fetissov S, Mathe AA, Jimenez PA, Bartfai T, Mortas P, Gaudet L, Moreau JL, Hökfelt T. Neuropeptide expression in rats exposed to chronic mild stresses. *Psychopharmacology (Berl)* 2005;178(2-3):115-124. doi: 10.1007/s00213-004-2015-3

[74] Shelton RC. The molecular neurobiology of depression. *Psychiatr Clin North Am* 2007;30(1):1-11. doi: 10.1016/j.psc.2006.12.005

[75] Shigeyuki Chaki, Taketoshi Okubo, Yoshinori Sekiguchi. Non-Monoamine-Based Approach for the Treatment of Depression and Anxiety Disorders. *Recent Pat CNS Drug Discov* .2006;1(1):1-27.

[76] Su K-P. Biological mechanism of antidepressant effect of Omega–3 fatty acids: How does fish oil act as a 'mind-body interface'? *Neurosignals* 2009;17(2):144–152. doi:10.1159/000198167

[77] Sun Y, Zupan B, Raaka BM, Toth M, Gershengorn MC. TRH-receptor-type-2-deficient mice are euthyroid and exhibit increased depression and reduced anxiety phenotypes. *Neuropsychopharmacology* 2009;34(6):1601-1608. doi: 10.1038/npp.2008.217

[78] Szeltner Z, Polgár L. Structure, function and biological relevance of prolyl oligopeptidase. *Curr Protein Pept Sci* 2008;9(1):96-107.

[79] Tardito D, Perez J, Tiraboschi E, Musazzi L, Racagni G, Popoli M. Signaling pathways regulating gene expression, neuroplasticity, and neurotrophic mechanisms in the action of antidepressants: A critical overview. *Pharmacol Rev* 2006;58(1):115–134. doi:10.1124/pr.58.1.7

[80] Thompson MA, Ohnuma K, Abe M, Morimoto C, Dang NH. CD26/dipeptidyl peptidase IV as a novel therapeutic target for cancer and immune disorders. *Mini Rev Med Chem* 2007;7(3):253-273.

[81] Van Gool AR, Van Ojik HH, Kruit WH, Mulder PG, Fekkes D, Bannink M, Scharpé S, Stoter G, Eggermont AM, Maes M, Verkerk R. Serum activity of prolyl endopeptidase, but not of dipeptidyl peptidase IV, is decreased by immunotherapy with IFN-alpha in high-risk melanoma patients. *J Interferon Cytokine Res* 2004;24(7):411-415.

[82] Zolotov NN, Narkevich VB, Pozdnev VF, Prikhozhan AV, Voronina TA, Raevskiĭ KS. Psychotropic properties of brain proline endopeptidase inhibitors. *Dokl Akad Nauk* 1992; 322(4):776-779. [Russian]

In: Antidepressants: Types, Efficiency …
Editor: Jayden T. Van Leeuwen, pp.155-167

ISBN 978-1-61668-581-2

Chapter 6

BEYOND THE MONOAMINE HYPOTHESIS: THE QUEST FOR AN INTEGRATIVE ETIOLOGY OF DEPRESSION AND NEW THERAPEUTIC STRATEGIES

Barbara Di Benedetto[1]1, Rainer Rupprecht[1,2], and Gerhard Rammes[1,3]

[1]Max Planck Institute of Psychiatry, 80804 Munich, Germany
[2] Department of Psychiatry and Psychotherapy, Ludwig Maximilian University, 80336 Munich, Germany
[3] Department of Anaesthesiology, Technische Universität, 81675 Munich, Germany

ABSTRACT

Understanding the pathogenesis of depression and the mechanism of action of clinically effective antidepressants are of considerable interest. Early clinical observations pointed to a decreased monoamine function, which has resulted in the "monoamine hypothesis" of depression. However, as helpful as this hypothesis was for the development of amine-based potent antidepressants, crucial discrepancies, e.g., delayed clinical onset of mood-enhancing effects and the lack of major mood alteration after monoamines depletion, made it rather unlikely that the cause of depression is a simple deficiency of central monoamines. Furthermore, in recent years a growing body of evidence highlighted the possibility that genome regulation, epigenetic modifications or alterations in differential neuronal cell type responsiveness could play a key role in the origin and development of mood disorders.

Therefore, providing an integrative theory of the neurobiology of depression may help to explain some of the complexities of this disorder and discover novel pharmacological targets. On the basis of current knowledge we want to discuss an extended "monoamine hypothesis" and propose possible new fields/ideas/concepts which need to be explored for the development of more effective antidepressant treatments.

1 Correspondence should be addressed to Dr. Barbara Di Benedetto, Max Planck Institute of Psychiatry, Molecular Psychopharmacology, Kraepelinstraße 2, D-80804 München, Germany. Email: barbara@mpipsykl.mpg.de, Tel: +49-89-30622506, Fax: +49-89-30622402.

INTRODUCTION

Mood disorders characterized by emotional disturbances such as major depressive disorder (MDD) are serious medical illnesses that affect up to 10% of the adult population (Kaufman, 2000). It is difficult to calculate their financial burden on the world's health systems; for the US alone it is estimated to amount to $80 billion per year. Thus, a better understanding of the pathophysiology of these disorders and the development of novel therapeutic treatments are highly desirable. Depressive disorders are characterized in humans by the core symptoms of depressed mood and/or loss of pleasure or interest in most activities (anhedonia). Moreover, depression includes other characteristics such as changes in body weight, sleeping patterns, psychomotor behavior, energy level and cognitive functioning (DSM-IV, 1994). Despite the prevalence of depression and its high impact, knowledge about its etiology and pathophysiology remains still elusive. An explanation for this could be attributed to the techniques available up to now to document aberrancies occurring in human brain circuits that regulate mood responses and lead to MDD development when not working properly. In fact, until now most of the studies rely on post-mortem brain tissue to identify molecular alterations, and on neuroimaging techniques to reveal affected brain regions, with all their limitations, as they are based on detection of neuronal activity using indirect markers of activation (Phelps, 2005). Secondly, most of the studies are based on searching new possible molecular targets for the development of new therapies looking at the mode of action of already existing antidepressants. This limits the possible identification of novel depression susceptible genes, as done for other complex syndromes, as research is already biased by the intrinsic nature of these drugs, which act specifically on monoamine systems. Though on one hand this approach helped develop faster and safer drugs, unfortunately on the other hand it prevented finding out the contributions of non-monoamine mechanisms to the development of depression, thereby preventing the identification of new candidate targets for the development of novel therapeutic strategies.

THE "MONOAMINE HYPOTHESIS" OF DEPRESSION

The first antidepressants were discovered in the late 1950s by serendipity, after two structurally unrelated compounds developed for non-psychiatric conditions, iproniazid (a monoamine oxidase inhibitor, MAOI) and imipramine, were found to relieve depressive symptoms in humans. These compounds were later shown to exert their effects through the enhancement of synaptic serotonin and noradrenaline availability. Therefore, it was proposed that depression could be related to an impairment in monoamine transmission and that antidepressant therapy would act via the restoration of the physiological monoamine availability in the brain. This led to the development of more potent amine-based antidepressants such as new MAOI (e.g. moclobemide) or monoamine reuptake inhibitors (like selective serotonin reuptake inhibitors, SSRIs (e.g. fluoxetine), selective noradrenalin reuptake inhibitors, NRIs (e.g. reboxetine), or serotonin and noradrenaline reuptake inhibitors, SNRIs (e.g. venlafaxine or duloxetine)). These drugs act by enhancing in particular serotonergic (5-HT) and noradrenergic (NA) signalling through either the inhibition of monoamine oxidase A, an enzyme which triggers breakdown of monoamines in the synaptic cleft, or the inhibition of the plasma membrane serotonin/noradrenalin reuptake transporters (SERT/NAT, respectively) (Iversen, 2000) (Fig 1).

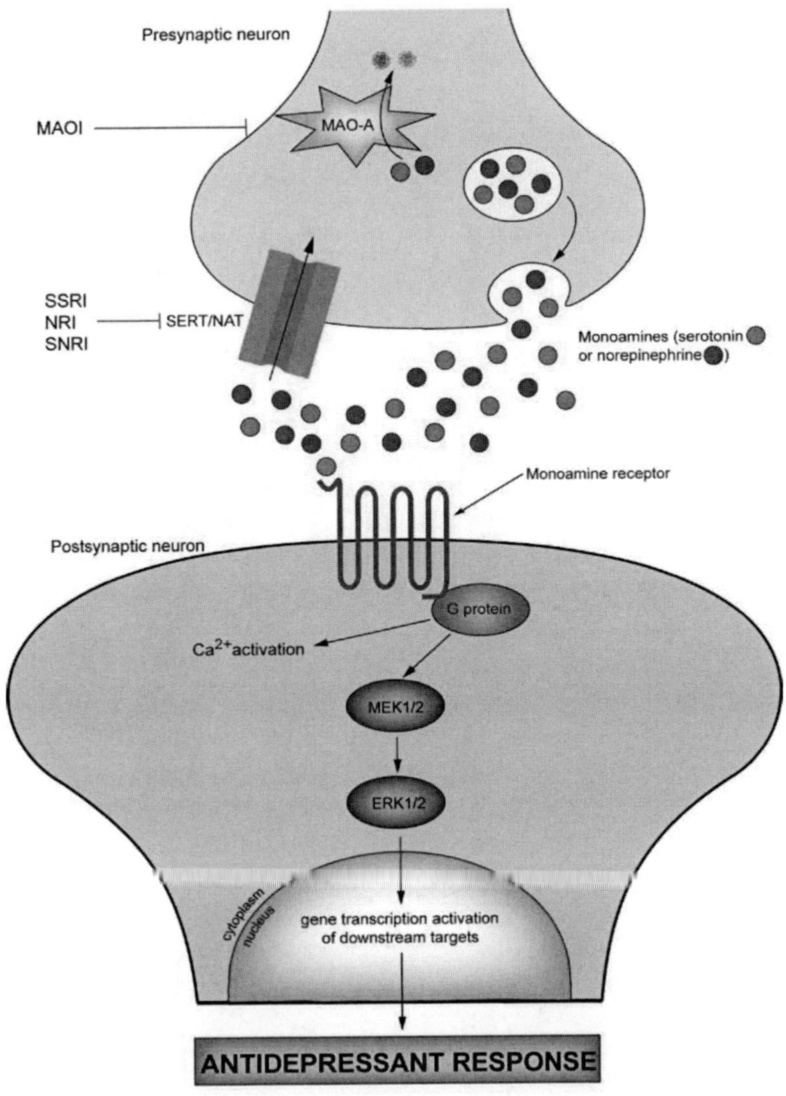

Figure 1. A simplified scheme of the general targets for conventional antidepressant therapies. Conventional treatments of depression affects neurotransmission of monoamines by increasing their synaptic availability. The antidepressant drugs in current clinical use include: (1) compounds that selectively block the reuptake of specific monoamines, such as selective serotonin (5-HT) reuptake inhibitors (SSRIs) (e.g. fluoxetine), compounds that selectively inhibit the reuptake of noradrenaline (NRIs) (e.g. reboxetine), compounds that selectively inhibit the reuptake of both 5-HT and noradrenaline (SNRIs) (e.g. venlafaxine and duloxetine); and (2) monoamine oxidase inhibitors (MAOI) (e.g. moclobemide), which increase synaptic concentrations of monoamines by inhibiting their degradation by MAO. Via the activation of G-protein coupled receptors and consequential regulation of Ca2+ modulation or ERK/MAPK cascade, these compounds can activate antidepressant responses. Abbreviations: SERT, serotonin transporter; NAT, noradrenaline transporter.

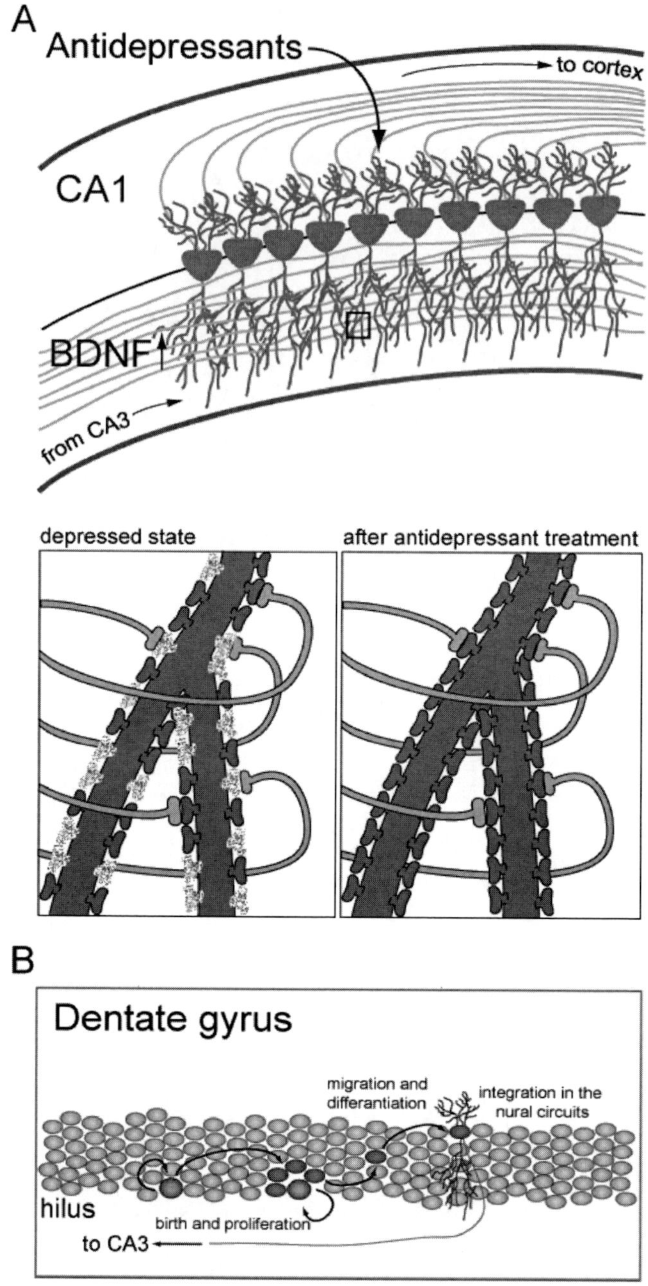

Figure 2. **The "neurotrophic hypothesis" of antidepressant** action proposes that antidepressants mediate their action by inducing an increase of BDNF availability in regions affected by MDD like the hippocampus (A). This would lead to neuroplastic changes like increased dendritogenesis and consequential increase of synaptic contacts, thereby restoring the physiological structure of neuronal networks. (B) a second hypothesis to explain the delayed onset of beneficial effects of antidepressant therapy proposes that neurogenesis in the hippocampal formation would be responsible for antidepressant responses, as the time required for newborn neurons to integrate into the already existing circuits correlates with the time needed for mood-enhancing effects of antidepressant therapy to become manifest.

Nevertheless, although amine-based agents have displayed fairly good antidepressant effects, several discrepancies have caused doubt that a simple deficiency in central monoamines in the brain could be the only cause of depression. Drugs of abuse, e.g., cocaine and amphetamines, though augmenting the concentration of serotonin, dopamine and norepinephrine do not have antidepressant effects and are therefore not useful for the treatment of depression. Similarly, studies dealing with monoamine depletion both in unmedicated depressive patients and in healthy controls led to inconclusive or equivocal results, showing that the sole depletion of serotonin or noradrenaline could only produce a mild additional reduction in mood in MDD patients and would not induce any of the core symptoms of MDD in healthy volunteers (Ruhe, 2007). Moreover, although these drugs act acutely in restoring monoamine availability, the mood-enhancing effects of treatment still require three to four weeks to become manifest. These observations encouraged the search for new theories about the mechanism of action of antidepressants and about the cause of MDD to identify possible new and more efficacious drugs for the treatment of MDD.

To explain the delayed onset of beneficial effects of antidepressant treatment, it has been proposed that the acute restoration of monoamine availability in the brain would activate neuroplastic changes, such as an increase in dendritic arborization and in the number of synaptic contacts. Therefore, research oriented in the direction of looking at the effects that these drugs could exert at the level of synapses has introduced a new hypothesis of depression and antidepressant action, namely the "neurotrophic hypothesis". Based on findings in animal models of stress-dependent depression, that showed a reduction of BDNF in the hippocampus, which could be reversed by antidepressant treatment (Duman, 2004; Duman, 1997), it has been suggested that such fluctuations in BDNF could explain at least in part the structural changes observed in the hippocampus of depressive patients.

Namely, post-mortem studies in MDD patients showed a marked reduction in dendritic arborisation complexity and consequently also in the number of synaptic contacts both in MDD patients and in the CA1 region of the hippocampus in animal models of stress-induced depression (Fig 2A).

This would also be in line with the memory and cognitive deficits observed in MDD; and would support the idea that the late onset of beneficial effects of antidepressants might correlate with the time needed to restore the physiological structure of neuronal networks in the hippocampal formation and in the prefrontal cortex, the two regions found to be mainly affected in depressive subjects (Brown, 1999; Hayley, 2005; McEwen, 2002). Indeed, it was demonstrated in mice that the three to four weeks needed to see the first effects of remission of depressive symptoms in the clinic correspond to the time needed for the induction of hippocampal neurogenesis and consequent birth/integration of new neurons in the already existing neural circuits (Santarelli, 2003) (Fig 2B).In particular in the study by Santarelli et al (2003), the authors elegantly showed that the widely used SSRI fluoxetine would induce neurogenesis after chronic treatment in the mouse hippocampal dentate gyrus. While ablation of hippocampal neurogenesis via low-dose x-irradiation of the heads of mice would prevent the antidepressant response to fluoxetine, as measured in the novel-suppressed feeding test. Although it is very interesting to explain the mechanism of action of antidepressants in part, this theory could not account for the differences observed in the response to antidepressant medication in different MDD patients. In fact, non response to treatment still remains a problem, since only about 70% of the patients respond to a first treatment.

EPIGENETIC MECHANISMS IN DEPRESSION

One of the ways in which experience can produce long-lasting alterations in the brain is through modifications, which can occur at the DNA level and influence gene expression without introducing changes in the DNA sequence itself. These belong to so-called epigenetic mechanisms and can be distinguished in two major groups: covalent changes on DNA, as methylations, or post-translational modifications (PTMs) of histone N-terminal tails, such as acetylations or methylations (Tsankova, 2007) (Fig 3). Histone proteins represent the core structures on which DNA is coiled up to regulate chromatin packaging, thereby controlling DNA availability to the transcription machinery. The tight control of the enzymes regulating histone acetylations/methylations (histone acetyltransferases, HAT, or deacetylases, HDAC, and histone methyltransferases, HMT, or demethylases) is therefore the mechanism which affects gene expression via chromatin remodeling. Recently two elegant studies on the direct implications of epigenetic mechanisms for antidepressant research showed that two HDACs, HDAC5 and HDAC2 are downregulated in the nucleus accumbens of animal models of chronic stress-induced depression-like phenotype (Covington, 2009; Renthal, 2007). In the first study, chronic administration of imipramine could reverse the effects of chronic stress on depression-like phenotype, restoring normal expression levels of HDAC5 in the nucleus accumbens of mice. In the second study, direct HDAC inhibitor infusion also in the nucleus accumbens reversed the effects of chronic defeat stress on measures of depression-like phenotype, with striking similarities to the effects of the standard antidepressant fluoxetine. Given that through epigenetic mechanisms so many variants can exist among individuals, depending on their individual life experiences, this led to the idea that some aspects of depression research, such as discordance rates in monozygotic twins and the resilience in relapse of symptoms among patients, could be explained by invoking epigenetic mechanisms (Mill, 2007). Moreover, it has been shown that for example, stress, a known precipitating factor in developing MDD, could induce suppression of BDNF expression via methylation of the BDNF promoter, thus inducing a depression-like phenotype. This could be reversed by chronic antidepressant treatment through the enhancement of histone acetyltransferase activity, thereby reactivating BDNF production (Tsankova, 2006). This would again be in line with the "neurotrophic theory" of depression and antidepressant action already introduced in the previous paragraph, providing the molecular mechanism suggesting such a theory. Due to the fact that environmental factors could also modify DNA methylation and histone modifications, it is therefore plausible to speculate that epigenetics would also explain how depression can become inheritable, as meiosis cannot completely cancel those modifications (Mill, 2007); this could also explain why monozygotic twins not only develop MDD with different clinical profiles, but also would not react to therapies with the same clinical response patterns (Fraga, 2005). Similarly, epigenetic modifications dependent on gene-environment interactions could account for the discrepancy that clinicians often have to face when treating MDD patients suffering of recurrent depression: these patients in fact will not necessarily respond to a drug in the same way as they did during previous episodes. Indeed, the modification patterns, which occur depending on the different lifespan experiences, can be so different, thereby inducing on one side a diverse susceptibility of individuals to the development of MDD even in monozygotic twins, and on the other side also provoking resilience in those patients, whose epigenetic modifications could counteract the respective mechanisms targeted by antidepressant treatment.

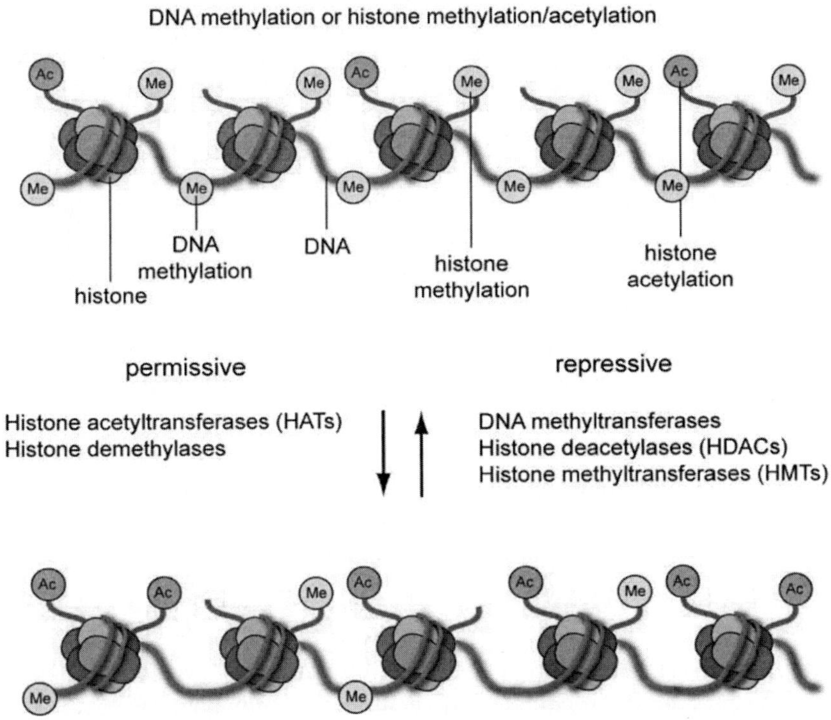

Figure 3. Epigenetic mechanisms regulating chromatin remodelling and DNA transcription. The transcription of genes potentially involved in neuroplastic responses to stress or antidepressant treatment can be regulated by specific enzymes which make transcriptional activation "permissive" or "repressive". Antidepressants were shown to play a role in the regulation of these enzymes, like HDACs.

Providing this, an approach, which would allow a screening for specific epigenetic modifications to be used as "personalized signature" like a marker of a defined depressive status or predictive for antidepressant response, would help the search for more potent amine-independent antidepressants and would strengthen the hope for the realization of "personalized therapies" for MDD patients. Moreover, the possibility to quantify and precisely detect such modifications would permit to bypass a high limit in psychiatry, where diagnostic categories are entirely based on verbal information, thereby representing a limited value for research (Hyman, 2007). Although very attractive, the attempt to screen patients´ proteomes might be too ambitious, due to the high number of proteins contained in the human body and their high fluctuations. Therefore, using animal models with phenotypes resembling some aspects of MDD for such screening approaches can help to find candidate proteins in rodent animal models. The recent development of technical tools like mass spectrometry-based quantitative proteomics (Aebersold, 2003), which could greatly advance the gain of information about PTMs, could for example help to identify new possible differentially regulated proteins comparing samples of depression-like vs controls animal models. For this, the introduction of the SILAC technology (Stable Isotopic Labeling by Amino Acids in Cell Culture) would increase the probability of finding new targets for the development of novel drugs for the treatment of psychiatric disorders. In SILAC experiments, two mammalian cell populations are grown in identical cell culture media deficient in some essential amino acids. One cell population is grown in medium with heavy (isotopic) amino acids while the other cell population is grown in medium with light (normal) amino acids. The natural metabolic machinery of the cells is utilized to label all cellular proteins with the heavy amino acid (Amanchy, 2005). After trypsin digestion, the peptides containing the light or heavy amino acids are chemically identical and can be processed together using any protein separation method eliminating quantification errors due to unequal sampling. Since the peptides are isotopically distinct, they can be easily distinguished by mass using MS analysis. Based on the relative peak intensity of the isotopic peptide pairs, you can quantitate differential protein expression and identify differential post-translational modifications between different samples. Moreover, the recent development of SILAC mice, a versatile tool by which it is possible to quantitatively compare different proteomes, thus determining protein functions under complex in vivo conditions (Kruger, 2008), in combination with behavioral manipulations for the induction of depression-like symptoms could support the search of PTMs that could represent a "fingerprint" for the development of MDD; and therefore represent good novel targets for drug discovery.

Depression and Astrocytes: The Glia Cells Hypothesis

Another important layer of complexity is introduced by the differences in cell-type specific responsiveness to drugs, due to the peculiar glia cells-neurons networking typical of different brain regions. Moreover, post-mortem studies in MDD patients have revealed that the cellular loss observed in hippocampus and cortical regions affects not only neuronal cells, but also glia cells, both with regard to their number and size (Cotter, 2002; Cotter, 2001; Ongur, 1998; Rajkowska, 1999; Stockmeier, 2004). This introduced the possibility that also glia cells, which turned out to be affected in MDD, could also be responsible for responding to antidepressant treatments. Indeed, in recent years it has become more and more clear that glial cells do not only play a structural role in the brain as protecting agents, but also actively participate in regulating signal transduction events (Ge, 2006; Navarrete, 2008; Parpura, 2000). Several reports have shown that glia cells have an impact on the surrounding neuronal environment (for review, see Araque et al, 1999). Astrocytes wrapping synapses are shown to participate in neurotransmitters uptake from synaptic cleft, in their synthesis from precursors, in supplying neurotransmitter precursors to neurons and in disposal of neurotransmitter excess (Danbolt, 2001; Hertz, 2004) (Fig 4i). In particular the role astrocytes play in the regulation of glutamate reuptake/release is important, as this neurotransmitter is known to exert neurotoxic effects in high concentrations.

In a recent review, Kugaya and Sanacora (2005) discussed the possibility that an impairment in glial cell function could contribute to the development of MDD, as their buffering action on glutamate system could be missing, thereby leading to a consequential (and not causal) neuronal loss frequently observed in MDD patients. They proposed that the action of antidepressants on the surviving glial cells would raise again their number and the correct proportion glia cells-neurons via enhancement of glia cell and neuron proliferation through release of glial neurotrophic factors (Kodama, 2004).

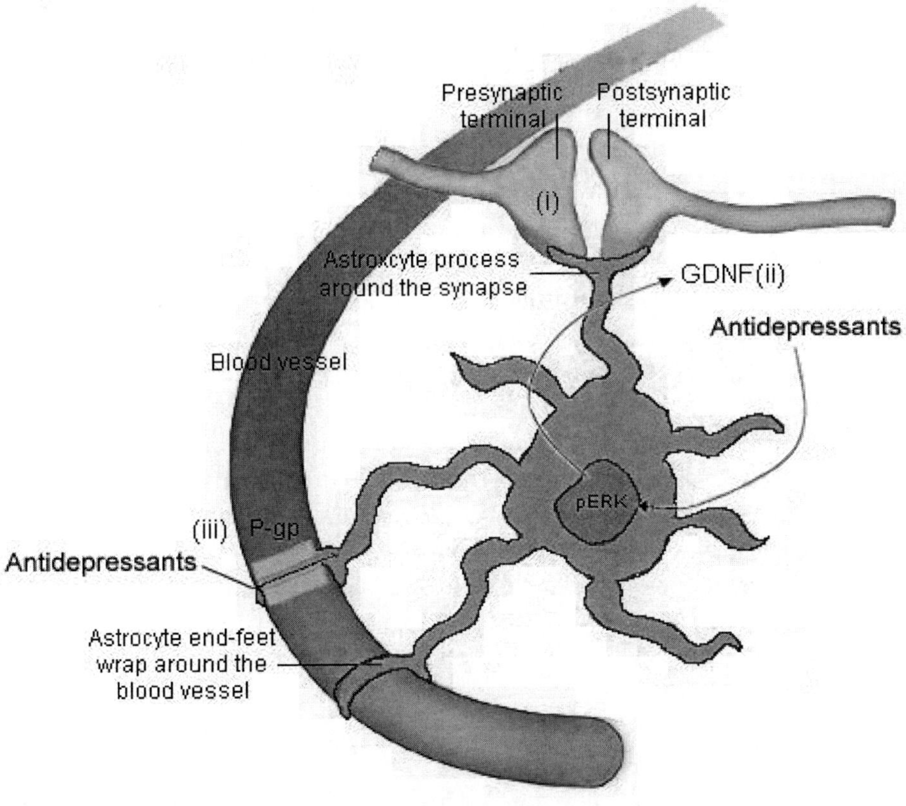

Figure 4. Astrocytes and neurons form an important network which regulates several brain functions. (i) Astrocytes wrapping synapses represent important key regulators supporting synaptic plasticity through modulation of neurotransmitter exchange between neurons; (ii) astrocytes can respond to several stimuli with the release of neurotrophic factors like GDNF; in particular it was shown that C6 glia cell line can release GDNF in response to ERK/MAPK activation upon antidepressant treatment; (iii) P-gp protein, which is localized on astrocyte end-feet to regulate the blood-brain-barrier, is an important mediator for the transfer of exogenous substances from blood vessels into the brain; mutations in this protein were shown to be positively correlated to the clinical response to antidepressants found to be its substrates.

Moreover, as the neurotransmitters released from astrocytes can signal back to neurons, these cells can regulate neuronal pre-synaptic activity through further increase or suppression of neuronal neurotransmitter release (Parpura, 2000). Indeed, astrocytes can release several factors which are responsible for maturation/survival of newly born neurons. Among these factors, GDNF is known to play an important role for the proliferation of neural progenitors in hippocampus and substantia nigra in the adult rodent brain (Chen, 2005). This suggests that also glia cells could play a fundamental role in the neurogenetic response of the brain to antidepressant treatment, as we discussed in the first paragraph. As it was shown for the neurotrophic factor BDNF, GDNF could also be beneficial to restore the physiological neuronal branching, which is found reduced in patients suffering from depression. Indeed, it has recently been demonstrated that glia cells respond with cell-autonomous cues to several antidepressants, activating specifically the ERK/MAPK signaling pathway (Hisaoka, 2007; Mercier, 2004) (Fig 4ii). Using C6 glioma cells and cultured astrocytes, these two groups showed independently that actually glia cells could activate specific responses to antidepressant treatments. Thus, it might be hypothesized that also in vivo such mechanisms could mediate antidepressant responses. In this case too, the late onset of clinical responses is in line with the idea that the release of neurotrophic factors needs a long time for restoring physiological networking.

As a further support of the role of glia cell in the response to antidepressant treatment, the efficiency of transportation of the clinically effective dosages of drugs into the brain is regulated by the blood-brain barrier; this is most tightly controlled by endfeets of astrocytes surrounding blood vessels, thereby controlling the passage of exogenous substances. It has been recently shown that, for example, the P-gp protein, which is also expressed on astrocytes (Fig 4iii), is responsible for controlling the active transport of substances in-out of the blood vessels via an ATP-dependent active-transport mechanism. Moreover, some, but not all antidepressants have been shown to be substrates of this protein. This study also revealed that the mutations within the gene encoding for P-gp positively correlated with the clinical response of patients to antidepressants that were found to be a substrate of this protein (Uhr, 2008). Therefore, further studies on P-gp protein would be highly needed to more deeply understand its mechanism of action. These would help the search for drugs that, acting on P-gp protein, would regulate the passage of antidepressants into the brain, thereby modulating the clinical responses of patients to treatments.

CONCLUSION

Despite several years of research, the exact neurobiological substrates of depression and the mechanisms of action of antidepressants still remain unclear. Many limitations in the techniques available up to now and the lack of standardization in the methods applied for the search of new pharmacological targets are still preventing the successful development of novel therapies for MDD. In this review we have discussed some of the aspects, which are currently under investigation for their efficacy in providing new fields, which need to be explored for a better understanding of the neurobiology of depression and the development of novel strategies for intervention. One of the major limitations in the field seems to rely on the fact that most studies are based on the hypothesis-driven approach that antidepressants act on the monoamine systems, therefore excluding the search for possible alternatively affected systems. Moreover, the non-hypothesis-driven approaches, such as the large-scale genome-wide analysis to search for specific possible susceptible genes affected in MDD, often lead to inconclusive results as they have been plagued by poor replication. This could be highly likely due to a lack of standardization in the procedures used for their performance or in the intrinsic difficulty by these screenings to detect also other genomic variations, such as epigenetic modifications. The analysis of epigenetic alterations in individuals affected by psychiatric disorders seems to be a very promising field for further studies: it would offer the possibility to ideally create "personalized" treatments for patients, based on their personal proteomic code which depends on the imprinting received by the specific life events. Although very promising, the latter is also limited by the difficulty of analyzing the whole human's proteome due to the high number and variations of protein content. Therefore, a combination of animal model studies, where the protein variability is less than in humans, and the new technologies available for proeteomic analysis, could improve our knowledge about the causes of depression and enhance the possibilities of finding new paths in drug discovery.

REFERENCES

Aebersold, R., and Mann, M. (2003). Mass spectrometry-based proteomics. *Nature 422*, 198-207.

Amanchy, R., Kalume, D.E., and Pandey, A. (2005). Stable isotope labeling with amino acids in cell culture (SILAC) for studying dynamics of protein abundance and posttranslational modifications. *Sci.STKE 2005*, pl2.

Araque, A., Parpura, V., Sanzgiri, R.P., and Haydon, P.G. (1999). Tripartite synapses: glia, the unacknowledged partner. *Trends Neurosci.22*, 208-215.

Brown, E.S., Rush, A.J., and McEwen, B.S. (1999). Hippocampal remodeling and damage by corticosteroids: implications for mood disorders. *Neuropsychopharmacology 21*, 474-484.

Chen, Y., Ai, Y., Slevin, J.R., Maley, B.E., and Gash, D.M. (2005). Progenitor proliferation in the adult hippocampus and substantia nigra induced by glial cell line-derived neurotrophic factor. *Exp.Neurol.196*, 87-95.

Cotter, D., Mackay, D., Chana, G., Beasley, C., Landau, S., and Everall, I.P. (2002). Reduced neuronal size and glial cell density in area 9 of the dorsolateral prefrontal cortex in subjects with major depressive disorder. *Cereb Cortex 12*, 386-394.

Cotter, D., Mackay, D., Landau, S., Kerwin, R., and Everall, I. (2001). Reduced glial cell density and neuronal size in the anterior cingulate cortex in major depressive disorder. *Arch.Gen.Psychiatry 58*, 545-553.

Covington, H.E., 3rd, Maze, I., LaPlant, Q.C., Vialou, V.F., Ohnishi, Y.N., Berton, O., Fass, D.M., Renthal, W., Rush, A.J., 3rd, Wu, E.Y., *et al.* (2009). Antidepressant actions of histone deacetylase inhibitors. *J.Neurosci.29*, 11451-11460.

Danbolt, N.C. (2001). Glutamate uptake. *Prog Neurobiol.65*, 1-105.

DSM-IV (1994). Diagnostic and Statistical Manual of Mental Disorders (DSM-IV): Washington D.C.: American Psychiatric Association.

Duman, R.S. (2004). Role of neurotrophic factors in the etiology and treatment of mood disorders. *Neuromol Med.5*, 11-25.

Duman, R.S., Heninger, G.R., and Nestler, E.J. (1997). A molecular and cellular theory of depression. *Arch.Gen.Psychiatry 54*, 597-606.

Fraga, M.F., Ballestar, E., Paz, M.F., Ropero, S., Setien, F., Ballestar, M.L., Heine-Suner, D., Cigudosa, J.C., Urioste, M., Benitez, J., *et al.* (2005). Epigenetic differences arise during the lifetime of monozygotic twins. *Proc.Natl.Acad.Sci.U S A 102*, 10604-10609.

Ge, W., Yang, XJ, Zhang, Z, Wang, HK, Shen, W, Deng, QD, Duan, S (2006). Long-term potentiation of neuron-glia synapses mediated by Ca2+-permeable AMPA receptors. *Science 312*, 1533-1537.

Hayley, S., Poulter, M.O., Merali, Z., and Anisman, H. (2005). The pathogenesis of clinical depression: stressor- and cytokine-induced alterations of neuroplasticity. *Neuroscience 135*, 659-678.

Hertz, L., and Zielke, H.R. (2004). Astrocytic control of glutamatergic activity: astrocytes as stars of the show. *Trends Neurosci.27*, 735-743.

Hisaoka, K., Takebayashi, M., Tsuchioka, M., Maeda, N., Nakata, Y., and Yamawaki, S. (2007). Antidepressants increase glial cell line-derived neurotrophic factor production through monoamine-independent activation of protein tyrosine kinase and extracellular signal-regulated kinase in glial cells. *J.Pharmacol.Exp.*Ther *321*, 148-157.

Hyman, S.E. (2007). Can neuroscience be integrated into the DSM-V? *Nat.Rev.Neurosci.8*, 725-732.

Iversen, L. (2000). Neurotransmitter transporters: fruitful targets for CNS drug discovery. *Mol.Psychiatry 5*, 357-362.

Kaufman, J., and Charney, D. (2000). Comorbidity of mood and anxiety disorders. *Depress Anxiety 12 Suppl 1*, 69-76.

Kodama, M., Fujioka, T., and Duman, R.S. (2004). Chronic olanzapine or fluoxetine administration increases cell proliferation in hippocampus and prefrontal cortex of adult rat. *Biol.Psychiatry 56*, 570-580.

Kruger, M., Moser, M., Ussar, S., Thievessen, I., Luber, C.A., Forner, F., Schmidt, S., Zanivan, S., Fassler, R., and Mann, M. (2008). SILAC mouse for quantitative proteomics uncovers kindlin-3 as an essential factor for red blood cell function. *Cell 134*, 353-364.

Kugaya, A., and Sanacora, G. (2005). Beyond monoamines: glutamatergic function in mood disorders. *CNS Spectr 10*, 808-819.

McEwen, B.S., Magarinos, A.M., and Reagan, L.P. (2002). Studies of hormone action in the hippocampal formation: possible relevance to depression and diabetes. *J.Psychosom.Res.53*, 883-890.

Mercier, G., Lennon, A.M., Renouf, B., Dessouroux, A., Ramauge, M., Courtin, F., and Pierre, M. (2004). MAP kinase activation by fluoxetine and its relation to gene expression in cultured rat astrocytes. *J.Mol.Neurosci.24*, 207-216.

Mill, J., and Petronis, A. (2007). Molecular studies of major depressive disorder: the epigenetic perspective. *Mol.Psychiatry 12*, 799-814.

Navarrete, M., and Araque, A. (2008). Endocannabinoids mediate neuron-astrocyte communication. *Neuron 57*, 883-893.

Ongur, D., Drevets, W.C., and Price, J.L. (1998). Glial reduction in the subgenual prefrontal cortex in mood disorders. *Proc.Natl.Acad.Sci.U S A 95*, 13290-13295.

Parpura, V., and Haydon, P.G. (2000). Physiological astrocytic calcium levels stimulate glutamate release to modulate adjacent neurons. *Proc.Natl.Acad.Sci. U S A 97*, 8629-8634.

Phelps, E.A., and LeDoux, J.E. (2005). Contributions of the amygdala to emotion processing: from animal models to human behavior. Neuron *48*, 175-187.

Rajkowska, G., Miguel-Hidalgo, J.J., Wei, J., Dilley, G., Pittman, S.D., Meltzer, H.Y., Overholser, J.C., Roth, B.L., and Stockmeier, C.A. (1999). Morphometric evidence for neuronal and glial prefrontal cell pathology in major depression. *Biol. Psychiatry 45*, 1085-1098.

Renthal, W., Maze, I., Krishnan, V., Covington, H.E., 3rd, Xiao, G., Kumar, A., Russo, S.J., Graham, A., Tsankova, N., Kippin, T.E., *et al.* (2007). Histone deacetylase 5 epigenetically controls behavioral adaptations to chronic emotional stimuli. *Neuron 56*, 517-529.

Ruhe, H.G., Mason, N.S., and Schene, A.H. (2007). Mood is indirectly related to serotonin, norepinephrine and dopamine levels in humans: a meta-analysis of monoamine depletion studies. *Mol. Psychiatry 12*, 331-359.

Santarelli, L., Saxe, M., Gross, C., Surget, A., Battaglia, F., Dulawa, S., Weisstaub, N., Lee, J., Duman, R., Arancio, O., *et al.* (2003). Requirement of hippocampal neurogenesis for the behavioral effects of antidepressants. *Science 301*, 805-809.

Stockmeier, C.A., Mahajan, G.J., Konick, L.C., Overholser, J.C., Jurjus, G.J., Meltzer, H.Y., Uylings, H.B., Friedman, L., and Rajkowska, G. (2004). Cellular changes in the postmortem hippocampus in major depression. *Biol. Psychiatry 56*, 640-650.

Tsankova, N., Renthal, W., Kumar, A., and Nestler, E.J. (2007). Epigenetic regulation in psychiatric disorders. *Nat. Rev. Neurosci. 8*, 355-367.

Tsankova, N.M., Berton, O., Renthal, W., Kumar, A., Neve, R.L., and Nestler, E.J. (2006). Sustained hippocampal chromatin regulation in a mouse model of depression and antidepressant action. *Nat. Neurosci. 9*, 519-525.

Uhr, M., Tontsch, A., Namendorf, C., Ripke, S., Lucae, S., Ising, M., Dose, T., Ebinger, M., Rosenhagen, M., Kohli, M., *et al.* (2008). Polymorphisms in the drug transporter gene ABCB1 predict antidepressant treatment response in depression. *Neuron 57*, 203-209.

In: Antidepressants: Types, Efficiency ...
Editor: Jayden T. Van Leeuwen, pp.169-198
ISBN 978-1-61668-581-2

Chapter 7

TIANEPTINE AND SERTRALINE: UNDERLYING NEUROCHEMICAL MECHANISMS OF ACTION

Rustem Uzbekov [1,2,3] ***and Irina Alieva*** [2,3]
[1]A. N. Belozersky Institute of Physico-Chemical Biology, Moscow State University, 119992 Moscow, Russian Federation
[2]Laboratoire Biologie Cellulaire et Microscopie Electronique, Faculte de Medecine, Universite Francois Rabelais, Tours, France
[3]Faculty of Bioengineering and Bioinformatics, Moscow State University, 119992 Moscow, Russian Federation

1. INTRODUCTION

According to the World Health Organization depression and anxiety are most frequently coexisted disturbances in the system of primary medical care (World Health Organization, 1999). These two conditions to a considerable extent overlap each other on clinical symptoms and a number of pathophysiological mechanisms (Nuller and Mikhalenko, 1988; Hamilton, 1988; Kasper, 2001). Hamilton marks that the anxiety at recurrent depression reveals in 96% of cases (1988). Clayton (1990), Cloninger (1990), Rodney et al. (1997), Tollefson et al. (1993) note that the anxiety can be found at 44-91% of patients with depression.

Depressed patients with symptoms of anxiety represent a special case of treatment with necessity of a choice of medicinal preparations that have both thymoleptic and marked anxiolytic effects (Avrutski and Neduva, 1988; Bakish, 1999). Introduction in clinical practice of antidepressants with a selective spectrum of action on serotonergic system – selective serotonin reuptake inhibitors (SSRI) or activators – can considerably increase efficiency of treatment of patients and improve the quality of life. However it requires a specification of indication to prescription of either preparation, investigation of clinical and metabolic pictures during the treatment and neurochemical mechanisms of their action. As shows the analysis of the literature the neurochemical mechanism of action of antidepressants influencing on serotonin reuptake is investigated insufficiently. For example Ansseau (1993) writes that paradoxical finding that both tianeptine and selective serotonin reuptake inhibitors exhibit antidepressant activity despite clearly antagonistic mechanisms is rather puzzling.

Thus in this study we want to discuss from clinical and biochemical points of view some aspects of dynamics of anxious depression under the treatment with serotonergic antidepressants with different mechanisms of action on serotonin reuptake. Besides that as a consequence of the study there will be reviewed different problems such as interactions between monoaminergic and hormonal systems, contribution of endogenous intoxication in the pathophysiology of mental disorders, in particular depression. One of the main results of this study is the development of the hypothesis of neurochemical mechanism of tianeptine action – selective serotonin reuptake enhancer.

2. Clinical Changes in Patients with Anxious Depression Under Tianeptine and Sertraline Action.

The group of patients consists of 61 persons (41 women and 20 men) at the age of 16 till 50. They were examined in the Department of Affective Disorders and in the Department of Brain Pathology of Moscow Research Institute of Psychiatry. All patients gave an informed consent for participation in the study (Maximova et al., 2000; Uzbekov et al., 2004).

Duration of mental disease at the moment of investigation was from 2 weeks till 18 years, duration of depression – from 2 weeks till 10 years.

Patient's state according to ICD-10 criteria (World Health Organization, 1992) was defined as a depressive episode as an independent disease (F32.1) and in the structure of recurrent depressive disorder (F33.1). The anxiety in the structure of the depression was the main indication to inclusion in the investigation.

Criteria for exclusion were comorbidity of depression with hallucinatory – delirious disorders, chronic alcoholism, drug abuse, mental diseases accompanied with organic lesions of the central nervous system. None of the patients received any treatment with antidepressants for at least 2 weeks prior to admission.

Clinical severity of the illness was assessed using the Hamiltjn Depression Scale (21 items) and the Hamilton Anxiety Scale which are described elsewhere (Bech, 1992).

According to the aim of investigation all the patients were divided in two groups by the open randomized method. As a monotherapy, patients of the first group (31 person) received tianeptine in a doze of 37, 5 mg/day, patients of another group (30 patients) – sertraline in a doze of 50 mg/day. The patients in whom the total points on the Hamilton Depression Scale decreased more than for 50% were considered as responders, less than for 50% - as nonresponders.

The control group consists of 15 volunteers who according to the clinical-biochemical parameters could be referred to practically healthy persons and were comparable on age to the examined patients.

A significant reduction of all symptoms of depression and anxiety was observed in the group of responders receiving tianeptine at the end of the 2nd week of treatment. After 4 weeks of tianeptine treatment, all responders showed a complete reduction of all symptoms of depression and anxiety according to Hamilton Depression Scale and Hamilton Anxiety Scale (both psychic anxiety and somatic anxiety) (Fig 1; Table 1). Similar results were obtained for those treated with sertraline (Fig 2; Table 3). In all cases the points on the second and on the forth weeks of the treatment were significantly lower (P < 0, 01) as compared with initial values.

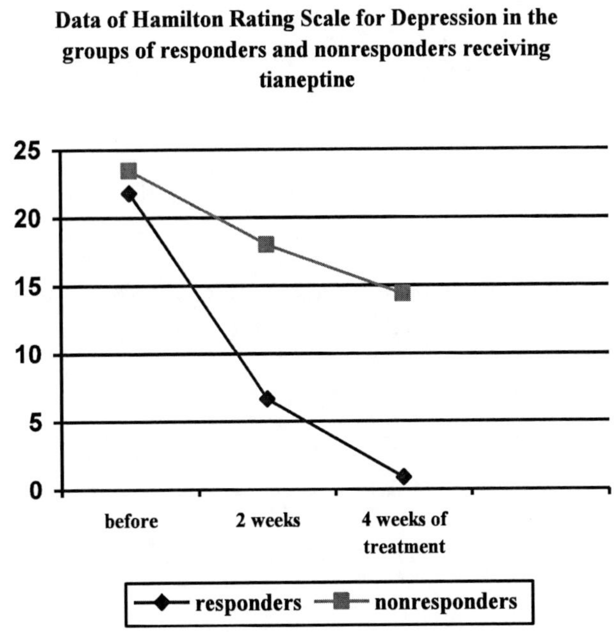

Figure 1.

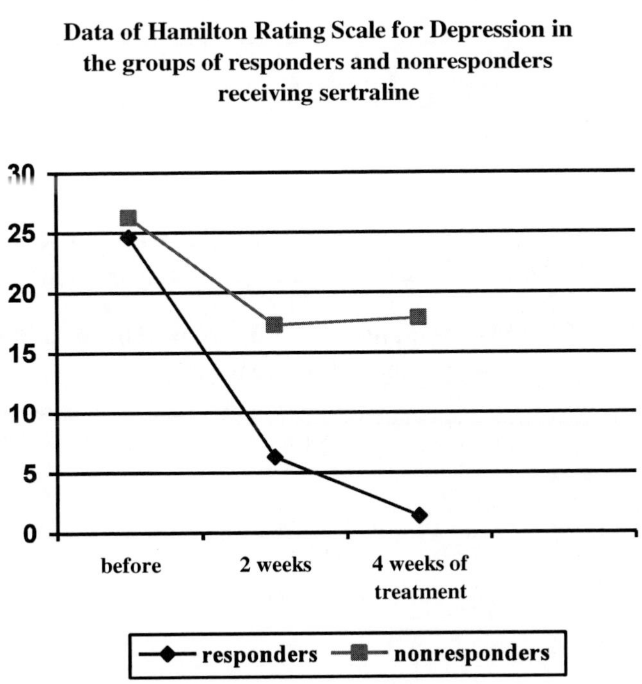

Figure 2.

Table 1. HAM-D and HAM-A total points changes for subgroup of responders under tianeptine treatment.

		Before treatment	2 weeks of treatment	P	4 weeks of treatment	P
Hamilton Rating Scale for Depression		21.85	6.65	p<0.01	0.87	p<0.01
Hamilton Rating Scale for Anxiety	Psychic Anxiety	18.43	5.52	p<0.01	0.30	p<0.01
	Somatic Anxiety	11.60	2.70	p<0.01	0.26	p<0.01

Table 2. HAM-D and HAM-A total points changes for subgroup of nonresponders under tianeptine treatment.

		Before treatment	2 weeks of treatment	P	4 weeks of treatment	P
Hamilton Rating Scale for Depression		23.50	18.00	p<0.05	14.38	n.s.
Hamilton Rating Scale for Anxiety	Psychic Anxiety	18.25	13.13	p<0.05	12.13	n.s.
	Somatic Anxiety	14.25	11.00	p<0.05	8.75	n.s

Table 3. HAM-D and HAM-A total points changes for subgroup of responders under sertraline treatment.

		Before treatment	2 weeks of treatment	P	4 weeks of treatment	P
Hamilton Rating Scale for Depression		24.61	6.30	p<0.01	1.35	p<0.01
Hamilton Rating Scale for Anxiety	Psychic Anxiety	17.91	3.00	p<0.01	0.43	p<0.01
	Somatic Anxiety	12.87	2.48	p<0.01	0.83	p<0.01

Table 4. HAM-D and HAM-A total points changes for subgroup of nonresponders under sertraline treatment.

		Before treatment	2 weeks of treatment	P	4 weeks of treatment	P
Hamilton Rating Scale for Depression		26.29	17.29	p<0.05	17.86	n.s.
Hamilton Rating Scale for Anxiety	Psychic Anxiety	19.43	11.86	p<0.05	12.57	n.s.
	Somatic Anxiety	12.71	6.86	p<0.05	6.86	n.s.

In the groups of nonresponders, receiving both tianeptine (Fig 1; Table 2) and sertraline (Fig 2; Table 4), after 2 weeks of the treatment there was a trend in reduction of depression and anxiety. At 4 weeks, those patients receiving tianeptine appeared to show a slightly greater improvement than those on sertraline (Fig 1 and 2; Tables 2 and 4, respectively).

At groups of nonresponders receiving both tianeptine and sertraline after 2 weeks of the treatment there were tendency to the reduction of the intensity of all components of depression and anxiety. However, at that time according to Hamilton Depression and Anxiety Scales the total points still did not reach significant differences with the initial points.

This investigation has shown a high, practically equal, antidepressive activity both of tianeptine and sertraline. There was revealed more pronounced anxiolitic effect of tianeptine whereas sertraline has shown equal analeptic and anxiolitic effects. Peculiarities in the action of investigated antidepressants make it possible to suppose that tianeptine can be recommended at anxious depression with pronounced psychic anxiety, astenic and sleep disorders whereas sertraline can be prescribed at anxious depression with pronounce depressive mood and psychomotor retardation.

3. Biochemical Changes in Anxious-Depressed Patients Under Antidepressant Therapy

Introduction in to clinical practice of antidepressants with a selective spectrum of action on serotonergic system [such as the selective serotonin reuptake inhibitors (SSRI) or serotonin reuptake enhancers] have considerably increased the efficacy of treatment of patients and improved their quality of life. Both tianeptine and sertraline are equally effective in patients with depression or depression associated with anxiety (Ansseau, 1993; Doogan and Caillard, 1992; Loo et al., 2001; Maximova et al., 2000, 2004).

Most investigations have been limited to studying the actions of these antidepressants on the serotonin reuptake and some routine biochemical parameters (Ansseau, 1993). Their effects on other biochemical parameters characterizing monoamine degradation, such as platelet monoamine oxidase or parameters reflecting the disturbances of homeostasis, such as middle-mass endotoxic molecules, semicarbazide-sensitive amine oxidase and albumin functional state, have been poorly investigated.

The aim of the study was to investigate the state of above mentioned parameters in patients with anxious depression. In addition, the biochemical profiles of patients with anxious depression following the treatment with tianeptine and sertraline were compared (Uzbekov et al., 2006).

43 out of 61 patients were investigated biochemically. Of these 21 patients received tianeptine and 22 patients - sertraline. Biochemical investigations were carried out by a double-blind method.

Biochemical parameters in all patients were estimated following the admission prior to any treatment and after two weeks of the therapy. The latter was done with the purpose to catch the initial stages of the reorganization of disturbed metabolism.

The activities of platelet monoamine oxidase (MAO) and serum semicarbazide-sensitive amine oxidase (SSAO) were estimated according to the method of McEwen and Cohen (1963) in modifications of Voloshina and Moskvitina (1985) and Balakleevski (1976), respectively.

Middle-mass endotoxic molecules (MMEM) represent a fraction of different blood plasma substances with the molecular mass of 300 - 5000 Dalton (Babb et al., 1972; Ringoir et al., 1987). The increase of the MMEM concentration in blood plasma is indicative of the aggravation of the degree of endogenous intoxication (Turianitsa et al., 1988; Chalenko, 1991; Umanskii et al., 1991; Uzbekov et al., 1995; Uzbekov and Misionzhnik, 2000; Uzbekov et al., 2006; Uzbekov et al., 2009). For the evaluation of the degree of endotoxicosis we have estimated MMEM concentration in blood plasma by method of Babb et al. (1972) in modification of Nikolaichik et al. (1991). Briefly, plasma, after consecutive protein precipitation with perchloric acid and ethanol, was centrifuged and the absorbtion of supernatant was read in spectrophotometer at 210 nm. For the evaluation of functional albumin properties we have used a fluorescence assay that permits to measure albumin binding capacity (Gryzunov et al., 1994; Moin et al., 1994). The method is based on the use of a new fluorescent probe K-35 (N-carboxyphenylimide of 4-dimethyl-ammo-l,8-naphthalenediearbonic acid). In the whole human serum we have estimated so called "effective albumin concentration" (EAC) and total albumin concentration (TAC) using specially developed method (Gryzunov et al., 1994; Moin et al., 1994; Gryzunov et al., 2000). Fluorescence of the samples was read with activation at 430 nm and fluorescence at 530 nm. Based on these parameters it is calculated the specific coefficient of albumin binding capacity that is called "reserve of albumin binding" (RAB) according by the following formula: RAB = EAC/TAC x 100%. RAB is the portion (in %) of albumin binding sites in serum or plasma that are not occupied by toxic metabolites. EAC and RAB values reflect the functional state of albumin molecules: decrease of these values indicate on the disturbances in albumin molecules (Gryzunov et al., 2000; Uzbekov and Misionzhnik, 2000) and increase of endogenous intoxication.

In a part of patients (20 persons, selection-randomized, estimation-double-blind) we have tried to elucidate the informative significance of the conventional biochemical indices (20 various parameters) of the serum measured on the standard automatic biochemical analyzers.

Prior to the beginning of the treatment all patients were characterized by a significant increase in platelet MAO activity (by 95%) and decrease of serum SSAO activity (by 43%) in comparison to the control group (Table 5). The MMEM concentration significantly exceeded control values (by 86%). Regarding the functional properties of serum albumin, EAC and RAB values were significantly reduced by 30 and 38%, respectively, as compared with the controls. At the same time the level of TAC did not differ from control values.

Table 5 shows that in responders after 2 weeks of the tianeptine treatment there were significant increase of EAC (by 10 %, $p=0,0391$ and $p<0,05$ according to U-test and K-S-test, respectively) and RAB (by 3 %, $p=0,0042$ and $p<0,025$) values. There were significant decrease of SSAO activity (by 7%, $p=0,0092$ and $p<0,01$) and in MMEM concentration (by 5%, $p=0,0308$ and $p<0,05$) as compared with background. MAO activity insignificantly decreased by 7 % ($p=0,0688$ and $p>0,10$). In the group of nonresponders EAC, RAB and MMEM values continued to decrease by 7%, 8% and 5%, respectively, MAO activity decreased by 23% whereas SSAO activity increased by 13% in comparison with background; all these changes were insignificant.

Table 5. activity and level of investigated parameters IN patients with anxious depression under tianeptine and sertraline treatment and in controls.

Investigated groups	MAO n mol benzaldehyde/ mg protein in hour	SSAO n mol benzaldehyde/ ml serum in hour	MMEM g/l	TAC g/l	EAC g/l	RAB %
Control (15 persons)	8.68±1.65	10.84±0.65	0.45±0.04	46.00±2.04	44.00±3.10	95.00±2.10
Background (43 patients)	* 16.91±3.50	** 6.22±0.82	** 0.84±0.08	49.53±2.82	** 30.95±2.82	** 64.76±2.96
Tianeptine Responders (13 patients)	* 15.80±2.40	** 5.82±0.91	** 0.80±0.04	51.6±2.68	** 33.85±1.63	** 66.70±3.29
Tianeptine Nonresponders (8 patients)	** 13.10±2.68	** 7.08±1.08	** 0.80±0.10	49.31±2.67	** 29.04±0.77	** 60.10±3.68
Sertraline Responders (15 patients)	** 19.11±2.61	** 6.56±0.68	** 0.93±0.07	** 54.00±2.80	** 33.29±2.70	** 61.81±4.58
Sertraline Nonresponders (7 patients)	** 27.72±3.82[§]	** 6.19±0.70	** 0.94±0.05	** 58.84±3.90	** 29.31±1.80	** 51.23±5.00[§]

*- p < 0, 05; **p < 0,001 –in comparison with control. [§] - p < 0, 05 – in comparison with background. MAO–monoamine oxidase, SSAO–semicarbazide-sensitive amine oxidase, MMEM–middle-mass endotoxic molecules, TAC–total albumin concentration, EAC-effective albumin concentration, RAB–reserve of albumin binding

After 2 weeks of sertraline treatment in patients-responders MMEM concentration continued to increase (by 11%, p=0,0308 and p<0,05) (Table 4). At the same time RAB value continued to decrease for 5% (p=0,0042 and p<0,025) in spite of that EAC value increased by 8% (p=0,0391 and p<0,05) and SSAO activity – by 17% (p=0,0092 and p<0,01) as compared with background. MAO activity increased insignificantly by 13 % (p=0,0688 and p>0,10). In nonresponders two weeks of sertraline treatment resulted in significant increase of MAO activity (by 64%, P < 0,05) and significant decrease of RAB value (by 21%, P < 0,05) in comparison with the background. MMEM concentration was increased insignificantly by 11% as compared with the background. After two weeks of the treatment the SSAO activity was unchanged.

The biochemical parameters determined were: total protein, albumin, alanine- and aspartate-aminotransferases, creatinine kinase, γ-glutamyltranspeptidase, acid and alkaline phosphatases, urea, creatinine, uric acid, cholesterol, triglycerides, bilirubin, glucose, inorganic substances (K, Ca, Ph, Fe, Cl) in the serum of 20 patients using biochemical automatic analyzer before and after two weeks of the treatment with the antidepressants (tianeptine - 9 patients, sertralme 11 patients). No differences were found in comparison with the controls.

The pharmacodynamics of both tianeptine and sertraline has received limited attention (Ansseau, 1993; Kato and Weitsch, 1988). There is, for example, practically no data about the influence of these serotonergic antidepressants on monoaminergic indices and on the degree of homeostasis disturbance.

For these reasons we have investigated some biochemical parameters reflecting above mentioned processes (Uzbekov et al., 2006). It was established that, in comparison with healthy controls, the patients with anxious depression were characterized by the significant increase of platelet MAO activity; this may reflect MAO activity in the brain (Stahl, 1985). The concentration of MMEM was significantly increased whereas EAC and RAB values, and SSAO activity, were significantly decreased. This implies that anxious depression is characterized by the strongly pronounced disturbances of monoaminergic metabolism and homeostasis as a whole.

Some time ago we have proposed (Uzbekov and Misionzhnik, 2000) that the degree of endogenous intoxication (endotoxicisis) can serve as a parameter of intensity of the disturbances of homeostasis and that the level of middle-mass endotoxic molecules in the blood reflects the degree of endotoxicosis. (Problems of endogenous intoxication will be discussed in part 4 of this chapter). We assume that during the development of psychic process the catabolic reactions are activated that is resulting in the increase of the concentration of different substances in the MM fraction (Turianitsa et al., 1988; Uzbekov et al., 1995). That took place at patients with anxious depression whose MMEM level was elevated almost twofold. The finding that in patients with anxious depression MMEM concentration was elevated almost twofold supports this thesis.

It is known that the monoamine oxidase is an integral component of the external mitochondrial membrane. The disturbance of MAO activity in anxious depression may be indicative of the fact that the pathological state is accompanied by the damage to the membrane structures resulting in the appearance in the blood of different toxic end products. A significant accumulation of the fluorescent Shiff-bases in the blood of depressed patients indicates oxidative membrane damage (Prilipko et al., 1987) that supports our supposition.

The functional state of serum albumin can serve as an objective parameter of degree of endotoxicosis in different pathological situations, and in particular in mental disorders (Gryzunov et al., 2000; Uzbekov et al., 1998; Uzbekov and Misionzhnik, 2000). Disturbance of albumin physic-chemical properties leads to the damage of its main functions – transport and detoxification. Decreased EAC and RAB values at anxious patients indicate to the disturbances in these two albumin functions and development of endotoxicosis.

Thus, besides the disturbances in monoaminergic metabolism patients with anxious depression are characterized by increased MMEM level, elevated MAO activity and decrease SSAO activity and functional properties of albumin that result in the development of endotoxicosis and disorder of homeostasis as a whole.

After 2 weeks of tianeptine treatment patients who responded were characterized by the decrease in MAO and SSAO activities, and the MMEM concentration together with an increase of EAC and RAB values. In responders to two weeks of sertraline medication there were opposite changes in MAO and SSAO activities and MMEM concentration and a decrease in RAB value (Tables 5). Thus antidepressant treatments appear to have the obvious influence on the indices of monoamine metabolism and parameters characteristic for endotoxicosis.

Analysis of the biochemical profiles has shown that in responders there were significant contrary directed changes of all investigated parameters under the treatment of antidepressnts possessing different mechanisms of action on serotonin reuptake (Fig. 3).

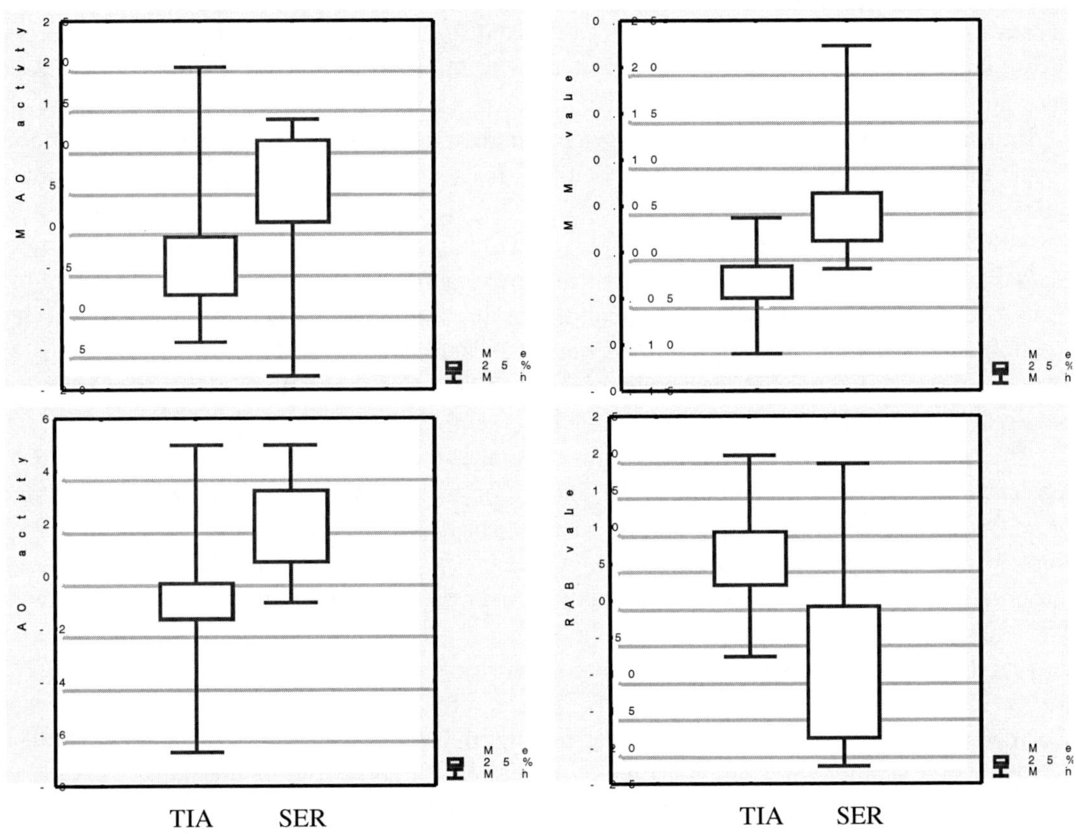

Left boxes – TIA (tianeptine), right boxes – SER (sertraline).

MAO - monoamine oxidase, AO - semicarbazide-sensitive amine oxidase, MMEM - middle-mass endotoxic molecules, RAB – reserve of albumin binding.

(Published with the permission of John Wiley & Sons, Ltd, Copyright © 2005. Biochemical profile in patients with anxious depression under the treatment with serotonergic antidepressants with different mechanisms of action. Hum Psychopharmacol Clin Exp 2006; 21: 109-115. Uzbekov M.G., Misionzhnik E.Y., Maximova N.M., Vertogradova O.P.)

Figure 3. Box and whisker plot of investigated groups under tianeptine and sertraline treatment.

The nonresponders following tianeptine treatment were characterized by the decrease in MAO activity and in the MMEM concentration, but, in contrast to the responders, the EAC and RAB values continued to decrease (Table 5). This implies a failure in the normalization of homeostasis (Uzbekov and Misionzhnik, 2000).

In nonresponders after two weeks of sertraline treatment MAO activity significantly increased whereas RAB value significantly decreased in comparison to the untreated state; the MMEM concentration continued to increase (Table 5). After two weeks of sertraline treatment in nonresponders was a worsening of the clinical status (Table 3).

In tianeptine responders decrease of MAO activity pointing out on the normalization of monoamine metabolism thaat is accompanied by the increase of parameters of functional albumin (EAC and RAB values) and decrease of MMEM level. All together are indicated to the decrease of the degree of endogenous intoxication and the improvement of homeostasis as a whole (Uzbekov and Misionzhnik, 2000; Uzbekov et al., 2006). In tianeptine nonresponders MAO activity is also started to decrease (Table 5). However this positive MAO activity dynamics under tianeptine treatment can not reveal itself on the clinical level because other investigated parameters do not exhibit a tendency to improvement. Thus a high MMEM level does not change and functional albumin parameters EAC and RAB continue to decrease. It possible to assume that nonresponders were characterized by more pronounced metabolic disturbances at a base line then responders. But it is necessary to emphasize that these patients did not have side effects.

Another metabolic picture was found in anxious patients under sertraline treatment (50 mg/day). The therapeutic effect under the treatment with this antidepressant is also manifested after two weeks of the medication. At that time there were changes in the activity or in the level of all investigated biochemical parameters (Table 1). It is seen that at responders the direction of all parameters (except EAC values) was quite opposite to what we have received in responders under tianeptine treatment.

Proceeding from our result we can conclude that there is another neurochemical mechanism under sertraline treatment. The latter as an inhibitor of serotonin reuptake promotes to the serotonin accumulation in the synaptic cleft and increases the efficacy of serotonin neurotransmission. Elevation (as a tendency) of MAO activity in responders gives the possibility to support serotonin concentration in the synaptic cleft on the optimal level. This enzyme deaminating the excess of the monoamine promote the supporting the positive clinical dynamics. But responders were also characterized by the tendency to the increase the degree of endotoxicosis (decrease of RAB value and increase of MMEM level). Besides that the increase of MAO activity is connected with the activation of H_2O_2 generation (as a product of the deaminating reaction) which promotes the activation of free radical reactions and lipid peroxidation (Gorkin, 1985; Beckman and Ames, 1998).

We think that in nonresponders under sertraline treatment inhibition of serotonin reuptake mechanisms is more pronounced then in responders. Possibly in the synaptic cleft serotonin is concentrated in excessive quantities. The significant increase of MAO activity (compensatory reaction directed to decrease of high serotonin concentration) supports this assumption (Table 5). But reuptake mechanisms are blocked by sertraline (inhibitor of serotonin reuptake). Because the normal accumulation of serotonin in the nerve ending is disturbed, the serotonin cell body by feedback mechanisms does not receive the blocking information and continues to synthesize and transport serotonin in the nerve ending. We suppose that it is one of the reasons of the excessive concentration of serotonin in the synaptic cleft. One can assume that in nonresponders under sertraline treatment the increase of serotonin concentration in the synaptic cleft is going more quickly then the elimination of its excess. All these exert negative influence on the metabolism in patients of this subgroup: the functional albumin parameters continue to decrease and the integral parameter of albumin functioning (RAB, reserve of albumin binding) already decreases significantly as compared with the initial level. At that time SSAO activity and MMEM level were stable on the initial pathological level. Thus in two weeks of sertraline therapy in nonresponders the monoamine metabolism begins to aggravate and the endotoxicosis to increase. On the clinical level in nonrespondesrs after two weeks of sertraline medication there were revealed negative side effects and their state even worsened (Maximova 2000, 2004).

Clinically in responders tianeptine and sertraline reveal practically equal positive effect. But the results of the biochemical investigation permit us to suppose that for the maintenance of positive therapeutic dynamics in responders under sertraline treatment the neurochemical mechanism must be in a very tense state because the degree of endogenous intoxication does not decrease. Also it is necessary to take into the account that SSRIs are blocking serotonin reuptake receptors (or serotonin transporter) that were earlier affected by the pathological depressive process (Bellivier et al., 2002). So it is possible to assume that during all medication period they are situated as if in "preserved pathological state". Any stressful condition can disturb this labile unstable equilibrium. We think that it may be one of the reasons why patients successfully stabilized in acute-phase treatment have a recurrent rate of 10% to 30% within one year, even if they continue to take medication with selective serotonin reuptake inhibitors (Ayuso-Gutierrz J., 2002; Hirshfeld R.M., 2001).

The results of this, and previous studies (Maximova et al., 2004), show that both tianeptine and sertraline are equally effective in the treatment of anxious depression. The present biochemical study, however, suggests that the underlying biochemical changes are more complete following tianeptine treatment. The precise significance of this awaits elucidation

4. The Role of Endogenous Intoxication in Pathogenetic Mechanism of Anxious Depression

Diseases that are followed by the increased activity of catabolic processes and intensity of hypoxia, with the disturbances in microcirculation, with necrosis of tissues and many others are accompanied with processes of intoxication. In spite of different etiological factors symptoms of intoxication have common features and clinical manifestations. Mechanisms of the development of these symptoms are almost identical. Commonness of pathogenesis and clinical manifestations permit us to state a presence of a syndrome of endogenous intoxication that not only accompanies practically all diseases but itself is a very important factor of pathogenetic mechanisms and in many cases predetermines inauspicious outcome. In any disease syndrome of endogenous intoxication aggravates the course of the main disease.

It is possible to subdivide the main causes of development of endogenous intoxication that leads to the impairments of homeostasis into several groups (Umansky et al., 1991; Uzbekov et al., 2000):

- destructive processes that are followed by the accumulation of excessive quantities of intermediate and end products of metabolism that exert toxic influences on different systems,
- impairments in membranes that in normal conditions regulate exchange of different substances between the cells and blood, prevent from penetration of toxic products in the cells,
- disturbances in detoxification processes,
- activation of cataboloic processes,

Numerous attempts to isolate specific for different diseases toxin or toxins are without success. We suppose that the possibility of clear differentiation of toxic substances is insignificant because there are not only disturbances but also distortions of metabolic processes at pathologic conditions.

Some time ago we have proposed (Uzbekov and Misionzhnik, 2000) that degree of endogenous intoxication can serve as a parameter of intensity of the disturbances of homeostasis. Endogenous intoxication (endotoxicosis) is a pathophysiological process that is characterized by the formation and accumulation in tissues and body fluids of different substances and metabolites, endotoxins in excessive concentrations or in forms that are not characteristic for the normal metabolism (Umanskii et al., 1991; Uzbekov and Misionzhnik, 2000).

We suppose that endogenous intoxication can reveals itself on the two levels – metabolic and clinical levels. Metabolic level of endotoxicosis is characterized by the excessive accumulation of the products of normal and distorted metabolism and can be discovered using different biochemical methods. Clinical level of endotoxicosis includes both metabolic disturbances and different clinical symptoms as complications of the disease and side-effects of the therapy (Uzbekov and Misionzhnik, 2000; Uzbekov et al., 2006).

Endogenous intoxication accompanies practically all diseases including mental disorders and plays an important role in their pathogenetic mechanisms (Malakhova et al., 2004; Umanski et al., 1991; Stober et al., 2009; Uzbekov and Misionzhnik, 2000; Uzbekov et al., 2006; Uzbekov et al., 2009).

Impairments in monoamine metabolism and functional albumin, free radical processes and lipid peroxidation, increased levels of middle-mass endotoxic molecules, disturbed platelet monoamine oxidase and serum semicarbazide-sensitive amine oxidase, etc, have contributed heavily to the development of endogenous intoxication.

Monoamine oxidase. Monoamine oxidase is the enzyme that catalyzes deamination of neurotransmitter catechol – and indoleamines – serotonin, noradrenaline and dopamine. Its activity reflects the state of monoaminergic neurotransmitter systems. Earlier it was shown by us that platelet MAO activity was increased by 100 and more % in patients with anxious depression (Uzbekov et al., 2006), in chronic schizophrenics (Mosolov et al., 1999), in first-episode drug-naïve schizophrenic patients (Uzbekov et al., 2009). According to S. Stahl (1985) platelet MAO can reflect MAO activity in the brain.

It is possible to consider the events that are connected with the increased MAO activity from several points of view. First, increased platelet MAO activity points out on the disturbances of monoamine metabolism. It is known (Gorkin, 1985) that MAO has different affinity for serotonin and noradrenaline and deaminates them with different velocities. It means that in patients with mental disorders, and in particular in patients with anxious depression, can be found changes not only in monoamine absolute concentrations but changes in the equilibrium between these two monoamines that is characteristic for healthy persons. Second, monoamine oxidase is an integral component of the external mitochondrial membrane. The disturbance of MAO activity in anxious depression may be indicative of the fact that the pathological state is accompanied by the damage to the membrane structures resulting in the appearance in the blood of different toxic end products. A significant accumulation of the fluorescent Shiff-bases in the blood of depressed patients indicates oxidative membrane damage (Prilipko et al., 1987) that supports our supposition. Accumulation of these substances in the blood promotes the increase of the level of MMEM and aggravates the degree of endogenous intoxication. Third, it is known (Beckman and Ames, 1998; Gorkin, 1985) that hydrogen peroxide formed in the reaction of deamination catalyzed by MAO represents the main source of free radicals (through the Fenton reaction) in the brain. Thus elevation of MAO activity can induce the activation of free radical processes and lipid peroxidation in patients with anxious depression as well as in patients with other mental disorders (Uzbekov et al., 2009; Yao et al., 2001). Fourth, the high MAO activity is followed by increase in the blood the level of toxic products (aldehyde and ammonia) that are formed in the reaction of deamination. Taken together these results suggest that an increased MAO activity precipitates a cascade of negative biochemical events.

Serum semicarbazide-sensitive amine oxidase. Serum semicarbazide-sensitive amine oxidase is considered to be an enzyme that is involved in the oxidation both xenobiotics and endogenous metabolites (Boomsma et al., 2003; Gong and Boor, 2006; Strolin Benedetti et al., 2006). The precise physiological and pathophysiological role of this enzyme is not known. We have found a decrease of SSAO activity in patients with anxious depression (Uzbekov et al., 2006). Also it has been reported a decrease of SSAO activity both in chronic schizophrenic patients (Baron et al., 1983) and in drug-naïve first-episode schizophrenic patients (Uzbekov et al., 2009). SSAO can convert some endogenous amines, such as methylamine and amineacetone, into highly toxic compounds – formaldehyde and methylglyoxal, respectively, as well as acrolein (Boomsma et al., 2003; Callingham et al., 1995; Gong and Boor, 2006). It is therefore possible that an increase in the blood concentrations of these substances following stressful life events for example, depression or schizophrenia, can exert harmful influences and endogenous intoxication can intensify. Callingham et al. (1995) have hypothesized that accumulation of above mentioned substances represents a danger to the organism. This danger can be diminished either physiologically by compensatory decrease of enzyme activity or pharmacologically using the inhibitors of this enzyme, for example aminoguanidin. We suppose (Uzbekov et al., 2009) that as the concentration of these toxic products increases there can turn on a compensatory mechanism of allosteric inhibition. As a result the enzyme activity and production of toxic products of enzymatic reaction can reduce. But these problems are awaiting their elucidation.

Serum albumin. One of universal mechanisms of organism's reaction on the increased level of metabolic reaction products is formation of complexes of different substances with proteins of blood (Gryzunov and Dobretsov, 1994, 1998). Serum albumin possesses unique properties and plays important role, besides others, in processes of detoxification and transport. For the evaluation of functional albumin properties we have used a fluorescence assay that permits to measure albumin binding capacity (Gryzunov et al., 1994; Moin et al., 1994). The method is based on the use of a new fluorescent probe K-35 (N-carboxyphenylimide of 4-dimethyl-ammo-l, 8-naphthalenediearbonic acid). Albumin is the only serum protein with which K-35 specifically binds. In the whole human serum we have estimated so called "effective albumin concentration" (EAC) and total albumin concentration (TAC) using specially developed method (Gryzunov et al., 1994; Moin et al., 1994; Gryzunov et al., 2000; Uzbekov et al., 2006). Based on these parameters it is calculated the specific coefficient of albumin binding capacity that is called "reserve of albumin binding" (RAB) according by the following formula: RAB = EAC/TAC x 100%. RAB is the portion (in %) of albumin binding sites in serum or plasma that are not occupied by toxic metabolites. EAC and RAB values reflect the functional state of albumin molecules: decrease of these values indicate on the disturbances in albumin molecules (Gryzunov et al., 2000) and increase of endogenous intoxication (Uzbekov and Misionzhnik, 2000; Uzbekov et al., 2006; Uzbekov et al., 2009).

Middle-mass endotoxic molecules. In the beginning of 70th Babb et al. (1972) have discovered in blood plasma of uremic patients the increased level of substances with molecular mass in the range of 500 - 5000 Dalton. They have called the fraction of these substances as a fraction of middle molecules and have proposed the hypothesis that middle molecules play a role in pathogenesis of uremia. After the hemodialysis there was the decrease of the concentration of middle molecules in the blood that was coincided with the improvement of patient's clinical status. The worsening of patient's status was followed with the elevation of these substances.

Later there were found elevation of MMEM content in plasma in different somatic (peritonitis, hepatitis, pneumonia, miocardial infarction, insult, etc) (Chalenko, 1991; Ringoir et al., 1987; Umanskii et al., 1991; Uzbekov and Misionzhnik, 2000) and nervous and mental (epilepsy, schizophrenia, depressions) (Turianitsa et al., 1988; Uzbekov et al., 1995; Mosolov et al., 1999; Uzbekov et al., 2006) diseases. It is considered that the increased MMEM level in the blood is the reflection of the aggravation of the degree of endotoxicosis (Nikolaichik et al., 1991; Parfenkova et al., 1987; Piradov et al., 1990; Umanskii et al., 1991; Ringoir et al., 1987; Uzbekov and Misionzhnik, 2000; Uzbekov et al., 2006; Uzbekov et al., 2009).

MMEM represents a fraction of different blood plasma substances with the molecular mass of 300 - 5000 Dalton (Ringoir et al., 1987). There are different short-and oligo-peptides, glycopeptides, degradation products of different blood proteins (albumin, fibrinogen, trombin, etc), lipid peroxidation products, some hormones, derivatives of glucuronic acids, di- and polyamines, products of pathologically distorted metabolism, etc, in this fraction. Different authors think that there are more then 30 biologically active substances (Chalenko, 1991; Nikolaichik et al., 1991; Ringoir et al., 1987; Tupikova, 1983). Many components of MMEM fraction are possessed of toxic properties and can inhibit different metabolic and physiologic processes such as energy production and membrane transport, erythropoiesis, microcirculation, reveal immunodepressive, cytotoxic and neuro- and psychotropic properties (Kovalevskii and Nifantieva, 1989; Ringoir et al., 1987; Tupikova, 1983;). Experimentally was proved that they exert toxic effects in concentrations much less then do it urea, uric acid or aromatic amines (Umanskii et al., 1991). It is necessary to mean that in normal condition MMEM fraction mainly reflects the catabolic processes whereas in pathologic conditions – combination of catabolic, destructive and distorted metabolic processes that take place in the organism.

In spite of that MMEM possess psychotropic properties (Ringoir et al., 1987; Tupikova, 1983; Umanskii et al., 1991) their role in the pathophysiology of mental disorders is investigated poorly.

The findings that in patients with anxious depression MM level was elevated almost twofold supports this thesis (Uzbekov et al., 2006). It is possible to assume that during the development of psychic process (depression and schizophrenia) there is activation of catabolic processes that resulted in the increase of the concentration of different substances in the MM fraction (Shikhov et al., 2000; Turianitsa et al., 1988.; Uzbekov et al., 1995; Uzbekov et al., 2006).

Possible pathogenetic mechanisms of the development of endogenous intoxication. The results of our investigations and literature data make it possible to propose pathogenetic mechanisms of the development of endogenous intoxication in endogenous disorders, in particular depression and schizophrenia (Uzbekov and Misionzhnik, 2000; Uzbekov et al., 2006; Uzbekov et al., 2009) (Fig. 4).

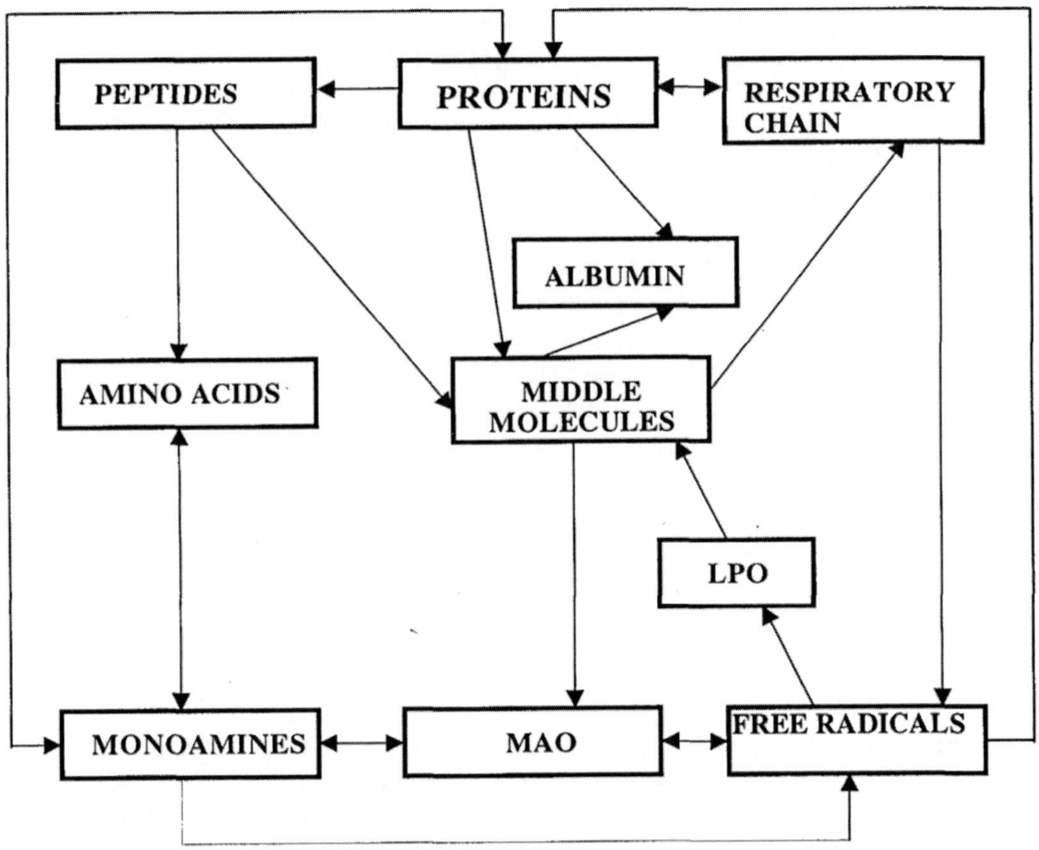

Figure 4. Middle molecules involvement in mechanisms of development of endotoxicosis in patients with schizophrenia resistant to psychopharmacotherapy

That is a closed chain of metabolic conversions in which disturbances in any unit initiates a cascade of subsequent pathological changes. Through the unit "MAO → monoamines" this pathological chain is interconnected with the general pathogenetic mechanisms of the development of endogenous disorders. For example, disturbances in monoamine metabolism and MAO activity promote activation of free radical production. It was known that catecholamines, and especially dopamine, take part in protein metabolism regulation; disturbances in dopamine metabolism induce imbalance in protein anabolic and catabolic processes with prevailing the latter reactions (Tret'jak and Arkhipova, 1992). Activation of catabolic processes promotes the increase of concentration of peptides with different molecular weight as well as "pathological" peptides as a consequence of metabolism distortion in endogenous disorders. As a result there is increase of concentration of MMEM fraction in the blood. Increased level of components of MMEM fraction containing "pathological" components can exert negative effects on the enzyme activity (MAO) and protein functions (Shikhov et al., 2000; Uzbekov and Misionzhnik, 2000).

Membrane damage and metabolic hypoxia in patients with endogenous disorders (Anders and Orlovskaya, 1982) is followed by disturbances of the mitochondrial oxidative phosphorylation (Marchbanks et al., 1995) that is induced the excessive free radical generation (Halliwell and Gutteridge, 2006). In its turn free radicals induce lipid peroxidation.

Lipid hydroperoxides changing albumin properties decrease its detoxification functions with subsequent aggravation of the degree of endogenous intoxication.

Progression of the main disorder (depression or schizophrenia) promotes the activation of the functioning of the "vicious circle" and increases of the degree of endogenous intoxication (Uzbekov and Misionzhnik, 2000).

We suppose that presented scheme (Fig. 4) explains not only the mechanisms of developing of endogenous intoxication but also points out some ways of the overcoming of this "circle" and decreasing of endogenous intoxication. There are theoretically some possible pharmacological treatments (Uzbekov and Misionzhnik, 2000):

- monoamine oxidase inhibitors – chain 'MAO-monoamines',
- antioxidants – chain 'free radicals- lipid hydroperoxides',
- inhibitors of proteolysis – chain 'peptides-proteins-middle-mass endotoxic molecules',
- correctors of oxidative phosphorylation.

5. Hormonal and Monoamine Interactions in Pathogenetic Mechanisms of Anxious Depression

There are several hypothesis of pathogenesis of depression and anxiety: monoamiergic (Nuller and Mikhalenko, 1988; Kasper, 2000), GABA-ergic (Hales et al., 1999), genetic (Hales et al., 1999), hormonal (Holsboer, 2001; Laakmann, 1991), imunne (Leonard, 2000) and some others.

The last 3 decades two hypothesis are elaborated the most intensively. One of them is monoaminergic hypothesis. According to this hypothesis pathogenetic mechanisms of depression and anxiety are connected with the deficit of serotonin and norepinephrine in the brain structures (Kasper, 2001; Ressler and Nemeroff, 2000).

The second hypothesis is hormonal according to which the main characteristic features of depression and anxiety are closely related with the disturbances in the hypothalamic-pituitary-adrenal (HPA) axis (Nuller and Mikhalenko, 1988; Laakmann, 1991). In this case the activity of hypothalamic corticotropine-releasing factor secretion is increased that is followed by the activation of АКТГ release from the pituitary. The letter activates the synthesis of glucocorticoids, in particular cortisol, in the adrenals which are secreted in blood. As a result cortisol concentration in blood is increased.

It may be assumed that all these and other factors in certain measures are involved in pathogenetic mechanisms of anxious depression, determine the pathochemical mechanisms of the disease and influence upon the stability of homeostasis.

From the other hand the existence of numerous hypothesis of the pathogenesis of depression indicate that a lot of aspects of this very difficult problem are not solved and requires the more profound investigation without restriction in the frame of only any one of the hypothesis.

In our investigations of anxious depression (Uzbekov et al., 2003) we have tried to elucidate some biochemical aspects of monoaminergic and hormonal systems interaction.

It was shown in the last 20-30 years that in 90 % of cases anxious depression is coincided by the activation of HPA axis (Leonard, 2000). The most available parameter for discovering the disturbances in this axis is the increased cortisol level in the patient's blood.

We have found almost 10 times increase of cortisol concentration in blood serum in anxious depressed patients in comparison with healthy volunteers (Uzbekov et al., 2003) (Table 6).

Table 6. Hormone content in the blood serum in patients with anxious depression.

		Cortisol μg/dl	Testosterone nmol/l	Estradiol pg/ml
Control	men	2.3 – 30.2	8.5 – 43.5	15 -60
	women		0.2 – 4.2	70 - 250
Patients	men	306.10±18.26***	9.64±4.52	73.38±9.49*
	women		15.37±4.93**	101.19±24.18

As it was indicated in the literature there is a deficit in serotonergic and noradrenergic activities in depression and anxiety (Bliss and Zwanziger, 1966; Kasper, 2001, Kelly and Cooper, 1998). Deficiency of these monoaminergic systems has injurious effects on cortisol homeostasis. Noradrenalin deficit leads to the increased cortisol level whereas serotonin deficit causes disturbances in the regulation of cortisol secretion. Insufficiency of both of these monoamines results in disturbances of circadian rhythms of cortisol srcretion. It means that increased in the morning cortisol level does not decrease in the evening and at night. It follows from this that increased cortisol level remains all the day and as consequence different enzyme and another systems are by the constant impact of glucocorticoids (Nuller and Mikhalenko, 1988).

Some time ago S. Kasper hypothesized that depression and anxiety are supervised by the equilibrium between serotonin and noradrenaline contents and their activities instead of their absolute levels (Kasper, 2001). It can mean that the anxiety and depression are connected with the disturbances in the regulation of the metabolism of these neurotransmitters. The concept of equilibrium is in accord with the fact that N. raphe, the center of serotonergic system, and Locus coeruleus, the center of noradrenergic system, are interconnected and mutually dependent structures.

We suppose that S. Kasper's concept is based on the theses that were stated and experimentally confirmed by E.A. Gromova in the middle of 70th of the last century. According to E.A. Gromova (1979) serotonergic and noradrenergic systems are in reciprocal interconnections, i.e. activation of one system leads to inhibition of the other and vice verse, and that emotional reactivity is determined by the equilibrium of their activities.

The question arises as what biochemical mechanisms are involved in the equilibrium disturbances between serotonergic and noradrenergic systems. Analysis of data that were received in clinical-biochemical and experimental investigations (Nuller and Mikhalenko, 1988) together with the results of our studies (Uzbekov et al., 2003; Uzbekov et al., 2006) permit us to propose a possible biochemical mechanism of these disturbances in anxious depression.

It is known that the increased cortisol level activates the enzyme, tryptophan – pyrrolase (Curzon, 1969), that switches tryptophan pathway of metabolism (precursor of serotonin synthesis) to another pathways of metabolism, in particular on kynurenin pathway (Lapin, 1996) that induces the decrease in serotonin biosynthesis. It is necessary to take in consideration that in normal conditions only about 5 % of all tryptophan content in the brain is used for serotonin biosynthesis. That is the reason why any disturbances in tryptophan – pyrrolase activity lead to changes in serotonin concentration. From the other hand, increased cortisol secretion induced activation of the enzyme, tyrosine aminotransferase, that can lead to the decrease of tyrosine concentration (Nemeth, 1978). This can be accompanied by the decrease in catecholamine biosynthesis and as consequence decrease in noradrenaline concentration (Fig. 5).

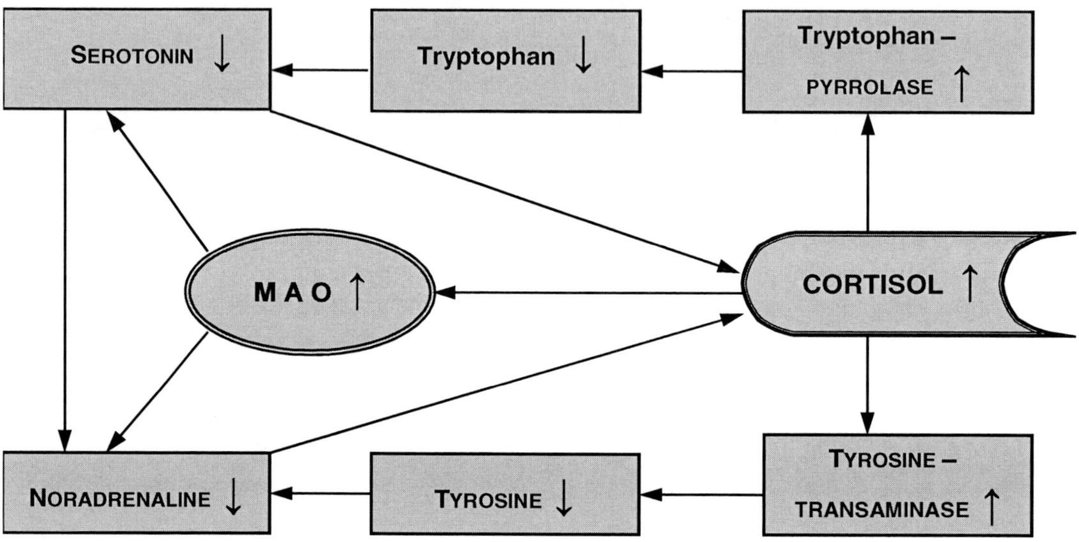

Figure 5.

Monoamine oxidase makes an important contribution in disturbances of serotonin and noradrenaline concentrations in the brain. It is possible to suppose that increased cortisol concentrations can induce elevation of MAO activity. Our supposition is supported by the results of our investigation (Uzbekov et al., 2006): in patients with anxious depression deaminating MAO activity was increased approximately in 2 times as compared with controls. It is necessary to note that MAO deaminating serotonin and noradrenaline with different velocities (Gorkin, 1985) not only decreases their levels to variable degree but also disturbs equilibrium between these monoamines.

All these disturbances finally lead to the formation of the vicious circle (Fig. 5). Increased cortisol level, from one side, activates monoamine oxidase that more actively deaminates monoamines; from the other side biosynthetic serotonin and noradrenaline pathways become impaired under the action of high cortisol.

The scheme on Fig. 5 indicates on, at least, three ways of the antidepressive therapy. The first two ways are directed on the normalization of monoamine metabolism: at first – inhibition of MAO activity with MAO inhibitors, and the second – normalization of serotonin and noradrenaline concentration in synaptic cleft using selective serotonin and noradrenaline reuptake inhibitors and serotonin reuptake enhancer. The third way – normalization of the state of HPA axis with the purpose of receiving the antidepressive effect – is the least investigated; such kind of therapy is followed with serious side effects and requested the further studies.

For a long it is known that monoamines and especially serotonin are involved in the regulation of sexual behavior (Gonzales et al., 1982) and that changes in serotonergic system activity can lead to changes in sexual sphere. Increase in the blood of the level of female hormone (estradiol) in men and the level of male hormone (testosterone) in women are the plausible reasons of the disturbances in the sexual sphere that is found in depressed patients. These and above mentioned changes are the evidence of profound disturbances of hormonal balance in anxious depression.

6. Neurochemical Mechanisms of Tianeptine and SSRIs Action: A Hypothesis.

Tianeptine is a serotonin (5-hydroxytryptamine, 5-HT) reuptake enhancer. It exhibits a mechanism of action totally opposite to selective serotonin reuptake inhibitors (SSRI), such as sertraline, but paradoxically both mechanisms of action are associated with a therapeutic efficacy in depressive disorders, in particular in anxious depressions. In spite of a numerous experimental and clinical trials the neurochemical mechanism of tianeptine action is not enough clear (Ansseau, 1993; Stahl, 1999; Kasper, 2006). Ansseau (1993) had analyzed the different effects of tianeptine and discussed the approaches, mainly clinical, which could help to understand "the paradoxical activity of tianeptine". But he did not express his views on the ways to solve the problem of the neurochemical and therapeutic mechanisms of action of this antidepressant. Stahl in his "Essential Psychopharmacology" (1999, p. 160) wrote: "Tianeptine is an example of an agent that allosterically modifies serotonin reuptake in a manner that is almost the opposite to that of the SSRIs. Although this might theoretically seem to have the potential to cause depression rather than treat it, tianeptine in fact appears to be antidepressant."

All these prompt us to carry out the comparative clinical-biochemical investigation of patients with anxious depression under the treatment of tianeptine and sertraline and on the basis of results of the study develop possible mechanism of tianeptine action. Clinical and biochemical aspects of this work are described above.

Anxious depression is characterized by the decrease in serotonergic activity (Kasper, 2001) and possibly by the decrease in serotonin concentration in the synapses. Twofold increased platelet MAO activity in anxious patients indirectly supported this view.

According to the literature (Avakjan, 1976; Hughes, 1972) it is supposed that at normal condition about 75% of serotonin released in the synaptic cleft undergoes functional inactivation by the reuptake in the presynaptic ending (neuron) by the reuptake mechanisms (reuptake receptor or serotonin transporter). Serotonin is accumulated in the synaptic vesicles and thus it becomes unavailable to the action of MAO localized in mitochondria of presynaptic ending. The remaining serotonin (approximately 25 %) undergoes chemical (irreversible) inactivation by MAO localized in mitochondria of glial cells (astrocytes and/or microglial cells) that close the synaptic cleft and where the neurotransmitter is taken up (Hughes, 1972; Avakjan, 1976; Whitaker et al., 1983). As serotonin uptake in neuronal and glial cells proceeds through the receptors (or transporters) it is possible to suppose that serotonin affinity for the receptors on presynaptic ending (neuron) and on glial cells correlates as 3 to 1 (75% and 25%, see above). It is necessary to note that receptors for serotonin on astrocytes differ from those on the neurons (Hertz and Tamir, 1981).

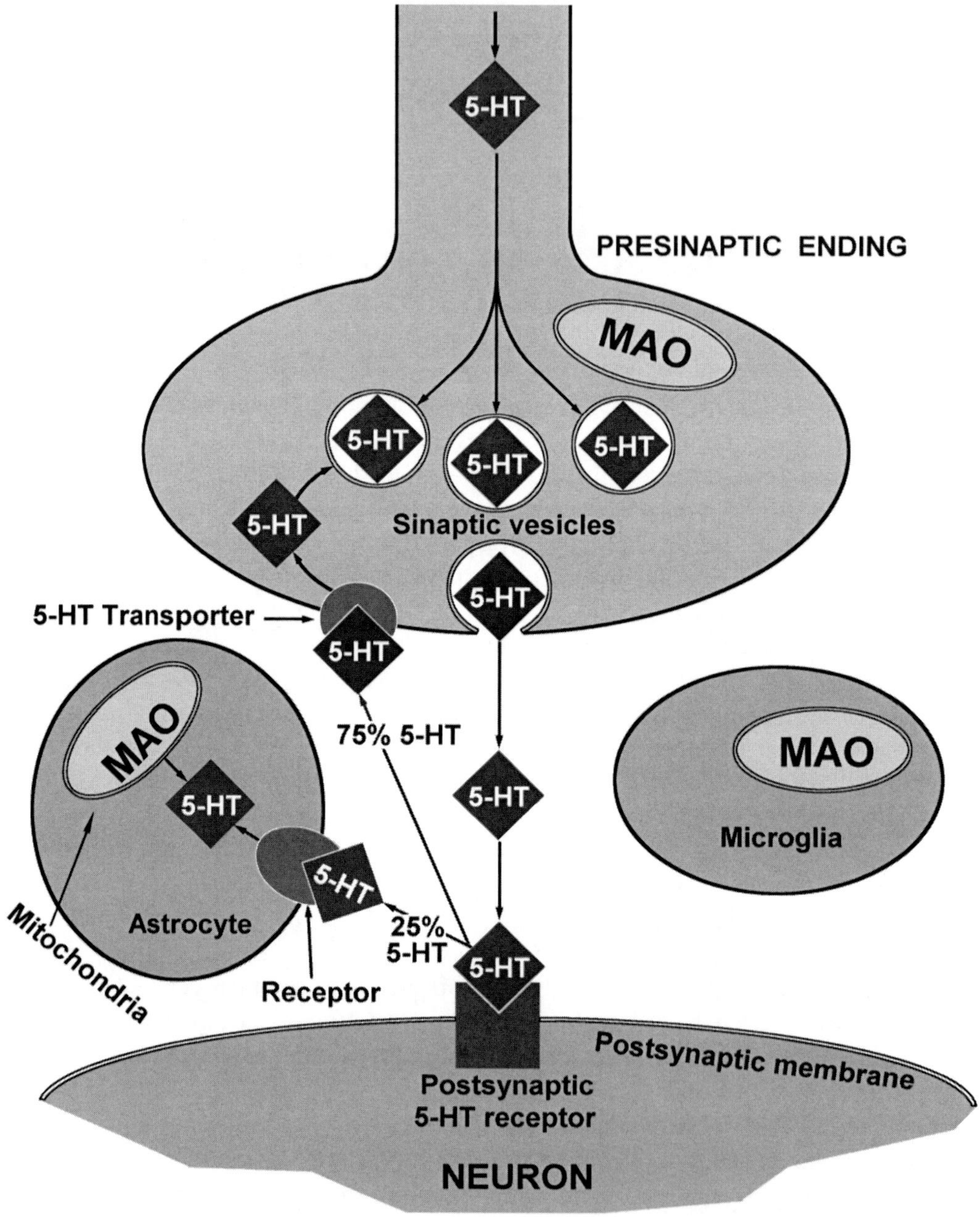

Figure 6.

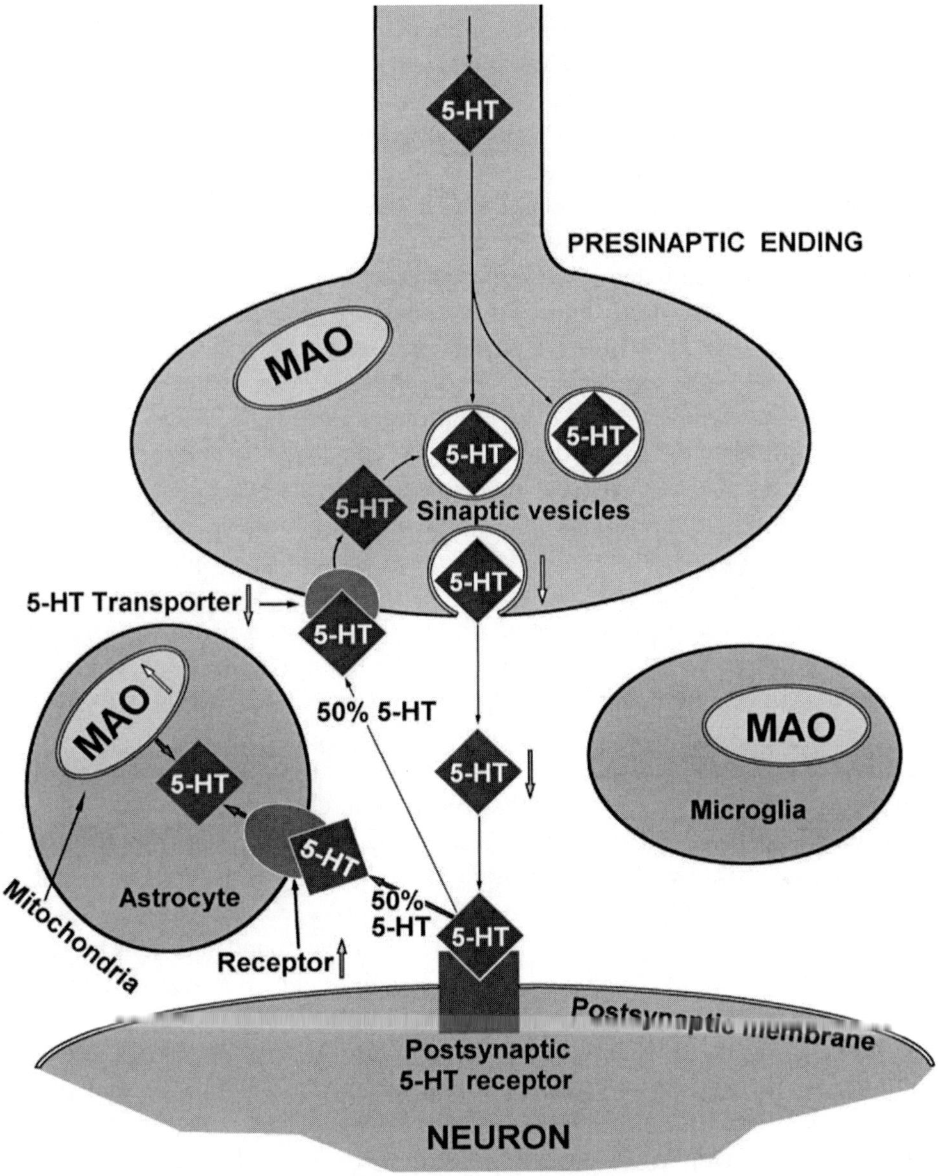

Figure 7.

It was earlier shown that in depressed patients the capacity (or activity) of the serotonin reuptake mechanisms were decreased (Bellivier et al., 2002; Slanley et al., 1982; Stahl, 1985). On the other hand in our study we have established that in anxious-depressed patients MAO activity was increased almost twofold (Uzbekov et al., 2006). The letter specifies that in this case serotonin is taken up more actively by the glial cells where MAO is localized. We can assume that the ratio – serotonin affinity for receptors on the presynaptic ending and the same on the glial cells in patients with anxious depression changes. The left part of the ratio is decreasing and the right part – is increasing, i.e. the ratio becomes, for example, 2 to 2 instead of 3 to 1 (as in norm). On the functional level it means that in anxious depression serotonin is taken up by glial cells in larger quantity where it chemically inactivated by MAO. Owing to this serotonin concentration in the synaptic cleft is reduced and as a result less quantity of serotonin is returned in the presynaptic ending. All this events lead to the disturbances in serotonergic activity and in particular serotonergic neurotransmission.

The therapeutic effects under tianeptine treatment (37,5 mg/day) is manifested after two weeks of therapy (Maximova et al., 2000; Uzbekov, 2006) that is supported by literature data (Quitkin et al., 1984; Kato and Weitsch, 1988; Ansseau, 1993). At that time we have found changes in activity or levels of all investigated biochemical parameters. These changes were not very pronounced although they were significant (Uzbekov, 2006).

Elucidation of the antidepressive mechanism of tianeptine action is one of the most difficult problems. The analysis of available data has shown the lack of any information that could explain neurochemical mechanism of action of this antidepressant. It is well known that tianeptine activates serotonin reuptake in the presynaptic ending. Thus promoting for the more "energetic withdrawal" of serotonin from the synaptic cleft. In spite of all existing theories tianeptine on the clinical level reveals antidepressive, anxiolytic effects. Ansseau writes about this situation in such words: "The paradoxical finding that both tianeptine and selective 5-HT reuptake inhibitors exhibit antidepressant activity despite clearly antagonistic mechanisms is rather puzzling" (1993).

We think that the problem of tianeptine action is necessary to consider from the point of view of structural-functional unity of the synapse. Based on this thesis the synapse has to be considered as a complex, multiple biological system but not only as a structure with "reuptake receptor".

According to our working hypothesis tianeptine, enhancing serotonin reuptake, decreases serotonin level in the synaptic cleft. Simultaneously with this process in responders we have established that a very high MAO activity starts to decrease. It is possible to suppose that tianeptine decreasing affinity of glial receptors for serotonin reduces activity of glial cells in serotonin uptake. That is followed by the inhibition of MAO activity. Our supposition is supported by results of Marinesco et al. (1996) who have found that tianeptine decreases serotonin availability to MAO which localized in glial cells. Because of that the ratio – serotonin affinity for the receptors on presynaptic endings and on glial cells changes. The left part of the ratio is increased (neuron) and the right part – decreased (glia), i. e. we have the ratio not 2 to 2 (peak of anxious depression) but, for example, 2,5 to 1,5 (beginning of the remission). Under tianeptine action two processes take place in the synaptic region –a) enhancing of serotonin reuptake in the synaptic ending and b) inhibition of MAO activity that is followed by increase of serotonin concentration in the synaptic cleft. But in a whole it is possible to assume that serotonin concentration in the synaptic cleft appeared to be dropped because process (a) is more active then process (b). That is the "paradox" of the action of this antidepressant.

What is the fate of serotonin, which continues to take up in the presynaptic ending? Here it is necessary to make an assumption. Tianeptine is characterized by one more property that has a principle meaning. Carlsson et al. (1969) had described that 4-methyl-alpha-meta-tyramine caused the depletion of serotonin from the intraneuronal stores. They also had found that tianeptine markedly potentiated this type of serotonin depletion. Later Fattaccini et al. (1990) and Labrid et al. (1992) have shown *in vivo* and *in vitro* that tianeptine had significantly increased serotonin depletion from its intraneuronal stores. Based on these data we can make the assumption that tianeptine directly or indirectly through any unknown mechanisms activates serotonin release from presynaptic ending in the synaptic cleft then.

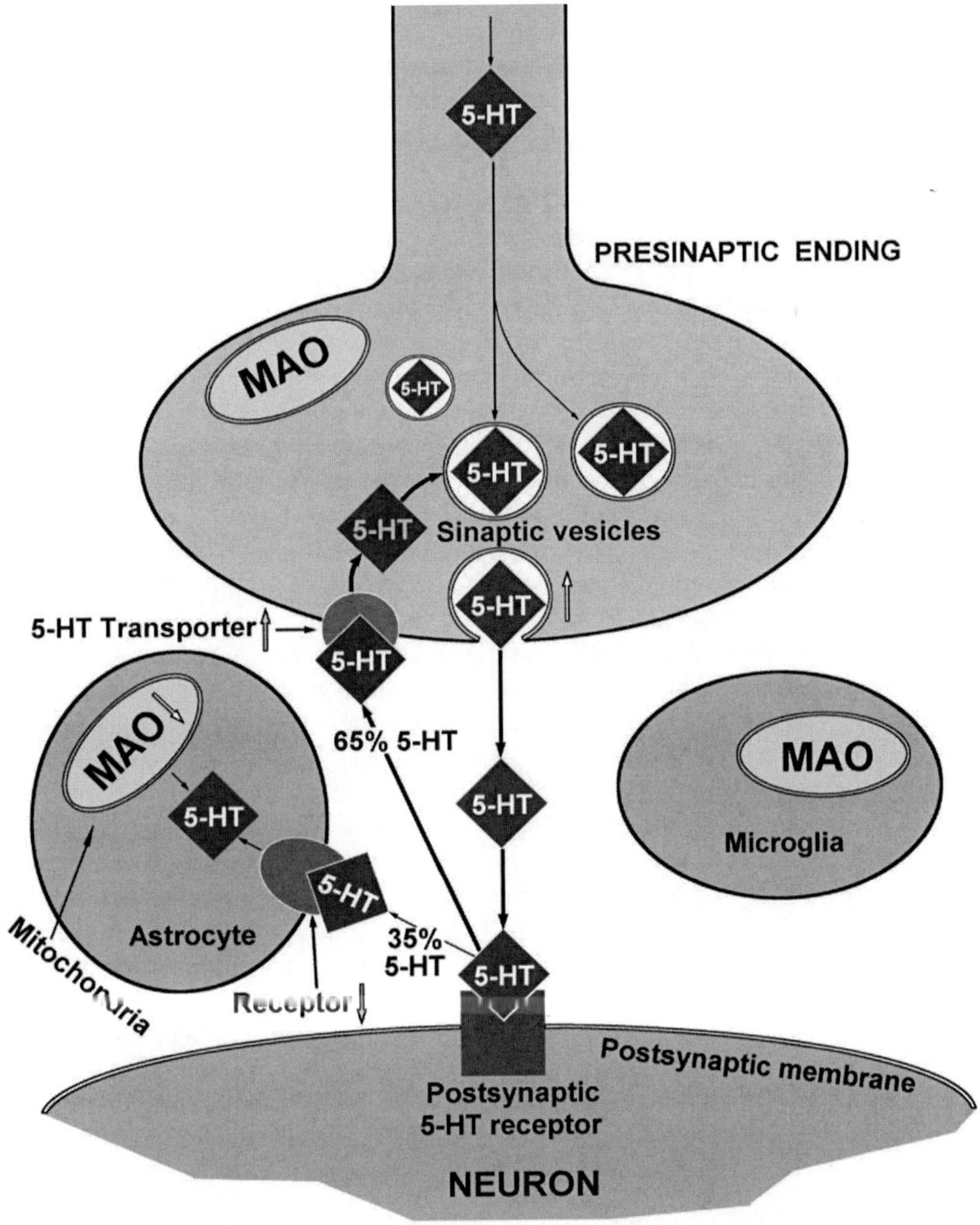

Figure 8.

Thus, tianeptine enhances not only serotonin reuptake but also it activates its surge from the ending into the synaptic cleft. So it is possible to conclude that under tianeptine action serotonin turnover rate in the synapse is increased that promotes the increase in the unit of time serotonin concentration on postsynaptic receptors. Decreasing MAO activity supports serotonin concentration in the synaptic cleft on the minimally allowable level to display its neurotransmitter functions.

Proceeding from the offered neurochemical mechanism of tianeptine action it is possible to hypothesize of the interrelation between the dynamics of MAO activity and the clinical status of anxious depressed patients. In responders activation of serotonin turnover rate in the synapse is accompanied by decrease of MAO activity that allows on the minimally allowable serotonin level in the synaptic cleft to achieve pronounced therapeutic effects. The increase of the parameters of functional albumin activity and decrease of MMEM level are indicated to the decrease of degree of endogenous intoxication and the improvement of homeostasis as a whole (Uzbekov et al., 2006).

Analysis of our own and literature data make it possible to suppose that tianeptine antidepressant effects are characterized by two-phase action.

In the first, acute phase of its action there take place the neurochemical processes on the synaptic level, i.e. processes that were described as stated above. They lead to a relative normalization of serotonergic neurotransmission, moreover tianeptine does not induce the decrease of 5-HT_{1A}–receptors sensitivity for serotonin (Leonard, 1999).

The second phase of tianeptine action begins, possibly, after a relative normalization of serotonergic neurotransmission. It is connected with such properties of this antidepressant as ability to decrease of degree of endogenous intoxication (Uzbekov et al., 2006) and mobilization and activation of compensatory and plastic mechanisms of the central nervous system. Thus, tianeptine reduces stress-induced atrophy of neuronal dendrites (Wagstaff et al., 2001; Watanabe et al., 1992), in stressed animals tianeptine attenuates the activation of the hypothalamo-pituitary-adrenal axis (Delbende et al., 1994; Droste et al., 2006), increases neuronal electric activity (Pineyro et al., 1995). It was shown that tianeptine prevents or reverses stress-associated structural and cellular changes in the brain and normalizes disrupted glutamatergic neurotransmission. In hippocampus, amygdala and cortex it prevents stress-induced dendritic atrophy, improves neurogenesis, reduces apoptosis and normalizes metabolite levels (Lucassen et al., 2004; Kasper and McEwen, 2008).

The latent period for about 2 weeks, that is necessary to reveal tianeptine therapeutic effect, possibly is connected with the reorganization of different pathologically disturb brain system (Ansseau, 1993; Hirschfeld, 2001; Uzbekov et al., 2006). The results of our investigations indicate that indeed as early as in two weeks of tianeptine treatment we have revealed the improvement of investigated biochemical parameters; although these changes were not very pronounced they were significant (Maximova et al., 2000; Uzbekov et al., 2006).

In conclusion, the first time in the literature we have proposed the hypothesis about neurochemical mechanism of tianeptine action. According to our hypothesis tianeptine not only activates serotonin reuptake but also activates serotonin release in synaptic cleft thus accelerating serotonin turnover in the synapse. Proposed mechanism mainly refers the first, acute phase of its action directed on the normalization of serotoninergic neurotransmission.

References

Anders VN, Orlovskaia DD. 1982. Enzynes involved in energy metabolism in the braind of schizophrenic patients (electron-cytochemical study). *Zh Nevropatol Psikhiatr Im SS Korsakova* 82(7): 111-117.

Ansseau M, 1993. The paradox of tianeptine. *Eur. Psychiatry* 8 (suppl 2): 89-93.

Avakjan OM. 1976. Up-to-date data about the mechanisms of the release and reuptake of catecholamines; possibilities and perspectives of their pharmacological regulation. *Mendeleev Zh Vsesouznogo Khimicheskogo Obshchestva* 21: 165-171.

Avrutski GYa, Neduva AA. 1988. *Therapy of Mental Diseases*. Meditzina: Moscow, (in Russian)

Ayuso-Gutierrez JL. 2002. Old and new antidepressants: where are we? *World J Biol Psychiatry* 3: 112-114.

Babb AL, Farrell PC, Uvelli DA, Scribner BH. 1972. Hemodialyzer evaluation by examination of solute molecular weight spectra. *Trans Amer Soc Artif Int Organs* 18: 98-105.

Bakish D. 1999. The patient with comorbid depression and anxiety: the unmet need. *J.Clin. Psychiatry* 60 (suppl 6): 20-24.

Balakleevski AI. 1976. Colorimetric method of estimation of serum monoamine oxidase activity. *Lab Delo* № 3: 151-153.

Baron M, Asnis L, Gruen R, Levitt M. 1983. Plasma amine oxidase and genetic vulnerability to schizophrenia. *Arch Gen Psychiatry* 40: 275-279.

Bech P. 1992. Acute therapy of depression. *J. Clin. Psychiat* 54 (suppl 8): 19-28.

Beckman KB, Ames BN. 1998. The free radical theory of aging matures. *Physiol Rev* 78: 547-581.

Bellivier F, Roy I, Leboyer M. 2002. Serotonin transporter gene polymorphisms and affective disorder-related phenotypes. *Curr Opin Psychiatry* 15: 49-58.

Bliss EL, Zwanziger J. 1966. Brain amines and emotional stress. J Psychiat Res 4: 189-198.

Boomsma F, Bhaggoe UM, van der Houwen AMB, van der Meiracker AH. 2003. Plasma semicarbazide-sensitive amine oxidase in human(patho)physiology . *Biochim Biophys Acta* 1647: 48-54.

Callingham BA, Crosbie AE, Rous BA. 1995. Some aspects of the pathophysiology of semicarbazide-sensitive amine oxidase enzymes. *Prog Brain Res* 106: 305-321.

Carlsson A, Corrodi H, Fuxe K, Hokfelt T. 1969. Effect of antidepressant drugs on the depletion of intraneuronal brain 5-hydroxytryptamine stores caused by 4-metyl-alfa-ethil-metatyramine. *Eur. J. Pharmacol* 5: 357-366.

Chalenko VV. 1991. Possible causes of the increase of concentration of molecules of middle mass in pathologic states. *Pathol Physiol and exp Therap* 4: 13-14.

Clayton PJ. 1990. The co-morbidity factor: establishing the primary diagnosis in patients with mixed symptoms of anxiety and depression. *J Clin Psychiatry* 51 (Suppl. 11): 35-39.

Cloninger CR. 1990. Co-morbidity of anxiety and depression. *J Clin Psychopharmacol* 10: 43S-46S.

Curzon G. 1969. Tryptophan pyrrolase – a biochemical factor in depressive illness. Br J Psychiatry 115: 1367-1374.

Delbende C., Tranchand Bunel D., Tarozzo G., Grino M., Oliver C., Mocaer E., Vaudry H. 1994. Effect of chronic treatment with the antidepressant tianeptine on the hypothalamo-pituitary-adrenal axis. *Eur J Pharmacol* 251: 245-251.

Doogan DP, Caillard V. 1992. Sertraline in the prevention of depression. *Br.J. Psychiatry* 160: 217-222.

Droste S.K., Schweizer M.C., Ulbricht S., Reul J.M. 2006. Long-term voluntary exercise and the mouse hypothalamic-pituitary-adrenocortical axis: impact of concurrent treatment with antidepressant drug tianeptine. *J Neuroendocrinol* 18: 915-925.

Fattaccini C.M., Bolanos-Jimenez F., Golzan H., Hamon M. 1990. Tianeptine stimulates uptake of 5-hydroxytryptamine in vivo in the rat brain. *Neuropharmacology* 29: 1-8.

Gong B, Boor PJ. 2006. The role of amine oxidases in xenobiotic metabolism. *Expert Opin Drug Metab Toxicol* 2: 559-571.

Gonzales G, Mendoza L, Ruiz J, Torrejon J. 1982. A demonstration that 5-hydroxytryptamine administrered peripherally can affect sexual behavior in male rats. *Life Sci* 31: 2775-2781.

Gorkin VZ. 1985. Studies on the nature and specific inhibition of monoamine oxidases. In Neuropharmacology'85, Keleman K, Magyar K, Visi ES (eds). Akademiai Kiado: Budapest.

Gromova EA. 1979. Functional relationship of catecholaminergic and serotoninergic systems of the brain – antagonism or reciprocity? In *Catecholaminergic Neurons*, Turpaev TM, Budantzev AU (eds). Nauka: Moscow; 97 – 105 (in Russian).

Gryzunov YA, Dobretsov GE. Serum albumin in clinical medicine. 1994. Book 1. Irius:Moscow.

Gryzunov YA, Dobretsov GE. Serum albumin in clinical medicine. 1998. Book 2. Irius:Moscow.

Gryzunov YA, Miller YI, Dobretsov GE, PestovaAB. 1994. Fluorescent assay for the determination of human serum albumin mass concentration. *Clin Lab Diagnostica* № 5: 27-31 (in Russian).

Gryzunov YuA, Smolina NV, Uzbekov MG, Dobretsov GE, Misionzhnik EYu, Maximova NM, Kurmysheva NYa, Syrejshchikova TI, Komar AA. 2008. Conformational changes of serum albumin in mental disorders. In *Advanced Information and Telemedicine Technologies for Health(II International Conference)*, Kovalev V, Tuzikov A, Ablameyko S, Aleinikova O (eds). United Institute of Informatics Problems: Minsk; 158-163.

Gryzunov YA, Syrejshchikova TI, Komarova MN, Misionzhnik EY, Uzbekov MG, Molodetskich AV, Dobretsov GE, Yakimenko MN. 2000. Serum albumin binding sites properties in donors and in schizophrenia patients: the study of fluorescence decay of the probe K-35 using S-60 synchrotron pulse excitation. *Nucl Instr and Meth A* 448: 478-482.

Hales RE, Yudofsky SC, Talbott JA (Eds.). 1999. *Textbook of Psychiatry*, 3rd Edition. Washington: American Psychiatric Press.

Halliwell B, Gutteridge JMC. 2007. *Free Radicals in Biology and Medicine.* Oxford, Oxford University Press, 851 p.

Hamilton M, 1988. Distinguishing between anxiety and depressive disorders. In *Handbook of Anxiety Disorders*, Last CA, Hersen M (eds). Pergamon Press: Oxford; 143-155.

Hertz L, Tamir H. 1981. Some properties of an astrocyte protein fraction that binds serotonin. *J. Neurochem* 37: 1331-1334.

Hirschfeld RM. 2001. Clinical importance of long-term antidepressant treatment. *Br J Psychiatry* 42 (Suppl): S4 – S8.

Holsboer F. 2001. Antidepressant drug discovery in the postgenomic era. World J *Biol Psychiatry* 2: 165-177.

Hughes J.1972. Evaluation of mechanisms controlling the release and inactivation of the adrenergic transmitter in the rabbit portal vein and vas deferens. *Br. J. Pharma* 44*:* 472-491.

Kasper S. 2001. Depression and Anxiety - Separate or Continuum. *World J Biol Psychiatry* 2: 162-163.

Kasper S. 2006. Neuroplasticity and the treatment of depression. *Neuropsychiatric Disease and Treatment* 2, Suppl 2: 15-20.

Kasper S., McEwen B.S. 2008. Neurobiological and clinical effects of the antidepressant tianeptine. *CNS Drugs* 22: 16-26.

Kato G, Weitsch AF. 1988. Neurochemical profile of tianeptine, a new antidepressant drug. *Clin. Neuropharmacol* 11 (suppl 2): S43-S50.

Keller CB, Cooper SJ. 1998. Differences and variability in plasma noradrenaline between depressive and anxiety disorders. *J Psychopharmacol* 12: 161-167.

Korobeinikova EN. 1989. A modified technique for measuring lipid peroxidation products in the thiobarbituric acid test. *Lab Delo* 7, 8-10.

Labrid C., Mocaer E., Kamoun A. 1992. Neurochemical and pharmacological properties of tianeptine, a novel antidepressant. *Br J Psychiatry Suppl* 15: 56-60.

Leonard BE. 1999. Neuropharmacology of antidepressants that modify central noradrenergic and serotonergic function: a shot review. *Hum Psychopharmacol Clin Exp* 14: 75-81.

Leonard B. 2000. Stress, Depression and the Activation of the Immune System. *World J Biol Psychiatry* 1: 17-25.

Kovalevskii AN, Nifantieva OE. 1989. About the screening method of the estimating of middle mass molecules. *Lab delo*, № 10:13-18.

Laakmann G. 1991. Psychopharmacoendocrinology and depression research. Springer: Berlin.

Lapin IP. 1996. Kynurenins and anxiety. *Adv Exp Med Biol* 398: 191-194.

Loo H, Saiz-Ruiz J, Costa e Silva JA, Ansseau M, Herrington R, Vaz-Serra A, Dilling H, DeRisio S. 2001. Efficacy and safety of tianeptine in the treatment of depressive disorders in comparison with fluoxetine. *Hum Psychopharmacol Clin Exp* 16: S31-S38.

Lucassen P.J., Fuchs E., Czeh B. 2004. Antidepressant treatment with tianeptine reduces apoptosis in the hippocampal dentate gyrus and temporal cortex. *Biol Psychiatry* 55: 789-796.

Malakhova MYa, ZubatkinaOV. 2004. *Metabolic criterion of homeostasis*. Pomorskii Universitet: Arkhangel'sk (in Russian).

Marchbanks RM, Mulcrone J, Whatley SA. 1995. Aspects of oxidative metabolism in schizophrenia. Brit J Psychiatr 167: 293-298.

Marinesco S, Poncet L, Debilly G, Jouvet M, Cespuglio R. 1996. Effects of tianeptine, sertraline and clomipramine on brain serotonin metabolism: a voltammetric approach in the rat. *Brain. Res* 736: 82-90.

McEwen CM, Cohen JD. 1963. An amine oxidase in normal human serum. *J Lab Clin Medicine* 62: 766-776.

Maximova NM, Vertogradova OP, Uzbekov MG. 2004. Dynamics of anxious depression under tianeptine and sertraline treatment: comparative clinical-biochemical investigation. *World Psychiatry* 3 (Suppl. 1): 277.

Maximova NM, Misionzhnik EY, Vertogradova OP, Uzbekov MG. 2000. Therapeutic efficacy and metabolic peculiarities in patients with depressive disorders under tianeptine (TIA) and sertraline (SER) treatment. *Eur Psychiatry* 15 (Suppl. 2): 379S.

Moin VM, Misionzhnik EY, Kuznetsova ZI, Gryzunov YA, Kirkovski VV, Uzbekov MG, Zubovski DI. 1994. Some characteristics of the method and reagents for the fluorescent determination of effective and total serum albumin concentration. *Clin Lab Diagnostica* №5: 33-35 (in Russian).

Mosolov SN, Uzbekov MG, Saikin MA, Misionzhnik EY, Tsukarzi EE, Molodetskikh AV. 1999. Use of intravenous low-intensity helium and neon laser therapy and alteration of biochemical parameters in schizophrenic patients resistant to pharmacotherapy. *Social and Clinical Psychiatry* 9: 57-62.

Nemeth S. 1978. The effect of stress or glucose feeding on hepatic tyrosine aminotransferase activity and liver and plasma tyrosine levels of intact and adrenalectomized rats. Horm Metabol Res 10: 144-147.

Nikolaichik VV, Moin VM, Kirkovski VV, Mazur LI, Lobacheva GA, Bichko GN, Baratashvili GG. 1991. The method of estimation of «middle molecules». *Lab. Delo* 10: 13-18 (in Russian).

Nuller YL, Mikhalenko IA. 1988. *Affective psychoses*. Nauka: Leningrad (in Russian).

Parfenkova GA, Chermiad'eva IF, Sitina VK. 1987. Middle molecules – a marker of endogenous intoxication (a review of the literature). *Vrach Delo* 4: 71-77.

Pineyro G., Deveault L., Blier P., Dennis T., de Montigny C. 1995. Effect of acute and prolonged tianeptine administration on the 5-HT transporter: electrophysiological, biochemical and radioligand binding studies in the rat brain. *Naunyn Schmiedebergs Arch Pharmacol* 351: 111-118.

Piradov MA, Gabrieliaan NI, Levchenko NI, Laeskii EG, Sevost'ianova OA. 1990. Endogenous toxemia in acute disorders of cerebral circulation. *Zh Nevropatol Psikhiatr Im SS Korsakova* 90(7): 16-19.

Prilipko LL, Erin AN, Beliaev BS, Piatnitskii AN, Siuniakov SA. 1987. Activation of lipid peroxidation in the bodies of schizophrenic and manic-depressive patients. *Zh Nevropatol Psikhiatr Im SS Korsakova* 87: 100-103.

Quitkin FM, Rabkin JG, Ross D, Mc Grath PJ. 1984. Duration of antidepressant drug treatment. What is an adequate trial? *Arch. Gen. Psychiatry* 41: 238-245.

Ressler KJ, Nemeroff CB. 2000. Role of serotonergic and noradrenergic systems in the pathophysiology of depression and anxiety disorders. *Depression and Anxiety* 12 (Suppl 1): 2-19.

Ringoir S, VanholderR, Massry SG (eds). 1987. *Uremic Toxins*. Plenum Press: New York-London.

Rodney J, Prior N, Cooper B, Theodoros M, Browning J, Steinberg B, Evans L. 1997. The comorbidity of anxiety and depression. *Austral and New Zealand J Psychiatry* 31: 700-703.

Shikhov SN, Uzbekov MG, Malin DI. 2000. Composition of middle-mass endotoxic molecules is changed in patients with depressive disorders under the treatment of plasmapheresis. *Proceedings of XIII Congress of psychiatrists of Russia*, Moscow, 373-373.

Stahl SM. 1985. Peripheral models for the study of neurotransmitter receptors in man. *Psychopharmacol. Bull* 21: 663-671.

Stahl SM. 1999. Essential Psychopharmacology. Neuroscientific Basis and *Clinical Applications*. Cambridge University Press: Cambridge.

Stanley M, Virgilio J, Gershon S. 1982. Tritiated imipramine sites are decreased in the frontal cortex of suicides. *Science* 216: 1337- 1339.

Stober G, Ben-Shachar D, Cardon M, Falkai P, Fonteh AN, Gawlik M, Glenthoj BY, Grunblatt E, Jablensky A, Kim Y-K, Kornhuber J, McNeil TF, Muller N, Oranje B, Saito T, Saoud M, Schmitt A, Schwartz M, Thome J, Uzbekov M, Durany N, Riederer P. 2009. Schizophrenia: From the brain to peripheral markers -A consensus paper of the WFSBP Task Force on biological markers. *World J Biol Psychiatry* 10(2): 127-155.

Strolin Benedetti M, Whomsley R, Baltes E. 2006. Involvement of enzymes other than CYPs in the oxidative metabolism of xenobiotics. *Expert Opin Drug Metab Toxicol* 2: 895-921.

Tollefson GD, Souetre E, Thomander L, Potvin JH. 1993. Comorbid anxious signs and symptoms in major depression impact on functional work capacity and comparative treat outcomes. *Int Clin Psychopharmacol* 8: 281-293.

Tupikova ZA. 1983. Middle-molecular uremic toxins (review of the literature). *Vopr Med Khim* 29(1): 2-10.

Turianitsa IM, Mishanich II, Rostoka LM. 1988. Middle molecule spectrum of the blood serum in patients with a continuously progressive paranoid form of schizophrenia undergoing treatment. *Zh Nevropatol Psikhiatr* 88: 109-111 (in Russian).

Umanskii MA, Pinchuk LB, Pinchuk VG. 1991. Syndrome of endogenous intoxication. Naukova Dumka: Kiev.

Uzbekov MG. 2004. Structural-functional approaches to the understanding of neurochemical mechanisms of action of psychotropic preparations: serotonergic antidepressants. *Social and Clinical Psychiatry* 14: 172-178.

Uzbekov MG, Misionzhnik EY. 2000. Nonspecific syndrome of endogenous intoxication as an integral component of patogenesis of psychic disorders. *Russian Journal of Psychiatry* № 4: 56-65.

Uzbekov MG, Misionzhnik EY, Neduva AA, Malin DI. 1995. Dynamics of the level of middle molecules and activity of some enzymes of neurotransmitter metabolism in patients with resistant endogenous psychosis under plasmapheresis. *Behavioural Pharmacol* 6 (Suppl 1): 61.

Uzbekov M.G., Misionzhnik E.Y., Maximova N.M., Vertogradova O.P. 2006. Biochemical profile in patients with anxious depression under the treatment with serotonergic antidepressants with different mechanisms of action. *Hum Psychophrmacol Clin Exp* 21: 109-115.

Uzbekov MG, Maximova NM, Misionzhnik EY, Vertogradova OP. 2002. About the neurochemical mechanism of tianeptine (coaxil) action in anxiety-depressed patients. *Social and Clinical Psychiatry* 12: 43-45.

Uzbekov MG, Misionhznik EY, Maximova NM, Vertogradova OP, Rizhov AM, Shikhov SN. 2003. Some aspects of metabolic disturbances in anxious depression. *Russian Journal of Psychiatry* № 6: 58-62.

Uzbekov MG, Misionzhnik EY, Molodetskich AV, Gryzunov YA, Komarova MN, Syrejshchikova TI, Yakimenko MN. 1998. Physic-chemical changes of albumin binding sites in schizophrenic patients. *Neirokhimia* 15 : 215-216 (in Russian).

Uzbekov MG, Misionzhnik EYu, Shmukler AB, Gurovich IYa, Gryzunov YuA, Smolina NV, Kalinina VV, Sokolova TN, Moskvitina TA, Shevchenko VA. 2009. Disturbances of monoamine oxidase activity and indices of endogenous intoxication in patients with the first episode of schizophrenia. *Zh Nevropatol Psikhiatr Im SS Korsakova* 109(5): 48-52.

Voloshina ON, Moskvitina TA. 1985. Method of estimation of platelet monoamine oxidase activity. *Lab.Delo* 5: 289-291 (in Russian).

Wagstaff A.J, Ormrod D., Spencer C.M. 2001. Tianeptine: a review of its use in depressive disorders. *CNS Drugs* 15: 231 – 259.

Watanabe Y., Gould E., Daniels D.C., Cameron H., McEwen B.S. 1992. Tianeptine attenuates stress-induced morphological changes in the hippocampus. *Eur J Pharmacol* 222: 157-162.

Whitaker P.M., Vint C.K., Morin R. 1983. Imipramine labels sites on brain astroglial cells not related to serotonin uptake. *J. Neurochem* 41: 1319-1322.

World Health Organization. 1992. *The Tenth Revision of the International Classification of Diseases and Related Health Problems.* WHO: Geneva.

World Health Organization. 1999. *"Composite International Diagnostic Interview (CIDI), Version I.O."*: Geneva.

Yao JK, Reddy RD, van Kammen DP. 2001. Oxidative damage and schizophrenia: an overview of the evidence and its therapeutic implications. *CNS Drugs* 15:287–310.

In: Antidepressants: Types, Efficiency …
Editor: Jayden T. Van Leeuwen, pp.199-219

ISBN 978-1-61668-581-2

Chapter 8

GENDER DIFFERENCES IN RESPONSE TO ANTIDEPRESSANTS*

***Shigeru Morishita*[†,1], *Toshihiko Kinoshita*[2] *and Seizaburo Arita*[3]**

[1]Depression Prevention Medical Center,
Kyoto Jujo Rehabilitation Hospital, Kyoto, Japan
[2]Department of Psychiatry, Kansai Medical University, Osaka, Japan
[3]Department of Mathematics and Biostatistics,
Kansai Medical University, Osaka Japan

ABSTRACT

Epidemiological studies have consistently shown that depression is approximately twice as common in females as in males. There is also some evidence that there are gender differences in the clinical manifestations. Some studies have addressed the epidemiological and pharmacological implications of gender-associated differences in the overall treatment response to antidepressants in clinical practice. Recently, several new antidepressants have become available. However, antidepressants do not have the same effect in all patients all the time. It is important to be able to predict which patients would most likely benefit from particular antidepressants. To examine gender differences in treatment remission in depressed patients treated with fluvoxamine, paroxetine, sertraline, milnacipran, or maprotiline, a retrospective cohort analysis was carried out. Three hundred and sixty-eight patients were identified who had been treated with one of fluvoxamine, paroxetine, sertraline, milnacipran, or maprotiline for depression. This study was done to explore the gender differences in the effect of these antidepressants. It was found that there was no difference in the overall treatment response among these antidepressants in male patients (x^2=7.650, df=4, P=0.1053). However, there was a

* A version of this chapter was also published in *Major Depression in Women,* edited by P. R. Bancroft and L. B. Ardley published by Nova Science Publishers, Inc. It was submitted for appropriate modifications in an effort to encourage wider dissemination of research.

† Corresponding author: Shigeru Morishita, Depression Prevention Medical Center, Kyoto Jujo Rehabilitation Hospital, 32 Kisshoinhattandacho, Minami-ku, Kyoto 601-8325, Kyoto, JAPAN. Phone: +81-75-671-2351; Fax: +81-75-671-2961 ; E-mail: s.morishita31@r9.dion.ne.jp

significant difference in the overall treatment response among these antidepressants in female patients (x^2=17.959, df=4, P=0.0013). Among female patients with depression, the remission rate was higher with sertraline and maprotiline than with fluvoxamine, paroxetine, and milnacipran. Furthermore, there was no difference in the treatment response among these antidepressants for males with their first episode of depression (x^2=6.194, df=4, P=0.1851), males with a recurrent episode of depression (x^2=9.101, df=4, P=0.0586), and females with their first episode of depression (x^2=3.725, df=4, P=0.4446). However, there was a significant difference in the treatment response among these antidepressants in females with a recurrent episode of depression (x^2=19.528, df=4, P=0.0006). Among females with a recurrent episode of depression, the remission rate was higher with sertraline and maprotiline than with fluvoxamine, paroxetine, and milnacipran. Therefore, sertraline and maprotiline are more effective than fluvoxamine, paroxetine, and milnacipran, particularly in females with a recurrent episode of depression. Thus, gender should be considered when selecting antidepressants. These results will be useful for helping guide clinicians treating female depression.

Keywords: women, depression, antidepressant, gender.

INTRODUCTION

Depression has become one of the most common psychiatric disorders in the world. Epidemiological studies have consistently shown that depression is approximately twice as common in females as in males [1, 2.3, 4], and the lifetime risk of a depressive episode is 21% in females versus 13% in males [5]. There is also some evidence that there are gender differences in the clinical manifestations of depression. Some authors have reported that depression in females tends to be more severe and is associated with increased functional impairment [6, 7]. Several studies have shown that females are likely to have a chronic and recurrent disease course [8]. In fact, recurrent depression, as well as seasonal affective disorder, appears to be markedly more common among females [9,10]. Females are more likely than males to attempt suicide, though males are more likely to actually succeed [11]. It has also been reported that depressed females appear to have a greater number of symptoms such as sleep disturbance, psychomotor retardation, feelings of worthlessness or guilt, anxiety, and somatization than males. Furthermore, females are more likely to present reverse vegetative or atypical symptoms, such as hypersomnia, hyperphagia, carbohydrate craving, and weight gain [12, 13]. Females have a greater risk than males of a depressive episode following a stressful life event [14]. Co–morbidities, including anxiety disorders and eating disorders, are more frequent in females [15, 16]. These findings suggest that there may be other gender differences in the etiology and pathogenesis of depression; thus, there could also be gender differences in the efficacy of antidepressant treatment.

Selective serotonin reuptake inhibitors (SSRIs) and dual serotonin and noradrenaline reuptake inhibitors (SNRIs) are the most commonly prescribed class of antidepressants. Compared to tricyclic antidepressants (TCAs), these antidepressants are characterized by a more favorable effect profile, simpler dosing, and less toxic effects in the event of an overdose [17, 18]. Although all SSRIs and dual SNRIs have been shown to be effective, there are few clinical trials supporting the superiority of one over another. In addition, all SSRIs and dual SNRIs do not have the same effect in all patients at any time or by gender. The authors have previously published studies dealing with the characteristics of SSRIs, dual SNRIs, and other antidepressants [19, 20, 21, 22, 23, 24, 25, 26, 27]; it is important to compare the characteristics of each SSRI and dual SNRI.

In the older literature, female gender was sometimes mentioned as a risk factor for treatment-resistant depression; however, there is little evidence to support this assertion. In any sample of patients with depression, including patients with refractory depression, there will always tend to be a preponderance of females due to the gender difference in the prevalence of depression [28]. Up to 2000, few studies dealt with the relationship between gender and antidepressant response [29, 30]. An earlier study of gender differences in the response to TCAs showed that older females had similar response rates to males, but that younger females responded preferentially to treatment with monoamine oxidase inhibitors (MAO inhibitors) compared to TCAs [29]. A meta-analysis published in 1996 reviewed 35 studies that compared the responses of 342 males and 711 females to imipramine; males had a significantly greater response [30]. Furthermore, more recent evidence published since 2000 indicates that gender may be a factor in predicting the response to one antidepressant versus another, especially with SSRIs and SNRIs. In 2000, Kornstein et al. [31] reported on gender differences in the response to sertraline, as a representative SSRI, versus imipramine, as a representative TCA, in patients with chronic major or double depression; females responded significantly better to sertraline than to imipramine, while males responded significantly better to imipramine. Furthermore, premenopausal females responded better to sertraline, but there was no difference in response to the two drugs in postmenopausal females. Subsequently, in 2004, Baca et al. [32] examined gender differences in the acute antidepressant response to sertraline and imipramine in nonmelancholic depression. The results showed that females were significantly more likely to respond to sertraline than to imipramine, while males respond similarly to sertraline and to imipramine. Fluoxetine is a popular SSRI, and, in 2001, Martenyi et al. [33] compared the clinical efficacy of fluoxetine and maprotiline in patients with severe unipolar depression to evaluate the effect of gender and age on antidepressant response. A significant difference was observed in females (more females responded to fluoxetine than to maprotiline), but not in males. However, this difference in females was only significant in females younger than 43 years of age; it was not significant in those older than 44 years. Joyce et al. [34] also reported gender and age differences in the response to fluoxetine. Their results showed that melancholic depressed patients 40 years or older, especially males, had a markedly superior response to nortriptyline compared to fluoxetine. Conversely, melancholic depressed patients, aged 18-24 years, especially females, had a marked response to fluoxetine. Berlanga and Flores-Ramos [35] reported that females treated with citalopram showed a significantly greater response than females treated with reboxetine (noradrenergic reuptake inhibitor); in males, no differences were observed for both drugs. Grigoriadis et al. [36] reported that, compared to postmenopausal females, premenopausal females had significantly lower Hamilton Depression Rating Scale (HAM-D) scores after 8 weeks of SSRI (fluoxetine, paroxetine, sertraline, and citalopram) treatment and had a significantly higher remission rate. Thase et al. [37] also reported similar findings; depressed females, 50 years or older, had a low chance of remission with SSRI treatment (fluoxetine, paroxetine, fluvoxamine), while depressed males of both age groups and depressed females 49 years or younger had significantly higher remission rates. Khan et al. [38] analyzed a total of 15 randomized, placebo-controlled trials that included 323 depressed patients with respect to gender differences in antidepressant treatment response. They found that females had a significantly greater response than males to SSRIs (fluoxetine, paroxetine, sertraline, citalopram). Gender differences in the response to SNRIs have also been examined. Some studies have found that depressed males tended to have a higher response rate than depressed females to milnacipran, an SNRI [23]. Gender differences for other SNRIs, venlafaxine and nefazodone, have also been investigated [35]. Venlafaxine and nefazodone were found to have a higher response rate in younger depressed females than in older depressed females. These findings suggest that females, especially young females, benefit from SSRIs, especially, sertraline, fluoxetine, and/or citalopram. However, the characteristics of female patients that are associated with response to treatment with SSRIs, SNRIs and/or other antidepressants have not been completely delineated.

In Japan, maprotiline, a selective noradrenaline reuptake inhibitor, has been prescribed for over 25 years to treat depression. However, fluvoxamine was introduced in 1999 as the first antidepressant SSRI. The SSRIs paroxetine and sertraline were introduced in 2000 and 2006, respectively, and milnacipran was introduced as an antidepressant SNRI in 2000. The aim of this study was to compare the clinical efficacy of SSRIs (fluvoxamine, paroxetine, sertraline), an SNRI (milnacipran), and a selective noradrenaline reuptake inhibitor (maprotiline) in the treatment of depression, and to evaluate the effect of gender and the frequency of episodes on antidepressant response.

METHOD

Patients

A retrospective cohort analysis involving outpatients treated in the Department of Psychiatry, Kawasaki Medical School Hospital, Kurashiki, The Depression Prevention Medical Center, Kyoto, Jujo Rehabilitation Hospital, Kyoto, Takeda Hospital, Kyoto, and Rakuto Clinic, Yamashina, Japan, was conducted. The antidepressants that were studied were selected based on the following considerations. Fluvoxamine, paroxetine, and sertraline are the only SSRIs available in Japan, and milnacipran is the only SNRI available in Japan. Maprotiline, a selective noradrenaline reuptake inhibitor, is used as a conventional antidepressant in Japan. For inclusion in this study, patients diagnosed with depression that were being treated with fluvoxamine, paroxetine, sertraline, milnacipran, or maprotiline were required to meet all of the following criteria.

Inclusion Criteria

Based on a review of the medical records of outpatients receiving fluvoxamine, paroxetine, sertraline, milnacipran, or maprotiline to treat depression, patients who met the DSM-IV criteria for major depressive disorder and who had been evaluated using the 21-item HAM-D [39] were included. Furthermore, prior to treatment, patients were required to have a total HAM-D score of 20-32 when they had been off psychotropic medications for at least 14 days. One antidepressant was given orally without any augmentation drugs, such as other antidepressants, lithium, mood stabilizers, or tryptophan. The daily dose of fluvoxamine was

50-150 mg, that of paroxetine was 20-40 mg, that of sertraline was 50-100 mg, that of milnacipran was 50-100 mg, and that of maprotiline was 50-100 mg. These daily doses are the recommended treatment doses in Japan. Patients were observed for 3 months. Based on the HAM-D scores, the clinical symptoms were evaluated as either in remission or in non-remission before and every week after antidepressant treatment. Remission was defined as a HAM-D score less than 7 and the absence of a depressed mood (defined as a HAM-D depressed mood item score of 0); all other patients were considered to be in non-remission.

Exclusion Criteria

Patients were excluded from the study if they had a history of seizure or myoclonus, combined anxiety disorder, obsessive-compulsive disorders, manic states, mixed state, rapid-cycling bipolar disorder, or other psychiatric disorders just before the antidepressants were given.

Statistical Analyses

The chi-square test (x^2-test) was used to compare the total remission rate of these antidepressants, the gender remission rate (male and female) of these antidepressants, the gender remission rate (male versus female) in each antidepressant treatment group, and the total first episode and recurrent episode depression remission rate among these antidepressants, as well as the remission rate (male and female) and the gender-recurrence in each antidepressant treatment group. To compare differences in the baseline characteristics of the five antidepressants treatment groups, the x^2-test and the F-test were used. A computer software program (StatView for Macintosh version 5.0, SAS Institute Inc.) was used for the analysis. The level of significance was set at $P<0.05$.

RESULTS

Three hundred sixty-eight patients met the above criteria and were included in the analyses.

1. The Baseline Characteristics of the Patients Treated with Fluvoxamine, Paroxetine, Sertraline, Milnacipran, and Maprotiline Are Shown in Table 1

Ninety-seven patients were taking fluvoxamine for treatment of depression. Forty-one (42.3%) were male and fifty-six (57.7%) were female; 44 patients (45.4%) had a first depression episode, and 53 patients (54.6%) had a recurrent depression episode. The patients' mean age±2SD was 49.5±16.5 years. The HAM-D score ranged from 20 to 32 (mean, 25.1).

Table 1. Baseline characteristics of the antidepressant treatment groups

	Fluvoxamine	Paroxetine	Sertraline	Milnacipran	Maprotiline
Male / Female	41/56	45/38	18/20	40/35	32/43
First / Recurrence	44/53	37/46	25/13	37/38	44/31
Mean age	49.5	47.6	43.0	59.9	53.7

Eighty-three patients were taking paroxetine for treatment of depression. Forty-five (54.2%) were male, and thirty-eight (45.8%) were female; 37 patients (44.6%) had a first depression episode, and 46 patients (55.4%) had a recurrent depression episode. The patients' mean age±2SD was 47.6±14.7 years. The HAM-D score ranged from 20 to 32 (mean, 27.2).

Thirty-eight patients were taking sertraline for treatment of depression. Eighteen (47.4%) were male, and 20 (52.6%) were female; 25 patients (65.8%) had a first depression episode, and 13 patients (34.2%) had a recurrent depression episode. The patients' mean age±2SD was 43.0±13.9 years. The HAM-D score ranged from 20 to 32 (mean, 26.9).

Seventy-five patients were taking milnacipran for treatment of depression. Forty (53.3%) were male, and 35 (46.7%) were female; 37 patients (49.3%) had a first depression episode, and 38 patients (50.7%) had recurrent depression episode. The patients' mean age±2SD was 45.9±13.4 years. The HAM-D score ranged from 20 to 32 (mean, 27.7).

Seventy-five patients were taking maprotiline for the treatment of depression. Thirty-two (42.7%) were male, and forty-three (57.3%) were female; 44 patients (58.7%) had a first depression episode, and 31 patients (41.3%) had a recurrent depressive episode. The patients' mean age±2SD was 53.7±14.3 years. The HAM-D score ranged from 20 to 32 (mean, 25.4).

Among the five antidepressants treatment groups, there was no difference in the number of males and females (x^2=4.274, df=4, P=0.3702), in the number of patients with a first episode of depression and those with a recurrent episode of depression (x^2=7.771, df=4, P=0.1003), and no difference in the mean age (using the F-test). All patients had similar levels of HAM-D scores.

2. Total Remission Rate (Figure 1)

At the end of a treatment period, remission was achieved in 64 (66.0%) of 97 patients in the fluvoxamine treatment group, 46 (55.4%) of 83 patients in the paroxetine treatment group, 29 (76.3%) of 38 patients in the sertraline treatment group, 55 (73.3%) of 75 patients in the milnacipran treatment group, and 62 (82.7%) of 75 patients in the maprotiline treatment group. There was a significant difference in the remission rate among the five treatment groups (x^2=15.833, df=4, P=0.0033). The post hoc cell index showed that the paroxetine treatment group had a lower remission rate than the other antidepressant groups.

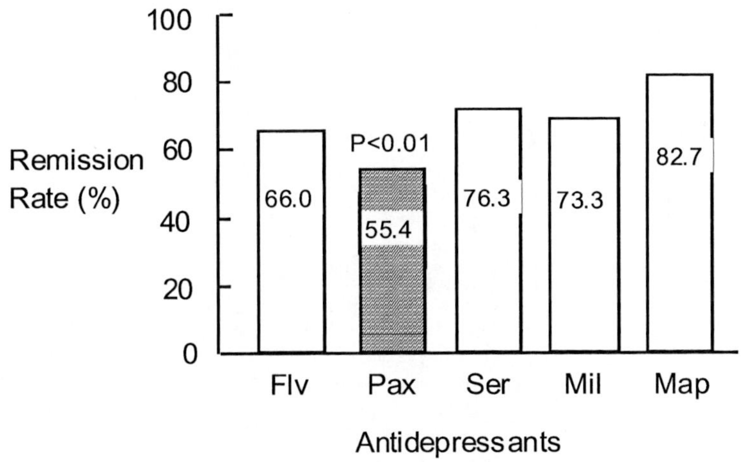

Figure 1. Total remission rates. Paroxetine shows lower remission than other antidepressants (P<0.01). Fluvoxamine (Flv), Paroxetine (Pax), Sertraline (Ser), Milnacipran (Mil), Maprotiline (Map).

3. Gender Remission Rate (Figures 2 and 3)

Figure 2 shows the male remission rate. At the end of a treatment period, remission was achieved in 28 (68.3%) of 41 male patients in the fluvoxamine treatment group, 26 (57.8%) of 45 male patients in the paroxetine treatment group, 10 (55.6%) of 18 male patients in the sertraline treatment group, 32 (80.0%) of 40 male patients in the milnacipran treatment group, and 25 (78.1%) of 32 male patients in the maprotiline treatment group. There was no difference in the remission rates in males among the five treatment groups (x^2=7.650, df=4, P=0.1053).

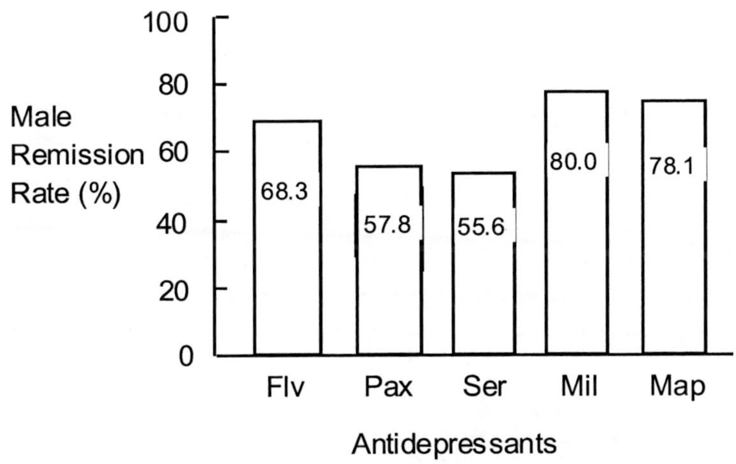

Figure 2. Male remission rates. There are no differences remission rates among five antidepressants. Fluvoxamine (Flv), Paroxetine (Pax), Sertraline (Ser), Milnacipra (Mil), Maprotiline (Map).

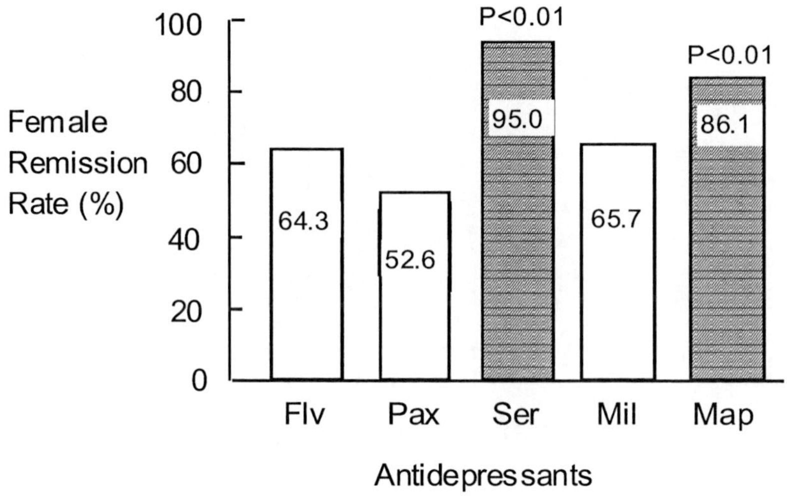

Figure 3. Female remission rates. Sertraline and maprotiline are significantly higher remission rates than fluvoxamine, paroxetine and milnacipran. Fluvoxamine (Flv), Paroxetine (Pax), Sertraline (Ser), Milnacipran (Mil), Maprotiline (Map).

Figure 3 shows the female remission rate. At the end of a treatment period, remission was achieved in 36 (64.3%) of 56 female patients in the fluvoxamine treatment group, 20 (52.6%) of 38 female patients in the paroxetine treatment group, 19 (95.0%) of 20 female patients in the sertraline treatment group, 23 (65.7%) of 35 female patients in the milnacipran treatment group, and 37 (86.1%) of 43 female patients in the maprotiline treatment group. There was a significant difference in the remission rate in females among the five antidepressants treatment groups (x^2=17.959, df=4, P=0.0013). The post hoc cell index showed that, in females, the sertraline and maprotiline treatment groups had higher remission rates than the fluvoxamine, paroxetine, and milnacipran treatment groups.

4. Gender Remission Rate for Each Individual Antidepressant (Figure 4)

Figure 4 shows the remission rates of males and females for each individual antidepressant.

Fluvoxamine

At the end of a treatment period, remission was achieved in 28 (68.3%) of 41 male patients and 36 (64.3%) of 56 female patients in the fluvoxamine treatment group. There was no difference between males and females in the remission rate (x^2=0.687, df=1, P=0.6807).

Paroxetine

At the end of a treatment period, remission was achieved in 26 (57.8%) of 45 male patients and 20 (52.6%) of 38 female patients in the paroxetine treatment group. There was no difference between males and females in the remission rate (x^2=0.221, df=1, P=0.6384).

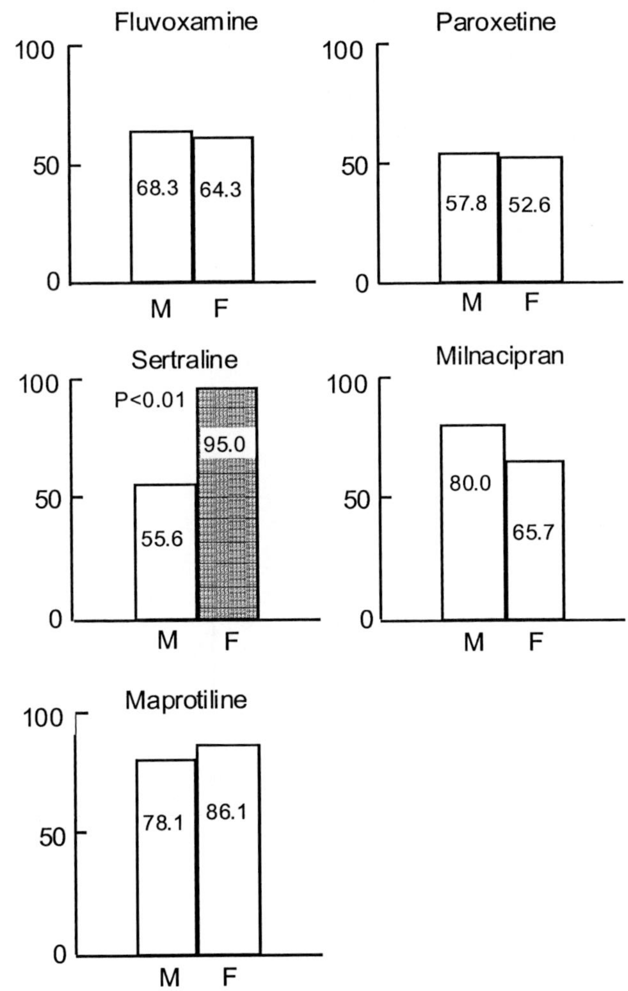

Figure 4. Gender remission rates in each individual antidepressant. Sertraline is significantly more likely to show a favorable remission to female than to male (P=0.0043). Milnacipran is tendency morelikely to show a good remission to male than to female (P=0.1628). Male (M), Female (F).

Sertraline

At the end of a treatment period, remission was achieved in 10 (55.6%) of 18 male patients and 19 (95.0%) of 20 female patients in the sertraline treatment group. There was a significant difference between males and females in the remission rate (x^2=8.155, df=1, P=0.0043); females were more likely than males to achieve remission.

Milnacipran

At the end of a treatment period, remission was achieved in 32 (80.0%) of 40 male patients and 23 (65.7%) of 35 female patients in the milnacipran treatment group. There was no difference between males and females in the remission rate (x^2=1.948, df=1, P=0.1628). However, based on the P-value (0.1628), there was a trend for male patients to show a more robust response to milnacipran than female patients.

Maprotiline

At the end of a treatment period, remission was achieved in 25 (78.1%) of 32 male patients and 37 (86.1%) of 43 female patients in the maprotiline treatment group. There was no difference between males and females in the remission rate (x^2=0.803, df=1, P=0.3701).

5. Remission Rates of Males with First Episodes and Recurrent Episodes (Figure 5)

Figure 5(A) shows the remission rates of male first episode depression patients in the five antidepressants treatment groups.

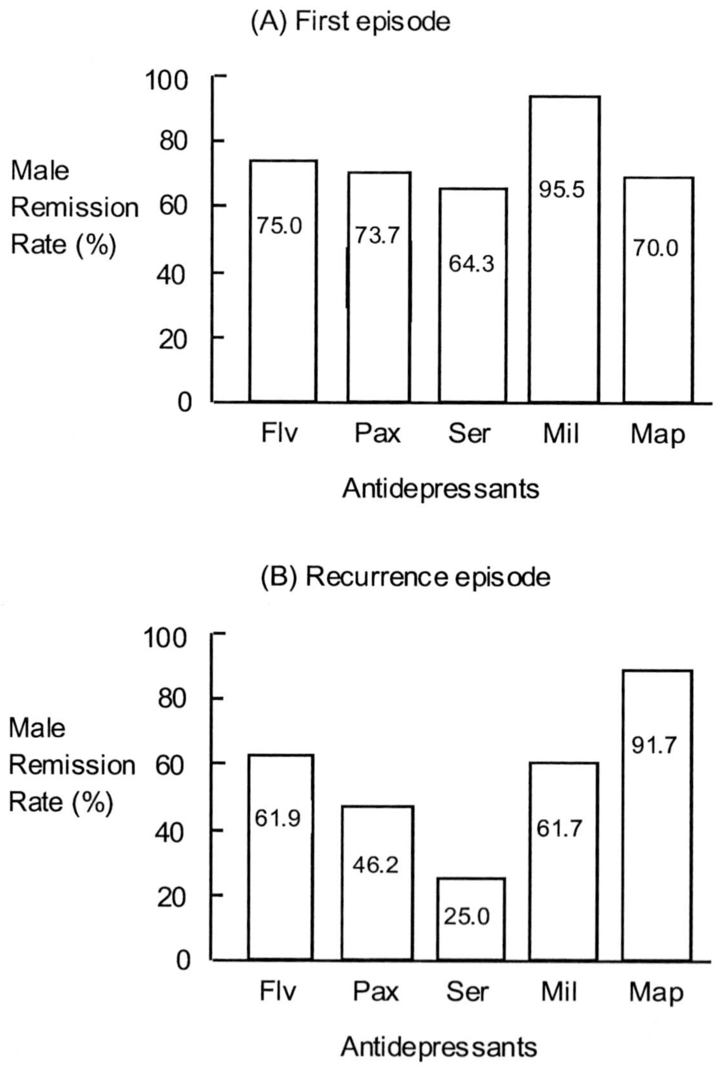

Figure 5. Remission rates of first episode and recurrence episode in male. There are no differences remission rates in male first episode and recurrence episode among five antidepressants treatment groups.

At the end of a treatment period, for male first episode depression patients, remission was achieved in 15 (75.0%) of 20 patients in the fluvoxamine treatment group, 14 (73.7%) of 19 patients in the paroxetine treatment group, 9 (64.3%) of 14 patients in the sertraline treatment group, 21 (95.5%) of 22 patients in the milnacipran treatment group, and 14 (70.0%) of 20 patients in the maprotiline treatment group. There was no difference in the remission rate of male first episode patients in the five antidepressants treatment groups (x^2=6.194, df=4 P=0.1851).

Figure 5(B) shows the remission rate of male patients with recurrent episodes of depression in the five antidepressants treatment groups. At the end of a treatment period, among the male recurrent episode patients, remission was achieved in 13 (61.9%) of 21 patients in the fluvoxamine treatment group, 12 (46.2%) of 26 patients in the paroxetine treatment group, 1 (25.0%) of 4 patients in the sertraline treatment group, 11 (61.1%) of 18 patients in the milnacipran treatment group, and 11 (91.7%) of 12 patients in the maprotiline treatment group. There was no difference in the remission rate of males with a recurrent episode of depression among the five antidepressants treatment groups (x^2=9.101, df=4 P=0.0586).

6. Remission Rates of Females with First Episodes and Recurrent Episodes (Figure 6)

Figure 6(A) shows the remission rates of females with a first episode of depression in the five antidepressants treatment groups. At the end of a treatment period, among the females with a first episode, remission was achieved in 20 (83.3%) of 24 patients in the fluvoxamine treatment group, 14 (77.8%) of 18 patients in the paroxetine treatment group, 11 (100%) of 11 patients in the sertraline treatment group, 14 (93.5%) of 15 patients in the milnacipran treatment group, and 20 (83.3%) of 24 patients in the maprotiline treatment group. There was no difference in the remission rate of females with a first episode among the five antidepressants treatment groups (x^2=3.725, df=4 P=0.4446).

Figure 6(B) shows the remission rates of females with a recurrent episode of depression in the five antidepressants treatment groups. At the end of a treatment period, among the females with a recurrent episode, remission was achieved in 16 (50.0%) of 32 patients in the fluvoxamine treatment group, 6 (30.0%) of 20 patients in the paroxetine treatment group, 8 (88.9%) of 9 patients in the sertraline treatment group, 9 (45.0%) of 20 patients in the milnacipran treatment group, and 17 (89.5%) of 19 patients in the maprotiline treatment group. There was a significant difference in the remission rate in the female patients with a recurrent episode among the five antidepressants treatment groups (x^2=19.528, df=4 P=0.0006). The post hoc cell index showed that patients treated with sertraline and maprotiline had higher remission rates than those treated with fluvoxamine, paroxetine, or milnacipran.

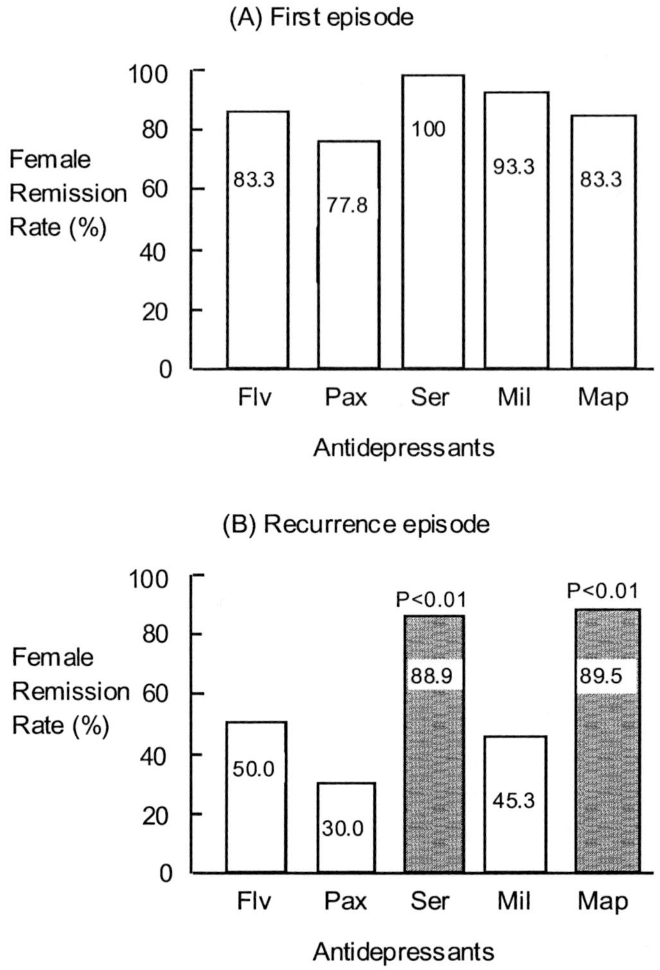

Figure 6. Remission rates of first episode and recurrence episode in female. There are no differences remission rates female first episode among five antidepressants treatment groups. However, sertraline and maprotiline are significantly more likely to show a favorable remission than fluvoxamine, paroxetine and milnacipran in female recurrence episode patients.

7. Gender-Frequency of Remission Rates for Each Individual Antidepressant (Figure 7)

Figure 7 shows the gender-frequency of the remission rates for each individual antidepressant.

Fluvoxamine

At the end of a treatment period, remission was achieved in 15 (75.0%) of 20 male first episode patients and 20 (83.3%) of 24 female first episode patients in the fluvoxamine treatment group, as well as 14 (73.7%) of 19 male recurrent episode patients and 16 (50.0%) of 32 female recurrent episode patients. There were no differences in the remission rates among first episode and among recurrent episode patients (first episodes: χ^2=0.466, df=1 P=0.4950; recurrent episodes: x^2=0.725, df=1 P=0.3944).

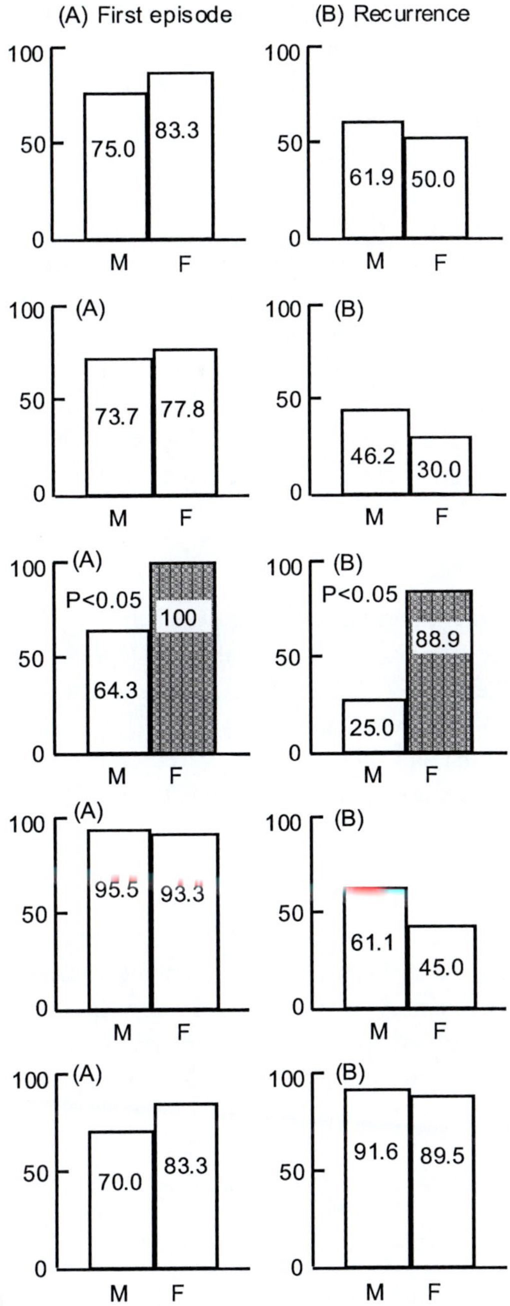

Figure 7. Gender-frequency of episode remission rates in each individual antidepressant. There are no differences remission rates between male and female in fluvoxamine, paroxetine, milnacipran and maprotiline treatment. However, sertraline is significantly more likely to show a favorable remission rate to female than to male in both first episode depression and recurrence episode depression. (A); first episode group, (B); recurrence episode group, Male (M), Female (F).

Paroxetine

At the end of a treatment period, remission was achieved in 14 (73.7%) of 19 male first episode patients and 14 (77.8%) of 18 female first episode patients in the paroxetine treatment group, as well as 12 (46.2%) of 26 male recurrent episode patients and 6 (30.0%) of 20 female recurrent episode patients. There were no differences in the remission rates among the first episode patients and among the recurrent episode patients (first episode: x^2=0.084, df=1 P=0.7718; recurrent episode: x^2=1.238, df=1 P=0.2658).

Sertraline

At the end of a treatment period, remission was achieved in 9 (64.3%) of 14 male first episode patients and 11 (100%) of 11 female first episode patients in the sertraline treatment group. There was a significant difference between genders in the remission rate (x^2=4.911, df=1 P=0.0267). At the end of a treatment period, remission was achieved in 1 (25.0%) of 4 male recurrent episode patients and 8 (88.9%) of 9 female recurrent episode patients in the sertraline treatment group. There was a significant difference between genders in the remission rate (x^2=5.306, df=1 P=0.0212). Both first episode and recurrent episode female depression patients were significantly more likely than males to show a favorable response to sertraline treatment.

Milnacipran

At the end of a treatment period, remission was achieved in 21 (95.5%) of 22 male first episode patients and 14 (93.3%) of 15 female first episode patients in the milnacipran treatment group, as well as in 11 (61.1%) of 18 male recurrent episode patients and 9 (45.0%) of 20 female recurrent episode patients. There were no differences between the genders in the remission rates among first episode and among recurrent episode patients (first episode: x^2=0.078, df=1 P=0.7794; recurrent episode: x^2=0.986, df=1 P=0.3206).

Maprotiline

At the end of a treatment period, remission was achieved in 14 (70.0%) of 20 male first episode patients and 20 (83.3%) of 24 female first episode patients in the maprotiline treatment group, as well as in 11 (91.6%) of 12 male recurrent episode patients and 17 (89.5%) of 19 female recurrent episode patients. There were no differences between genders in the remission rates among first episode and among recurrent episode patients (first episode: x^2=1.104, df=1 P=0.2933; recurrent episode: x^2=0.040, df=1 P=0.8406).

DISCUSSION

This study assessed gender differences in the response to treatment with SSRIs (fluvoxamine, paroxetine, and sertraline), an SNRI (milnacipran), and a selective noradrenaline reuptake inhibitor (maprotiline) in patients with depression. A significant interaction between gender and response was found; among patients taking sertraline, females had a higher remission rate than males. This result may be important in helping physicians choose an appropriate antidepressant. Table 2 shows the major reports that have studied the relationship between gender and response to antidepressants.

Table 2. The interaction of gender and antidepressants in depression

Authors and References No.	Results
Raskin et al.(1974)[29]	Young female: MAOI > Benzodiazepines
Hamilton (1996)[30]	Imipramine: Male > Female
Kornstein et al.(2000)[31]	Male: Sertraline < Imipramine
	Female: Sertraline > Imipramine
Martenyi et al.(2001)[33]	Male: Fluoxetine = Maprotiline
	Old female: Fluoxetine = Maprotiline
	Young female: Fluoxetine > Maprotiline
Quitkin et al.(2002)[43]	TCA, Fluoxetine: Male = Female
	Young female: MAOI > TCA
Hildebrandt et al.(2003)[40]	Citalopram, Paroxetine: Male = Female
Morishita et al.(2003)[23]	Milnacipran: Male > Female
	Fluvoxamine, Paroxetine: Male = Female
Joyce et al.(2003)[34]	Male: Nortriptyline > Fluoxetine
	Female: Nortriptyline < Fluoxetine
Grigoriadis et al.(2003)[36]	SSRIs, SNRIs: Young female > Old female
Wohlfarth et al.(2004)[44]	Imipramine, Amitriptyline: Male = Female
Baca et al.(2004)[32]	Male: sertraline = Imipramine
	Female: Sertraline > Imipramine
Thase et al.(2005)[37]	SSRIs: Male = young female
	SSRIs: Young female > Old Female
	Venlafaxine: Male = Female
Khan et al.(2005)[38]	SSRIs: Male < Female
	SNRIs: Male = Female
Pinto-Meza et al.(2006)[41]	SSRIs: Male = Female
Berlanga et al.(2006)[35]	Male: Citalopram = Reboxetine
	Female: Citalopram > Reboxetine
Kornstein et al.(2006)[42]	Duloxetine: Male = Female
Papakostas et al.(2007)[45]	Bupropion, SSRIs: Male = Female

SSRI

Sertraline

Kornstein et al. were the first to report gender differences in treatment response to sertraline [31] in a trial involving 235 males and 400 females with major depression who were treated for 12 weeks with either sertraline (50-200 mg/day) or imipramine (50-300 mg/day). Analysis of the intent-to-treat study population at the 12-week study endpoint showed that males and females with depression responded differently to sertraline than to imipramine. Females were more likely to respond to sertraline, while males were more likely to respond to imipramine. It was also found that premenopausal females responded significantly better to sertraline than to imipramine (57% versus 41%, P=0.01). Subsequently, Baca et al. [32] reported that, among patients with nonmelancholic depressive disorders, there were gender differences in the acute antidepressant response to sertraline and imipramine. Their trial involved 50 male and 184 female patients with nonmelancholic depression or dysthymia who were treated with an 8-week course of either sertraline (50-200 mg/day) or imipramine (75-225 mg/day). Among males, there were no differences in the response or remission rates between sertraline and imipramine, while among females, there were significant differences in either the response or remission rates between sertraline and imipramine. Females were significantly more likely to respond to sertraline than to imipramine (75% versus 52.1%, P=0.008). Moreover, compared to males, females taking sertraline showed statistically significant greater reduction in anxiety symptoms and in clinical global impression severity. The present retrospective study also showed that, among females, sertraline had a significantly higher remission rate than other SSRIs (fluvoxamine and paroxetine) and SNRIs (milnacipran), and that among sertraline-treated patients, females had significantly higher remission rates than males. Furthermore, the present study also found that, among female recurrent episode patients, sertraline had a significantly higher remission rate than other SSRIs (fluvoxamine and paroxetine) and SNRIs (milnacipran). These findings suggest that sertraline has a specific effect in female patients with depression.

Fluoxetine

Gender differences in the response to fluoxetine treatment have also been reported in patients with depression. A randomized, double-blind, 6-week study by Martenyi et al. [33] evaluated gender differences in response to fluoxetine (20 mg/day) or maprotiline (100-200 mg/day) in 105 (44 male and 61 female) depressed patients. Females, but not males, responded better to fluoxetine than to maprotiline (P=0.017). The analysis of response rates in females by age showed that females aged younger than 44 years (P=0.023), but not females aged 44 years and older, had a significantly higher response to fluoxetine than to maprotiline. Subsequently, Joyce et al. [34] reported on the effect of age and gender on the antidepressant response to fluoxetine and nortriptyline in patients with melancholic depression; 113 patients with major depression were randomized to receive either fluoxetine (mean dose 27 mg/day) or nortriptyline (mean dose 100 mg/day) as their initial antidepressant for a 6-week period. There was a significant difference between the treatment groups; young females (18-24 years of age), but not young males (18-24 years of age), showed a better response to fluoxetine. Furthermore, older males (40 years and older), but not older females (40 years and older) responded significantly more favorably to nortriptyline.

Citalopram

One report has shown that there are gender differences in the pharmacological response to citalopram and reboxetine, which are selective noradrenaline reuptake inhibitors [35]. Eighty-six depressed patients (38 male and 58 female), 18 to 40 years of age, participated in an 8-week, double-blind, clinical trial. Among females, 80% responded to citalopram (20 mg/day) and 56% responded to reboxetine (4.0 mg/day). ANOVA showed a statistically significant interaction between citalopram and reboxetine (P=0.029).

Paroxetine and Fluvoxamine

Both paroxetine and fluvoxamine are SSRIs; there is no evidence to suggest that there are significant gender differences in the pharmacological response to these SSRIs [23,40,41].

SNRI

Milnacipran

A previous retrospective analysis of 18 female and 28 male patients with depression suggested that there are gender differences in the response to milnacipran; among these patients, males tended to have greater improvement (82.4%) than females (62.1%) (P=0.076).

Venlafaxine and Duloxetine

Thase et al. [37] analyzed eight randomized, controlled trials of patients with major depression. Eight hundred and fifty-one patients were treated with venlafaxine. The remission rate with venlafaxine ranged from 41% to 48%; the rate did not differ significantly by age and gender, and there were no significant interactions involving age and gender. Kornstein et al. [42] analyzed seven randomized, controlled trials of patients with depression. Eight hundred ninety-six patients received duloxetine. Duloxetine had a significant advantage over placebo with respect to the HAM-D scores in both males and females (P<0.05). However, there was no significant difference in the reduction rate of the HAM-D score between males and females treated with duloxetine (P=0.894).

Selective Noradrenaline Reuptake Inhibitors

Maprotiline and Reboxetine

In the present study, it was found that females had a significantly higher remission rate (86.1%) with maprotiline than with fluvoxamine (64.3%), paroxetine (52.6%) or milnacipran (65.8%). However, the remission rate did not differ between males (78.1%) and females (86.1%) with maprotiline treatment. Berlanga and Flores-Ramos [35] showed that reboxetine was not as same as citalopram in females.

MAO inhibitors

Raskin et al. [29] compared diazepam (30 mg/day) and phenelzine (45 mg/day) to placebo in a total of 325 (107 male and 218 female) patients with depression. They reported that young females tended to have a better response to phenelzine treatment. Quitkin et al. [43] analyzed 1746 patients with depression who had been treated with TCAs, MAO inhibitors (phenelzine, tranylcypromine, L-deprenyl), fluoxetine, or placebo. Using the log-rank test, survival analysis showed that young females had a better response than young males (x^2=4.97, df=1, P=0.03) to MAO inhibitor treatment.

TCA

A meta-analysis by Hamilton published in 1996 reviewed 35 studies [30] involving 342 males and 711 females treated with imipramine and found that males had a statistically significantly greater response than females ($P<0.01$). However, another meta-analysis by Quitkin [43] showed that males and females, both younger and older than 50 years of age, had equivalent response rates to imipramine and desipramine, which are both TCAs. Hildebrandt et al. [40] also reported that males and females had similar remission rates when treated with clomipramine. A meta-analysis by Wohlfarth et al. [44], involving a total of 30 randomized, placebo-control trials that included 3886 patients (1555 males and 2331 females), was published in 2004; no gender differences in response to the TCAs imipramine and amitriptyline were found.

Others

Bupropion

Bupropion inhibits the reuptake of noradrenaline and dopamine. Pupakosta et al. [45] analyzed 10 double-blind studies including 943 male and 1179 female patients with depression and compared the effects of bupropion treatment and SSRI treatment. No difference between bupropion treatment and SSRI treatment in the improvement of the HAM-D scores was noted among females ($P=0.114$).

CONCLUSION

Females are twice as likely as males to suffer from depression. The paucity of research on gender-specific differences related to antidepressants is a significant public health issue and represents an understudied yet necessary research area. Reports published to date, as well as the data presented in the present study, suggest that there are gender differences in the responses to some antidepressants. Females, particularly young females, appear to have a favorable response to the SSRIs sertraline, fluoxetine, and citalopram, but there do not appear, at least at the present time, to be any gender differences in the responses to other SSRIs. There may be gender differences in the response to SNRIs, particularly milnacipran, and females may have a better response to MAO inhibitors than males. There appear to be no gender differences in the response to TCAs.

With respect to the mechanisms responsible for the gender differences observed, Kornstein [31] suggests that gender differences may reflect the differential efficacy of SSRIs in treating different subtypes of depression (melancholic versus atypical features) that present in females and males; differential effects of sex hormones may also explain gender differences in the efficacy of various SSRIs. Other data suggest that female sex hormones may affect the response to treatment; estrogen enhances the response to SSRIs and inhibits the response to TCAs [46]. One recent study reported that the availability of serotonin 1A receptors decreased with age, with a particularly marked decrease in older males [47]. This decreased availability of serotonin 1A receptors in older males may be important with respect to explaining gender differences in the response to SSRIs. Fluoxetine increases tryptophan and decreases serum cortisol levels in females but not in males [48]. Estrogens inhibit MAO activity, which may explain the gender differences in response to MAO inhibitors [49]. However, the mechanisms of the gender differences in response to antidepressant treatments for depression are still unknown.

Although further studies are required to assess the gender differences in the response to antidepressant treatment, the results of the present study should help guide clinicians in determining the antidepressants that are suitable for female patients with depression.

References

[1] Regier, DA; Boyd, JH; Burker, JrJD; et al. One-month prevalence of mental disorders in the United States: based on five epidemiologic catchment area sites. *Arch. Gen. Psychiatry*, 1988;45:977-986.

[2] Weissman, MM; Band, R; Joycc, PR; et al. Sex differences in rates of depression: cross-national perspectives. *J. Affect. Disord.,* 1993;29:77-84.

[3] Kessler, RC; McGonagle, KA; Swartz, M; et al. Sex and depression in the National Comorbidity Survery: 1. lifetime, prevalence, chronicity, and recurrence. *J. Affect Disord.,* 1993;29:85-96.

[4] Maier, W; Gansicke, M; Rezaki, M; et al. Gender differences in the prevalence of depression: a survery in primary care. *J. Affect. Disord*., 1999;53:241-252.

[5] Kessler, RC; McGonagle, KA; Zhao, S; et al. Lifetime and 12-month prevalence of DSM-III-R psychiatric disorders in the United States. Results from the National Comorbidity Survery. *Arch. Gen. Psychiatry*, 1994;51:8-19.

[6] Thase, ME; Reynold, CF; Frank, E; et al. Do depressed men and women respond similsly to cognitive behavior therapy? *Am. J. Psychiatry,* 1994;151:500-505.

[7] Kornstein, SG; Schatzberg, AF; Yonkers, KA; et al. Gender differences in presentation of chronic major depression. *Psychopharmacol. Bull.*, 1996;31:711-718

[8] Sargeant, JK; Bruce, ML; Florio, LP; et al. Factors associated with 1^year outcome of major depression in the community. *Arch. Gen. Psychiatry*, 1990;47:519-526.

[9] Rasenthal, NE; Sack, DA; Gillin, JC; et al. Seasonal affective disorder. A description of the syndrome and preliminary findings with light therapy. *Arch. Gen. Psychiatry,* 1984;41:72-80.

[10] Leibenluft, E; Hardin, TA; Rosentahal, NE. Gender differences in seasonal disorder. *Depression*, 1995;3:13-19.

[11] Hirschfeld, RM, Russel, JM. Assessment and treatment of suicidal patients. *N. Engl. J. Med*., 1997;337:910-915.

[12] Kornstein, SG. Gender differences in depression: implication for treatment. *J. Clin. Psychiatry*, 1997;58(suppl. 15):12-18.

[13] Silverstein, B. Gender difference in the prevalence of clinical depression: the role played by depression associated with somatic symptoms. *Am. J. Psychiatry,* 1999;156:480-482.

[14] Nazroo, JY; Edward, AC; Brown, GW. Gender differences in the onset of depression following a shared life event: a study of couples. *Psychol. Med*., 1997;27:9-19.

[15] Rapaport, MH; Thompson,PM; Kelsoe, JR; et al. Gender differences in outpatient research subjects with affective disorders: a comparison of descriptive variables. *J. Clin. Psychiatry*, 1995;56:67-72.
[16] Fava, M; Abraham, M; Alpert, J et al. Gender differences in Axis I comobidity among depressed outpatients. *J. Affect. Disord.*, 1996;38:129-133.
[17] Nelson, JCN. Safety and tolerability of the new antidepressants. *J. Clin. Psychiatry*, 2003;18:34-35.
[18] Puech, A; Montgomery, SA; Prost,JF; et al. Milnacipran, a new serotonin and noradrenaline reuptake inhibitor: an overview of its antidepressant activity and clinical tolerability. *Int. Clin. Psychopharmacol.*, 1997;12:99-108.
[19] Morishita, S; Atita, S. Possible predictors of response to Fluvoxamine for depression. *Hum. Psychopharmacol. Clin. Exp.*, 2003;18:197-200.
[20] Morishita, S; Arita, S. Differential period of onset of action of Fluvoxamine, Paroxetine and Milnacipran for depression. *Hum. Psychopharmacol. Clin. Exp.*, 2003;18:479-482.
[21] Morishita, S; Arita, S. Induction of mania in depression by Paroxetine. *Hum. Psychopharmacol. Clin. Exp.*, 2003;18:565-568.
[22] Morishita, S; Arita, S. The clinical use of Milnacipran for depression. *Eur. Psychiatry*, 2003;18:34-35.
[23] Morishita, S; Arita, S. Differential effects of Milnacipran, Fluvoxamine and Paroxetine for depression, especially in gender. *Eur. Psychiatry*, 2003;18:418-420.
[24] Morishita, S; Arita, S. Differential effects of Fluvoxamine, Paroxetine and Milnacipran for depression, especially with regard to age. *Hum. Psychopharmacol. Clin. Exp.*, 2004;19:405-408.
[25] Morishita, S; Arita, S. Prevalence of induced mania in patients treatment with Milnacipran: a comparison with Paroxetine. *Eur. Psychiatry*, 2004;19:315-316.
[26] Morishita, S; Arita, S. Differential effects of Milnacipran, Fluvoxamine and Paroxetine for inhibited and agitated depression. *Eur. Psychiatry*, 2004;19:450-451.
[27] Morishita, S; Arita, S. Clinical characteristics as predictors of response to Fluvoxamine, Paroxetine and Milnacipran in patients with depression. *Curr. Psychiat. Rev.*, 2005;1:319-324.
[28] Kessler, RC; McGonagle, KA; Swartz, M; et al. Sex and depression in the National Comorbidity Survery I: lifetime prevalence, chronicity, and recurrence. *J. Affect. Disord.*, 1993;29:85-96.
[29] Raskin, A; Schulterbrandt, JG; Reating, N; et al. Depression subtype and response to phenelzine, diazepam, and a placebo: results of a nine-hospital collaborative study. *Arch. Gen. Psychiatry*, 1974;30:66-75.
[30] Hamilton, JA; Grant, M; Jensvold, MF. Sex, gender, and hormones. In: Jensvold, MF; Halbreich, U; Hamilton, JA, eds. *Psychopharmacology and Women*. Washington, DC: American Psychiatric Press; 1996; 241-257.
[31] Kornstein, SG; Schatzberg, AF; Thase, ME; et al. Gender differences in treatment response to sertraline versus imipramine in chronic depression. *Am. J. Psychiatry*, 2000;157:1445-1452.
[32] Baca, E; Garcia, M; Porras-Chavarino, A. Gender differences in treatment response to sertraline versus imipramine in patients with nonmelancholic depressive disorders. *Progr. Neuropsychopharmacol.,* 2000;28:57-65.

[33] Martenyi, F; Dossenbach, M; Mraz, K; et al. Gender differences in the efficacy of fluoxetine and Maprotiline in depressed patients: a double-blind trial of antidepressants with serononergic or norepinephriergic reuptake inhibition profile. *Eur. Neuropsychopharmacol. Biol. Psychiatry,* 2001;11:227-232.

[34] Joyce, PR; Mulder, RT; Luty, SE; et al. A differential response to nortriptyline and fluoxetine in melancholic depression: the importance of age and gender. *Acta Psychiatr. Scand.,* 2003;108:20-23.

[35] Berlanga, C; Flores-Ramos, M. Different gender response to serotoneigic and noradrenergic antidepressants. A comparative study of the efficacy of citalopram and reboxetine. *J. Affect. Disord.*, 2006;1-3:119-123.

[36] Grigoriadis, S; Kennedy, SH; Bagby, RM. A comparison of antidepressant response in younger and older women. *J. Clin. Psychopharmacol.,* 2003;23:405-407.

[37] Thase, ME; Entsuah, R; Cantillon, M; et al. Relative antidepressant efficacy of venlafaxine and SSRIs: sex-age interactions. *J. Womens Health*, 2005;14:609-616.

[38] Khan, A; Brodhead, AE; Schwartz, KA; et al. Sex differences in antidepressant response in recent antidepressant clinical trials. *J. Clin. Psychopharmacol.*, 2005;25:318-324.

[39] Hamilton, M. A rating scale for depression. *J. Neurol. Neurosurg. Psychiatry,* 1960;23:56-62.

[40] Hildebrandt, MG; Steyerberg, EW; Stage, KB; et al. Are gender differences important for the clinical effects of antidepressant? *Am. J. Psychiatry,* 2003;160:1643-1650.

[41] Pinto-Meza, A; Usall, J; Berrano-Blanco, A; et al. Gender differences in response to antidepressant treatment prescribed in primary care. Does menopause make a difference? *J. Affect. Disord.*, 2006;93:53-60.

[42] Kornstein, SG; Wohlreich, MM; Mallinckrodt, CH; et al. Duloxetine efficacy for major depressive disorder in male vs. female patients: data from 7 randomized, double-blind, placebo-controlled trials. *J. Clin. Psychiatry,* 2006;67:761-770.

[43] Quitkin, FM; Stewart, JW; McGrath, PJ; et al. Are there differences between women's and men's antidepressant response? *Am. J. Psychiatry,* 2002;159:1848-1854.

[44] Wohlfarth, T; Storosum, JG; Elferin, AJA; et al. Response to tricyclic antidepressants. independent of gender? Am J Psychiatry, 2004;161:370-372.

[45] Papakostas, GI; Kornstein, SG; Clayton, AH; et al. Relativeantidepressant efficacy of bupropion and the selective serotonin reuptake inhibitors in major depressive disorder: gender-age interactions. *Int. Clin. Psychopharmacol.*, 2007;22:226-229.

[46] Halbreich, U; Kahn, LS. Role of estrogen in the etiology and treatment of mood disorders. *CNS Drugs,* 2001;15:797-817.

[47] Meltzer, CC; Drevents, WC; Price, JC; et al. Gender-specific aging effects on serotonin 1A receptor. *Brain Res.,* 2001;895:9-17.

[48] Bano, S; Akhter, S; Afridi, MI. Gender based response to fluoxetine hydrochloride medication in endogenous depression. *J. Coll Physicians Surg. Pak.*, 2004;14:161-165.

[49] Davidson, J; Pelton, S. Forms of atypical depression and their response to antidepressant drug. *Psychiatry Res*., 1986;17:87-95.

In: Antidepressants: Types, Efficiency … ISBN 978-1-61668-581-2
Editor: Jayden T. Van Leeuwen, pp.221-224

Expert Commentary

ADULT NEUROGENESIS AND DEPRESSION: A NOVEL THEORY FOR DEPRESSION?*

***Philippe Taupin*†**
National Neuroscience Institute, Singapore
National University of Singapore
Nanyang Technological University, Singapore

The recent confirmation that neurogenesis occurs throughout adulthood in mammals raises the question of the function of newly generated neuronal cells in the adult brain [1-2].

The hippocampus is an important memory center of the brain [3]. It is also involved in pathological processes, like Alzheimer's disease and epilepsy [4, 5]. Several lines of evidence further suggest that the hippocampus is involved in the etiology of major depressive disorders, like chronic stress and depression [6].

In the adult brain, neurogenesis occurs primarily in two regions, the subventricular zone (SVZ) and the dentate gurus (DG) hippocampus, in various species including human [7-9]. The hippocampus of patients with depression show signs of atrophy and neuronal loss [11-13]. This suggests that adult hippocampal neurogenesis may contribute to the etiology of depression.

Various classes of drugs are currently prescribed for the treatment of depression, like the selective serotonin reuptake inhibitors fluoxetine, the monoamine oxidase inhibitors tranylcypromine, the specific norepinephrine reuptake inhibitors reboxetine and the phosphodiesterase-IV inhibitors rolipram [14]. Chronic administration of these antidepressants increases neurogenesis in the DG, but not the SVZ in adult rats [15, 16]. This suggests that hippocampal neurogenesis contributes to the therapeutic effects of antidepressants. X-irradiation of the hippocampal region, but not other brain regions, like the

* A version of this chapter was also published in *Stem Cell Applications in Diseases*, edited by Jean Mikkel L. Sorensen published by Nova Science Publishers, Inc. It was submitted for appropriate modifications in an effort to encourage wider dissemination of research.

† Correspondence: 11 Jalan Tan Tock Seng, Singapore 308433. Tel. (65) 6357 - 7533. Fax (65) 6256 - 9178. Email obgpjt@nus.edu.sg

SVZ or the cerebellar region, prevents the behavioral effect of the antidepressants, like fluoxetine, in adult mice [17]. As X-irradiation of the hippocampal area in adult rats causes long-term reductions in cell proliferation in the DG [18]. These data show that adult hippocampal neurogenesis mediates the activity of antidepressants, like fluoxetine, in adult mice.

Stress is an important causal factor in precipitating episodes of depression, and decreases hippocampal neurogenesis in adult monkeys [19]. It is proposed that the waning and waxing of hippocampal neurogenesis are important causal factors in the precipitation and recovery from episodes of clinical depression [20]. In all, neurogenesis plays an important role in the etiology of depression and the activity of antidepressants [17, 21].

There are, however, controversies and debates over the involvement of the hippocampus and adult neurogenesis in the etiology of depression. Among them, 1) a link between neurogenesis, loss of nerve cells, atrophy and decrease of hippocampal volume in patients with depression or animal models remains to be demonstrated, 2) some studies show that hippocampal volume remains unchanged in depressive patients [22], 3) the hippocampal formation may not be the brain region primarily involved in depressive episodes, as other areas may play a critical role in depression [23], 4) there are questions over the validity of animal models of depression as representative of the human disorder, and 5) neurogenesis may be more a contributing factor of plasticity of the central nervous system, rather than of specific physiological or pathological processes [24]. The involvement of adult neurogenesis in depression remains therefore speculative [25, 26].

In all these data involved with the hippocampus, a structure classically involved in learning and memory, and adult neurogenesis in depression, anxiety disorders and the activity of antidepressants. However, the neurogenic theory of depression remains the source of controversies and debates, and must be further confirmed. More data and evidence are needed to confirm the involvement of adult neurogenesis in depression. Nonetheless, the evidence that increased neurogenesis contributes to the effects of antidepressants may hold the key for the understanding of the long-term consequences of the effects of antidepressants of the physiopathology of the central nervous system. It may lead to new drug design and new strategies to treat depressive disorders. To this aim, the mechanism underlying the involvement of adult neurogenesis in the etiology of depression and the activity of antidepressants remain to be fully understood [27].

REFERENCES

[1] Gage FH. (2000) Mammalian neural stem cells. *Science*. 287, 1433-8.

[2] Kaplan MS. (2001) Environment complexity stimulates visual cortex neurogenesis: death of a dogma and a research career. *Trends Neurosci*. 24, 617-20.

[3] Sweatt JD. (2004) Hippocampal function in cognition. *Psychopharmacology* (Berl). 174, 99-110.

[4] Panegyres PK. (2004) The contribution of the study of neurodegenerative disorders to the understanding of human memory. *QJM*. 97, 555-67.

[5] Sloviter RS. (2005) The neurobiology of temporal lobe epilepsy: too much information, not enough knowledge. *C. R .Biol*. 328, 143-53.

[6] Campbell S, Macqueen G. (2004) The role of the hippocampus in the pathophysiology of major depression. *J. Psychiatry Neurosci*. 29, 417-26.

[7] Taupin P, Gage FH. (2002) Adult neurogenesis and neural stem cells of the central nervous system in mammals. *J. Neurosci Res*. 69, 745-9.

[8] Eriksson PS, Perfilieva E, Bjork-Eriksson T, Alborn AM, Nordborg C, Peterson DA, Gage FH. (1998) Neurogenesis in the adult human hippocampus. *Nat. Med.* 4, 1313-7.

[9] Curtis MA, Kam M, Nannmark U, Anderson MF, Axell MZ, Wikkelso C, Holtas S, van Roon-Mom WM, Bjork-Eriksson T, Nordborg C, Frisen J, Dragunow M, Faull RL, Eriksson PS. (2007) Human neuroblasts migrate to the olfactory bulb via a lateral ventricular extension. *Science*. 315, 1243-9.

[10] Sheline YI, Wang PW, Gado MH, Csernansky JG, Vannier MW. (1996) Hippocampal atrophy in recurrent major depression. *Proc. Natl. Acad. Sci. USA*. 93, 3908-13.

[11] Campbell S, Marriott M, Nahmias C, MacQueen GM. (2004) Lower hippocampal volume in patients suffering from depression: a meta-analysis. *Am. J. Psychiatry*. 161, 598-607.

[12] Colla M, Kronenberg G, Deuschle M, Meichel K, Hagen T, Bohrer M, Heuser I. (2007) Hippocampal volume reduction and HPA-system activity in major depression. *J. Psychiatr. Res*. 41, 553-60.

[13] Brunello N, Mendlewicz J, Kasper S, Leonard B, Montgomery S, Nelson J, Paykel E, Versiani M, Racagni G. (2002) The role of noradrenaline and selective noradrenaline reuptake inhibition in depression. *Eur. Neuropsychopharmacol*. 12, 461-75.

[14] Malberg JE, Eisch AJ, Nestler EJ, Duman RS. (2000) Chronic antidepressant treatment increases neurogenesis in adult rat hippocampus. *J. Neurosci*. 20, 9104-10.

[15] Malberg JE, Duman RS. (2003) Cell proliferation in adult hippocampus is decreased by inescapable stress: reversal by fluoxetine treatment. *Neuropsychopharmacology*. 28, 1562-71.

[16] Santarelli L, Saxe M, Gross C, Surget A, Battaglia F, Dulawa S, Weisstaub N, Lee J, Duman R, Arancio O, Belzung C, Hen R. (2003) Requirement of hippocampal neurogenesis for the behavioral effects of antidepressants. *Science*. 301, 805-9.

[17] Tada E, Parent JM, Lowenstein DH, Fike JR. (2000) X-irradiation causes a prolonged reduction in cell proliferation in the dentate gyrus of adult rats. *Neurosci*. 99, 33-41.

[18] Gould E, Tanapat P, McEwen BS, Flugge G, Fuchs E. (1998) Proliferation of granule cell precursors in the dentate gyrus of adult monkeys is diminished by stress. *Proc. Natl. Acad. Sci. USA*. 95, 3168-71.

[19] Jacobs BL, Praag H, Gage FH. (2000) Adult brain neurogenesis and psychiatry: a novel theory of depression. *Mol. Psychiatry*. 5, 262-9.

[20] Malberg JE. (2004) Implications of adult hippocampal neurogenesis in antidepressant action. *J. Psychiatry Neurosci*. 29, 196-205.

[21] Campbell S, MacQueen G. (2006) An update on regional brain volume differences associated with mood disorders. *Curr. Opin. Psychiatry*. 19, 25-33.

[22] Ebmeier KP, Donaghey C, Steele JD. (2006) Recent developments and current controversies in depression. *Lancet.* 367, 153-67.

[23] Taupin P. (2006) Adult neurogenesis and neuroplasticity. *Restor. Neurol. Neurosci*. 24, 9-15.

[24] Taupin P. (2006) Neurogenesis and the Effects of Antidepressants. *Drug Target Insights*. 1, 13-17.

[25] Feldmann RE Jr, Sawa A, Seidler GH. (2007) Causality of stem cell based neurogenesis and depression - To be or not to be, is that the question? *J. Psychiatr. Res.* 41, 713-23.

[26] Djavadian RL. (2004) Serotonin and neurogenesis in the hippocampal dentate gyrus of adult mammals. *Acta Neurobiol. Exp.* (Wars). 64, 189-200.

INDEX

A

D

E

F

G

H

I

K

L

M

N

O

P

Q

R

S

T

U

V

W

X

Y